ASH-SAP: American Society of Hematology Self-Assessment Program

ASH™-SAP
American Society of Hematology Self-Assessment Program

THIRD EDITION

Editors

Marc J. Kahn, MD
Stephanie A. Gregory, MD

Chapter Authors

Thomas C. Abshire, MD
Kenneth C. Anderson, MD
George R. Buchanan, MD
Alan B. Cantor, MD, PhD
Mark A. Crowther, MD, MSC, FRCPC
Georgette A. Dent, MD
Henry C. Fung MD, FRCPE
Francis J. Giles, MD
Stephanie A. Gregory, MD
Jay H. Herman, MD
Teru Hideshima, MD, PhD
Meghan A. Higman, MD, PhD
Sima Jeha, MD
Marc J. Kahn, MD
Thomas R. Klumpp, MD, FACP
Cindy Leissinger, MD
Daniel C. Link, MD
Michael Linenberger, MD
Alice D. Ma, MD
Dana C. Matthews, MD
Keith R. McCrae, MD
Martha P. Mims, MD, PhD
Josef T. Prchal, MD
Robert E. Richard, MD, PhD
Paul G. Richardson, MD
Nita L. Seibel, MD
Jamile M. Shammo, MD, FASCP
Kevin Shannon, MD
Akiko Shimamura, MD, PhD
Don L. Siegel, PhD, MD
Jamie E. Siegel, MD
Lewis R. Silverman, MD
David P. Steensma, MD, FACP
F. Marc Stewart, MD
Wendy Stock, MD
Mark M. Udden, MD
Koen van Besien, MD
Parameswaran Venugopal, MD
Ted Wun, MD, FACP
Marc S. Zumberg, MD

Published by

AMERICAN SOCIETY OF HEMATOLOGY ®

American Society of Hematology
1900 M Street, NW, Suite 200
Washington, DC 20036
202-776-0544

ASH Customer Service Toll-Free (within U.S. only)
866-828-1231

First published 2003
Second edition 2005
Third edition 2007

ISBN-13: 978-0-9789212-0-0

ISBN-10: 0-9789212-0-8

Set in 10/13pt Minion by Cadmus Communications
Printed and bound by Cadmus Communications Lancaster, PA.

Contents

Authors

Thomas C. Abshire, MD
Professor of Pediatrics
Hemophilia of Georgia, Inc., Director's Chair in Hemostasis
AFLAC Cancer Center and Blood Disorders Service
Emory University
Atlanta, GA

Kenneth C. Anderson, MD
Chief of Division of Hematologic Neoplasia
Director of the Jerome Lipper Multiple Myeloma Center
Vice-Chair, Joint Program in Transfusion Medicine
Dana-Farber Cancer Institute
Boston, MA

George R. Buchanan, MD
Professor of Pediatrics
Director of Pediatric Hematology-Oncology
The University of Texas Southwestern Medical Center at Dallas
Dallas, TX

Alan B. Cantor, MD, PhD
Assistant Professor of Pediatrics
Children's Hospital Boston
Division of Hematology/Oncology
Boston, MA

Mark A. Crowther, MD, MSc, FRCPC
Professor and Chair, Division of Hematology
McMaster University
Director of Laboratory Hematology
Hamilton Regional Laboratory Medicine Program
Head of Service, Hematology
St. Joseph's Healthcare
Hamilton, Ontario, Canada

Georgette A. Dent, MD
Associate Professor of Pathology and Laboratory Medicine
Associate Dean for Student Affairs
University of North Carolina School of Medicine
Chapel Hill, NC

Henry C. Fung MD, FRCPE
Coleman Foundation Professor of Medicine
Director, Section of Stem Cell Transplantation
Division of Hematology, Oncology and Stem Cell Transplantation
Rush Medical College, Rush University
Chicago, IL

Francis J. Giles, MD
Professor of Medicine
Chief, Section of Developmental Therapeutics
Department of Leukemia
University of Texas
M.D. Anderson Cancer Center
Houston, TX

Stephanie A. Gregory, MD
The Elodia Kehm Professor of Medicine
Director, Section of Hematology
Rush Medical College/Rush University Medical Center
Chicago, IL

Jay H. Herman, MD
Professor
Departments of Medicine and Anatomy, Pathology and Laboratory Medicine
Director, Transfusion Medicine
Cardeza Foundation for Hematologic Research
Thomas Jefferson University
Philadelphia, PA

Teru Hideshima, MD, PhD
Principal Associate in Medicine
Jerome Lipper Myeloma Center
Dana-Farber Cancer Institute
Boston, MA

Meghan A. Higman, MD, PhD
Assistant Professor of Pediatric Hematology and Oncology
Children's Hospital of Buffalo and Roswell Park Cancer Institute
Buffalo, NY

Sima Jeha, MD
Director, Leukemia/Lymphoma Developmental Therapeutics
Associate Member, Hematology/Oncology
St. Jude Children's Research Hospital
Memphis, TN

Marc J. Kahn, MD
Professor of Medicine
Section of Hematology/Medical Oncology
Associate Dean for Admissions and Student Affairs
Tulane University School of Medicine
New Orleans, LA

Thomas R. Klumpp, MD, FACP
Professor of Medicine
Fox Chase-Temple University BMT Program
Philadelphia, PA

Cindy Leissinger, MD
Professor of Medicine
Director, Louisiana Center for Bleeding and Clotting Disorders
Tulane University School of Medicine
New Orleans, LA

Daniel C. Link, MD
Associate Professor of Medicine, Pathology and Immunology
Division of Oncology
Washington University School of Medicine
Saint Louis, MO

Michael Linenberger, MD
Associate Professor, Division of Hematology, Department of Medicine
University of Washington
Associate Member, Fred Hutchinson Cancer Research Center
Medical Director, Apheresis and Cellular Therapy
Seattle Cancer Care Alliance
Seattle, WA

Alice D. Ma, MD
Associate Professor of Medicine
Division of Hematology/Oncology
Assistant Fellowship Program Director for Research
University of North Carolina School of Medicine
Chapel Hill, NC

Dana C. Matthews, MD
Associate Professor, Hematology/Oncology
Department of Pediatrics
University of Washington School of Medicine
Director, Clinical Hematology
Children's Hospital and Regional Medical Center
Seattle, WA

Keith R. McCrae, MD
Professor of Medicine and Pathology
Division of Hematology-Oncology
Case Western Reserve University School of Medicine
Cleveland, OH

Martha P. Mims, MD, PhD
Associate Professor of Medicine
Division of Hematology and Oncology
Baylor College of Medicine
Houston, TX

Josef T. Prchal, MD
Professor of Hematology
Division of Hematology
University of Utah Health Sciences Center
Salt Lake City, UT

Robert E. Richard, MD, PhD
Assistant Professor
Division of Hematology, Department of Medicine
University of Washington School of Medicine
Seattle, WA

Paul G. Richardson, MD
Assistant Professor of Medicine
Division of Medical Oncology/Hematologic Malignancies
Harvard Medical School
Dana-Farber Cancer Institute
Boston, MA

Nita L. Seibel, MD
Professor of Pediatrics
George Washington University School of Medicine,
Director of Outreach Services
Department of Hematology/Oncology
Childrens National Medical Center
Washington, DC

Jamile M. Shammo, MD, FASCP
Assistant Professor of Medicine and Pathology
Director, Hematology Oncology Fellowship Program
Section of Hematology and Stem Cell Transplantation
Rush University Medical Center
Chicago, IL

Kevin Shannon, MD
Professor and Vice-Chair
Department of Pediatrics
Hematopoietic Malignancies Program Leader
Comprehensive Cancer Center
University of California
San Francisco, CA

Akiko Shimamura, MD, PhD
Assistant Professor of Pediatrics
Director, Bone Marrow Failure Program
Pediatric Hematology/Oncology
Children's Hospital Boston
Boston, MA

Don L. Siegel, PhD, MD
Professor and Vice-Chair, Pathology & Laboratory Medicine
Chief, Division of Transfusion Medicine
Director, Transfusion Medicine Clinical and Research Fellowship Training Programs
University of Pennsylvania Medical Center
Philadelphia, PA

Jamie E. Siegel, MD
Clinical Associate Professor of Medicine
Director, Cardeza Foundation Hemophilia Treatment Center
Medical Director, Cardeza Foundation Special Hemostasis Laboratory
Thomas Jefferson University
Philadelphia, PA

Lewis R. Silverman, MD
Mount Sinai School of Medicine
Director of Myelodysplastic Syndrome and Myeloproliferative Disease Center
Division of Hematology/Oncology
New York, NY

David P. Steensma, MD, FACP
Associate Professor of Medicine and Oncology
Division of Hematology, Department of Medicine
Mayo Clinic
Rochester, MN

F. Marc Stewart, MD
Medical Director, Seattle Cancer Care Alliance
Professor of Medicine, University of Washington
Member, Fred Hutchinson Cancer Research Center
Seattle, WA

Wendy Stock, MD
Associate Professor of Medicine
Director, Leukemia Program
University of Chicago Pritzker School of Medicine
Chicago, IL

Mark M. Udden, MD
Professor of Medicine
Chief, Hematology Service, Ben Taub General Hospital
Hematology/Oncology Section
Department of Medicine
Baylor College of Medicine
Houston, TX

Koen van Besien, MD
Professor of Medicine
Director Stem Cell Transplant and Lymphoma Programs
Section of Hematology/Oncology
University of Chicago
Chicago, IL

Parameswaran Venugopal, MD
The Samuel G. Taylor, III, MD Professor of Oncology
Associate Professor of Medicine
Co-Director, Section of Hematology
Rush University Medical Center
Chicago, IL

Ted Wun, MD, FACP
Professor of Medicine, Pathology and Laboratory Medicine
Division of Hematology and Oncology
Vice-Chief, Program Director
University of California – Davis
Sacramento, CA

Marc S. Zumberg, MD
Associate Professor
Director, Therapeutic Apheresis
University of Florida
Department of Medicine
Division of Hematology/Oncology
Gainesville, FL

CME information

Two versions of this self-assessment are available: one is the standard version for *AMA Category 1 PRA Credit*™, and one version awards lifelong learning points toward the American Board of Internal Medicine (ABIM) Maintenance of Certification program in addition to CME credits. The standard version includes a printed syllabus divided into chapters dedicated to specific topical areas in hematology, as well as a self-assessment exam book that includes case-based, multiple-choice questions and critiques. A Web-based multimedia component reflects the same information contained in the printed text and adds the platform for the online exam. For the *ASH-SAP* with Maintenance of Certification module, the printed question book is withheld, but access to the online hematology text and the online exam are included.

Accreditation

The American Society of Hematology (ASH) is accredited by the Accreditation Council for Continuing Medical Education to sponsor CME for physicians. ASH designates the standard version of this educational activity for a maximum of 50 *AMA PRA Category 1 Credits*™. Physicians should only claim credit commensurate with the extent of their participation in the activity. Physicians who participate in this CME activity but are not licensed in the United States are also eligible for *AMA PRA Category 1 Credits*™.

ASH designates the *ASH-SAP* with Maintenance of Certification module educational activity for a maximum of 50 *AMA PRA Category 1 Credits*™. Physicians should only claim credit commensurate with the extent of their participation in the activity.

Target audience

ASH-SAP is a high-quality educational product offering up-to-date information in the field of hematology for hematologists, medical oncologists, internists, pediatricians, and hematology-oncology fellows and trainees.

Educational objectives

The self-assessment's goals are:

1 to provide timely clinical updates on new developments in hematology

2 to help practicing physicians prepare for recertification

3 to serve as a tool for board review

Date of release:
May 1, 2007

Online access expires/Last date for users to claim CME credit for this edition:

May 1, 2010

Disclosures

As a provider accredited by the Accreditation Council for Continuing Medical Education (ACCME), the American Society of Hematology must ensure balance, independence, objectivity, and scientific rigor in all of the educational activities it sponsors. All authors are expected to disclose any financial relationships with any proprietary entity producing health care goods or services that have occurred within 12 months from the start of or during the production of the work and which are relevant to the author's content. If an author has such a financial interest, then s/he must disclose the name of the commercial interest and nature of the relationship (eg, consultant, grantee, etc.). If the author has no such financial relationship, s/he must declare that s/he has nothing to disclose. The intent of this disclosure is not to prevent an author with a significant financial or other relationship from making a presentation, but rather to provide readers with information on which they can make their own judgments. It remains for the audience to determine whether the author's interests or relationships may influence the work with regard to exposition or conclusion.

	Research support/ Research	Consultant	Major stockholder	Speakers' bureau	Scientific advisory board
Thomas C. Abshire, MD		Novo Nordisk, ZLB Behring, Bayer			Novo Nordisk, ZLB Behring, Bayer
Kenneth C. Anderson, MD	Millennium, Celgene, Novartis	Millennium, Celgene, Novartis		Millennium, Celgene, Novartis	
George R. Buchanan, MD					
Alan B. Cantor, MD, PhD					
Mark A. Crowther, MD, MSc, FRCPC	Pfizer, Leo Laboratories			Pfizer, Leo Laboratories, Calea	
Georgette A. Dent, MD					
Henry C. Fung MD, FRCPE				Biogen Idec, Genentech, Millennium, Celgene	
Francis J. Giles, MD					
Stephanie A. Gregory, MD	Biogen Idec, Celgene, Genentech, Amgen, Millennium, Ortho Biotech, GlaxoSmithKline, Ligand, Berlex, Merck	Biogen Idec, Genentech, Amgen, Ortho Biotech, GlaxoSmithKline			
Jay H. Herman, MD					
Teru Hideshima, MD, PhD		Keryx Biopharmaceuticals			
Meghan A. Higman, MD, PhD					
Sima Jeha, MD	sanofi aventis	Genzyme		Genzyme	
Marc J. Kahn, MD					
Thomas R. Klumpp, MD, FACP					
Cindy Leissinger, MD					
Daniel C. Link, MD					
Michael Linenberger, MD					
Alice D. Ma, MD					
Dana C. Matthews, MD		Wyeth			
Keith R. McCrae, MD		Baxter		GlaxoSmithKline	
Martha P. Mims, MD, PhD			Amgen, Biogen Idec		
Josef T. Prchal, MD					
Robert E. Richard, MD, PhD					

	Research support/ Research	Consultant	Major stockholder	Speakers' bureau	Scientific advisory board
Paul G. Richardson, MD		Celgene, Millennium		Celgene, Millennium	
Nita L. Seibel, MD				Astellas, Enzon, Pfizer	
Jamile M. Shammo, MD, FASCP	Amgen, Celgene, Pharmion	Celgene, Pharmion		Amgen, Ortho Biotech, Celgene, Pharmion	
Kevin Shannon, MD					
Akiko Shimamura, MD, PhD					
Don L. Siegel, PhD, MD					
Jamie E. Siegel, MD					
Lewis R. Silverman, MD					
David P. Steensma, MD, FACP					
F. Marc Stewart, MD					
Wendy Stock, MD	Berlex			Enzon	
Mark M. Udden, MD	Amgen				
Koen van Besien, MD	Millennium, Miltenyi Biotec, Genzyme	AnorMED		Millennium	
Parameswaran Venugopal, MD				Genentech, Berlex	
Ted Wun, MD, FACP	Icagen/McNeil Genentech	Genentech		Glaxo-Smith-Kline	
Marc S. Zumberg, MD					

In compliance with ACCME policy, the American Society of Hematology also requires all authors to disclose any discussion of off-label drug use.

Dr. Crowther will discuss the use of anticoagulants during pregnancy and outside of current licensed indications.

Dr. Higman will discuss multiple agents for pediatric oncology.

Dr. Jeha will discuss early-phase studies of different agents (published data).

Dr. Leissinger will discuss off-label dosing of epoetin alfa in HIV patients.

Dr. Linenberger will discuss the use of recombinant factor VIIa in non-hemophiliac patients.

Dr. Seibel will discuss chemotherapy used in treating children with ALL.

Dr. Shammo will discuss off-label uses of hematopoietic growth factors.

Dr. Steensma will discuss imatinib for HES/mastocytosis, 2C0A for HES, and anagrelide for non-ET thrombocytosis.

Dr. Stock will discuss the trials incorporating monoclonal antibodies, rituxan, and campath into front-line therapy for subsets of ALL.

Dr. Venugopal will discuss the use of rituximab in front-line therapy of lymphomas.

Dr. Wun will discuss the therapy of HLH, LCH, and mastocytosis that have not been labeled for that purpose.

Claiming CME and ABIM credit

Scores of 80% or better on the self-assessment exams are eligible to claim credit for the activity. On **May 1, 2010**, online access expires, and this is also the last date for users to claim credit for this edition. The remainder of this section details the types of credit available for completing this activity. For questions about credit, please contact the ASH Education & Training Department at *cme@hematology.org* or call toll-free 866-828-1231 (within United States only).

Category 1 CME Credits

Two versions of this self-assessment are available, and each version is designated for a maximum of 50 AMA PRA Category 1 Credits™. Physicians should only claim credit commensurate with the extent of their participation in the activity.

Standard Version

In order to receive AMA PRA Category 1 Credits for participation in this activity, you must first complete the self-assessment test. To receive 50 Category 1 CME Credits for the standard version, go to *www.ash-sap.org* to complete the exam for the standard version. The test can be taken all at once, or parts of it can be completed at the end of each chapter and saved until the entire program is completed.

ASH-SAP with Maintenance of Certification Module

In order to receive 50 AMA PRA Category 1 Credits for participation in the ASH-SAP with American Board of Internal Medicine (ABIM) Maintenance of Certification (MOC) Module version, you must first complete the ABIM-MOC self-assessment test online at *www.ash-sap.org*. The test can be taken all at once, or parts of it can be completed at the end of each chapter and saved until the entire program is completed.

ABIM Maintenance of Certification points

You may only receive lifelong learning points toward the ABIM Maintenance of Certification program if you are using the *ASH-SAP with ABIM Maintenance of Certification Module* version of this activity, and you must complete this exam **online** at *www.ash-sap.org*. You must also be currently enrolled in the ABIM Maintenance of Certification program to earn these points.

Please refer to the ASH-SAP Web site at *www.ash-sap.org* for further information about the number of lifelong learning points to be awarded and how these points are processed.

Claiming CME and ABIM credit

Scores of 80% or better on the self-assessment exams are eligible to claim credit for the activity. On **May 1, 2010**, online access expires, and this is also the last date for users to claim credit for this edition. The remainder of this section details the types of credit available for completing this activity. For questions about credit, please contact the ASH Education & Training Department at *cme@hematology.org* or call toll-free 866-828-1231 (within United States only).

Category 1 CME Credits

Two versions of this self-assessment are available, and each version is designated for a maximum of 50 *AMA PRA Category 1 Credits*™. Physicians should only claim credit commensurate with the extent of their participation in the activity.

Standard Version

In order to receive *AMA PRA Category 1 Credits*™ for participation in this activity, you must first complete the self-assessment test. To receive 50 Category 1 CME Credits for the standard version, go to *www.ash-sap.org* to complete the exam for the standard version. The test can be taken all at once, or parts of it can be completed at the end of each chapter and saved until the entire program is completed.

ASH-SAP with Maintenance of Certification Module

In order to receive 50 AMA PRA Category 1 Credits for participation in the *ASH-SAP* with American Board of Internal Medicine (ABIM) Maintenance of Certification (MOC) Module version, you must first complete the ABIM-MOC self-assessment test online at *www.ash-sap.org*. The test can be taken all at once, or parts of it can be completed at the end of each chapter and saved until the entire program is completed.

ABIM Maintenance of Certification points

You may only receive lifelong learning points toward the ABIM Maintenance of Certification program if you are using the *ASH-SAP with ABIM Maintenance of Certification Module* version of this activity, and you must complete this exam **online** at *www.ash-sap.org*. You must also be currently enrolled in the ABIM Maintenance of Certification program to earn these points.

Please refer to the *ASH-SAP* Web site at *www.ash-sap.org* for further information about the number of lifelong learning points to be awarded and how these points are processed.

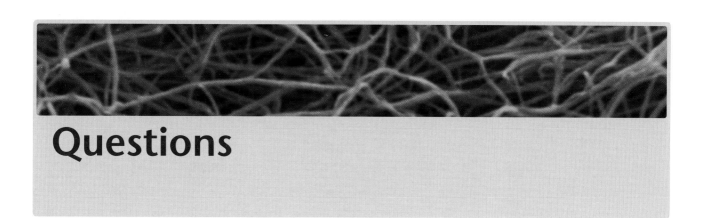

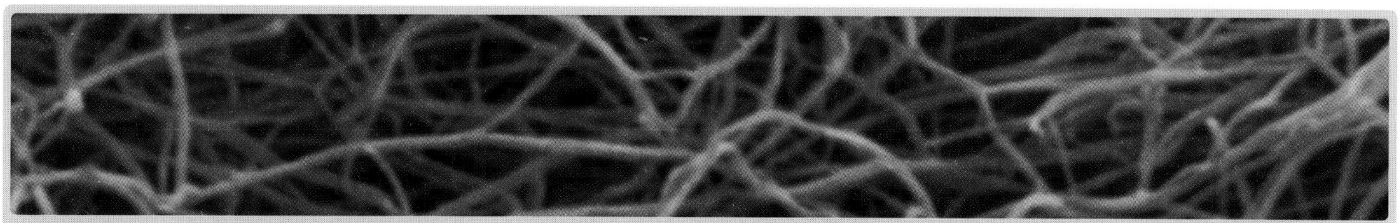

Questions

CHAPTER 01

Molecular basis of hematology

Question 1

A variety of treatments are available for the treatment of myelodysplastic syndrome.

Q Which of the following agents used to treat myelodysplastic syndromes acts at the level of gene expression?

A Cytarabine
B 5-Azacytidine
C Fludarabine
D Antithymocyte globulin

Question 2

Prior to embarking on the human genome project, it was estimated that approximately 100,000 genes would be found and sequenced. In fact, only about 30,000 genes were found.

Q Which of the following is the best explanation for this disparity?

A There are fewer genes than estimated because most human proteins have multiple functions
B Original estimates of the number of genes were based on extrapolations from gene-poor areas
C Many protein-encoding genes produce multiple protein products
D Many genes are duplicated throughout the genome

Question 3

A 25-year-old man is being evaluated for anemia. Hemoglobin electrophoresis suggests that the abnormality is in the β globin gene. Further evaluation reveals that the mutant β globin protein is shorter than normal β globin. Sequencing of the β globin gene reveals the patient to be heterozygous for a single nucleotide substitution in exon 2.

Q Which of the following is the most likely effect of the single nucleotide substitution?

A It causes a frameshift such that a new stop codon is created
B It results in creation of a new splice site such that a portion of exon 2 is spliced out of the mutant transcript
C It results in substitution of a polar for a nonpolar amino acid in the mutant β globin molecule
D It results in substitution of one polar amino acid for another

Question 4

You are asked to consult on a case of a 21-year-old woman who wishes to become pregnant with her first child. The patient reports that both a maternal uncle and her brother have hemophilia A, but the exact nature of the mutation is not known. The patient wants to know if she is a carrier. The patient and her brother are genotyped for a polymorphism that is tightly linked to the factor VIII gene; the patient is heterozygous for the polymorphism whereas the affected brother's X chromosome has the polymorphism.

Q Which of the following would be required to determine whether this patient is a carrier of the mutation?

A No further testing required
B Genotyping of both her parents
C Genotyping of her affected uncle
D Genotyping of her father

Question 5

A 61-year-old woman is being evaluated for an elevated white count. Bone marrow examination shows a hypercellular marrow; 65% of the nucleated cells are myeloid blasts based on flow cytometry. Cytogenetic examination of the marrow demonstrates normal female karyotype in 100 out of 100 cells. The patient is diagnosed with acute myeloid leukemia M2.

Q Which of the following would likely detect a cytogenetic abnormality in this patient?

A Fluorescence *in situ* hybridization for t(15;17)
B Repeat standard cytogenetics with more cells
C Repeat cytogenetics using peripheral blood rather than marrow
D Polymerase chain reaction of bone marrow to detect a microdeletion

Question 6

You are asked to see a patient with chronic myelogenous leukemia who has been on imatinib 400 mg per day for 3 years. The complete blood cell count has been normal since the fourth month of treatment, and the patient is told that she is in cytogenetic remission at her 6-month visit. The patient asks if the disease is likely to recur.

Q Which of the following tests is the most useful predictor of relapse in this patient?

A Real-time polymerase chain reaction assay for bcr-abl transcripts in peripheral blood
B Fluorescence *in situ* hybridization for the 9:22 translocation on a fresh bone marrow sample
C Cytogenetic analysis of a fresh bone marrow sample
D Flow cytometry examination of a fresh bone marrow sample

Question 7

One of your patients is interested in participating in a trial that will use DNA microarrays to investigate gene expression and response of follicular lymphoma to chemotherapy. The trial requires submission of a small piece of malignant lymph node tissue from each lymphoma patient prior to treatment and data on how the patient responds to treatment.

Q Which of the following statements is most accurate regarding the use of microarrays in this trial?

A Researchers plan to examine gene expression at the RNA level and compare the pattern in patients who do and do not respond to chemotherapy
B Evaluation of normal lymph node tissue from lymphoma patients would yield similar results
C Microarray data accurately predicts which proteins are over- or underexpressed, and this information will be used to develop drug targets
D Genes that are overexpressed in microarray experiments will be shown to harbor mutations that cause follicular lymphoma

Question 8

Your patients are participating in a research project that examines the correlation between immunoglobulin gene rearrangements in chronic lymphocytic leukemia and response to therapy. Using Southern blotting techniques, κ and λ light-chain rearrangements on chronic lymphocytic leukemia (CLL) cells from 10 patients are examined; granulocytes from each patient are used as germ line controls.

Q Which of the following would be a likely outcome of this experiment?

A In CLL cells with λ gene rearrangements, all κ genes will be germ line
B Granulocytes will have various κ and λ gene rearrangements
C CLL cells that have one germ line κ gene and one rearranged κ gene will have 2 germ line λ genes
D The most common pattern in CLL cells will be one germ line and one rearranged κ gene and one germ line and one rearranged λ gene

Question 9

Acquired deletion of microRNA genes have been implicated in the pathogenesis of chronic lymphocytic leukemia (CLL).

Q Which of the following is the most likely mechanism for the effect of microRNA genes on CLL cells?

A MicroRNA genes inhibit transcription of genes that regulate the cell cycle
B MicroRNA genes inhibit translocation of messenger RNA (mRNA)
C MicroRNA genes inhibit translation of specific mRNAs whose protein products inhibit apoptosis
D MicroRNA genes inhibit translation of gene transcripts from cell cycle products

Question 10

A 4-year-old girl develops visible cyanosis during the course of a severe episode of otitis media. Both the patient and her mother have ~50% normal activity of cytochrome b_5 reductase in red blood cells. Her physician suspects she has an acquired methemoglobinemia with some genetic predisposition based on enzyme studies of her and her mother's blood. Hemoglobin electrophoresis is normal. You propose that the patient and her mother are heterozygous for a mutation in the cytochrome b_5 reductase gene; however, sequencing of complementary DNA (cDNA) derived from patient mononuclear cells and those of her mother demonstrates no defects.

Q Which of the following is the most likely explanation for the failure to detect a molecular defect?

A The defect is a single-nucleotide substitution in the fourth exon and codes for a conservative amino acid change

B The defect is in an intron and causes abnormal splicing of exons 1 and 2, resulting in an early stop codon

C The defect is in glucose-6-phosphate dehydrogenase, not in cytochrome b_5

D The defect is in erythrocytes but not in other cells and can be detected only in reticulocyte cDNA

Question 11

A 7-year-old boy and his mother are referred to you for treatment of the boy's hemophilia B (factor IX deficiency). The patient's mother is quite interested in gene therapy for factor IX deficiency and asks about the risks of gene therapy. The trial she is considering uses a nonviral vector to insert the factor IX gene into the patient's cultured fibroblasts, followed by reintroduction of the cells into the patient.

Q Which of the following would represent the highest risk of participating in this trial?

A The gene could activate an oncogene

B Expression of the factor IX gene could be transient

C The patient will require immune suppression

D The gene could increase the possibility of birth defects in the patient's offspring

CHAPTER 02

Cellular basis of hematopoiesis and marrow failure syndromes

Question 1

An 18-year-old woman presents with pallor and fatigue. Her past medical history is significant for surgical correction of a thumb malformation. There are no recent medications. Her physical examination is notable for pallor, short stature, several café-au-lait spots, scattered petechiae, and 2 large bruises. Her complete blood cell count is notable for a white blood cell count of 3,000/μL with a neutrophil count of 800/μL, hemoglobin of 9 g/dL, mean corpuscular volume of 101 fL, and platelets of 50,000/μL. B_{12} and folate levels are normal. Her bone marrow examination shows 20% marrow cellularity with an otherwise normal differential. Marrow cytogenetics are normal. She has a healthy sister who is an HLA match. Peripheral blood is sent for diepoxybutane (DEB) testing and returns negative for Fanconi anemia.

Q Which of the following would be the most appropriate next step in the management of this patient?

A Allogeneic hematopoietic stem cell transplantation
B Serial blood counts
C Skin biopsy specimen for DEB testing
D Bone marrow sample for DEB testing

Question 2

A 25-year-old woman presents with fatigue. She has previously been healthy with normal blood counts. Her examination is unremarkable. Her current blood counts reveal a hemoglobin of 8.2 g/dL, white blood cell count of 3,000/μL, absolute neutrophil count of 950/μL, and platelet count of 70,000/μL. Her reticulocyte count is low. Bone marrow examination is consistent with myelodysplasia. Marrow cytogenetics reveals a clonal population with complex cytogenetic abnormalities. Her sister, who is an HLA match, is healthy. Her brother, who is not an HLA match, has a horseshoe kidney, mild thrombocytopenia, and macrocytosis and is quite short compared with the rest of the family.

Q What is the most appropriate next step in the management of this patient?

A Send blood on the patient for diepoxybutane testing
B Send the patient for an allogeneic bone marrow transplant
C Perform a renal ultrasound
D Initiate a search for a matched unrelated donor

Question 3

A 20-year-old woman presents with fatigue. She has been treated with antithymocyte globulin (ATG) and cyclosporin for severe aplastic anemia at the age of 15 but has been stable off of all medications for the past 4 years. Her white blood cell counts and neutrophil counts have been normal. Her hemoglobin has been around 12.5 g/dL, and her platelet counts are typically in the 120,000–130,000/μL range. Her physical examination is unremarkable. Her blood counts today are remarkable for a white blood cell count of 5,000/μL with a neutrophil count of 1,700/μL, a hemoglobin of 8 g/dL with a low reticulocyte count, a mean corpuscular volume of 101 fL, and a platelet count of 70,000/μL. You recheck the counts 1 week later, and the neutrophil count is 1200/μL, hemoglobin 7.5 g/dL, and platelets 50,000/μL.

Q What is the most appropriate next step in the management of this patient?

A Bone marrow aspirate and biopsy with cytogenetics
B Thyroid function tests
C Treatment with cyclosporin
D Treatment with ATG and cyclosporine

Question 4

A 30-year-old man presents with pallor and fatigue. He has been previously healthy and has not been on any medications for the past 3 months. Family history is unremarkable. His examination is remarkable only for pale mucous membranes and a few scattered petechiae on his ankles. His blood counts reveal a white blood cell count of 2,000/μL, an absolute neutrophil count of 250/μL, hemoglobin of 8.5 g/dl, platelets of 15,000/μL, low reticulocyte counts, and a mean corpuscular volume of 103. Aspartate aminotransferase, alanine aminotransferase, bilirubin, lactate dehydrogenase, serum urea nitrogen, and creatinine were all normal. His marrow examination showed 5% marrow cellularity with no significant dysmorphic or megaloblastic features or malignant cells. Tests for human immunodeficiency virus and paroxysmal nocturnal hemoglobinuria were negative.

Q Which of the following would be the most appropriate next step in the evaluation of this patient?

A Cytogenetic analysis of bone marrow specimen
B Measurement of serum vitamin B_{12}
C Measurement of serum folate
D Measurement of serum thyroid-stimulating hormone and thyroxine (T_4)

Question 5

A 25-year-old man presents with fatigue and petechiae. He had been healthy until 3 months ago when he developed fever, jaundice, and transaminitis. Tests of hepatitis A, B, and C were negative. His symptoms gradually resolved, and his transaminases are now normal with normal liver function. Previously, he drank an average of 2 alcoholic beverages per week but stopped after his illness. His family history is unremarkable. This examination is notable for pallor and scattered petechiae. Laboratory studies are significant for a leukocyte count of 3,000/μL with a neutrophil count of 450/μL, a hemoglobin of 8 g/dL with a low reticulocyte count, and a platelet count of 15,000/μL. His human immunodeficiency virus test was negative.

Q Which of the following would be the most appropriate next step in the evaluation of this patient?

A Bone marrow aspirate and biopsy
B Serologic test for cytomegalovirus
C Serologic test for parvovirus
D Liver biopsy

Question 6

A 19-year-old woman is evaluated for therapy after a recent diagnosis of severe aplastic anemia. She has been otherwise healthy. She has not been on any medications over the past 3 months other than an occasional Tylenol. Her examination is remarkable only for a few scattered petechiae and small bruises. Human immunodeficiency virus testing, Fanconi anemia testing, and paroxysmal nocturnal hemoglobinuria testing are all negative. She has 2 healthy siblings, a 20-year-old sister who is an HLA match and a 15-year-old brother who is not an HLA match.

Q Which of the following would be the most appropriate management for this patient?

A Allogeneic bone marrow transplant with her sister as the donor
B Antithymocyte globulin and cyclosporin
C Blood count monitoring and transfusion support
D Erythropoietin and granulocyte colony-stimulating factor

Question 7

You are following a 1-year-old boy with a history of severe thrombocytopenia since birth. Blood counts at this time reveal the following:

White blood count	6.9 k/mm^3
Absolute neutrophil count	3.2 k/mm^3
Hematocrit	38%
Platelet count	17 k/mm^3

The mean platelet volume is within the normal range. Radiographs demonstrate the presence of radii bilaterally, and evaluation for Fanconi anemia is negative. Bone marrow examination at this time reveals a normocellular marrow with normal morphology, but markedly reduced numbers of megakaryocytes. You continue to follow the patient with serial blood counts over the next several years. By 4 years of age, the hematocrit has declined to 16% and absolute neutrophil count to 300/mm^3. Repeat bone marrow examination reveals a markedly hypocellular marrow with no evidence of dysplastic forms. Cytogenetic studies are normal.

Q Mutational analysis of which of the following genes would be the most useful next diagnostic step?

A Thrombopoietin
B Wiskott–Aldrich gene
C *GATA-1*
D c-*mpl*
E *MYH9*

Question 8

You are asked to provide consultation on a 3-year-old girl with a history of severe thrombocytopenia since birth with average platelet counts of about 10 k/mm^3. The platelet volume is within the normal range. There are no physical anomalies. A bone marrow examination earlier revealed a normocellular bone marrow with a markedly reduced number of megakaryocytes. Her other blood counts had been in the normal range, but now her absolute neutrophil count has declined to 800/mm^3, and her hemoglobin has decreased to 8.0 g/dL with a reticulocyte count of 0.3%. Repeat bone marrow studies show a moderately hypocellular marrow with absent megakaryocytes but no dysplastic changes. Chromosome breakage studies are negative, and the cytogenetic analysis is normal. Serum thrombopoietin levels are markedly elevated. She has 2 siblings from the same biologic parents. They are reported to have normal blood counts.

Q Which of the following would be the most appropriate next step in the management of this patient?

A Prednisone
B HLA-typing of siblings
C Intravenous immunoglobulin
D Recombinant pegylated thrombopoietin
E Desmopressin (DDAVP)

Question 9

You are asked to evaluate a 2-month-old female infant with worsening pallor and lethargy. Initial complete blood cell count reveals the following:

White blood cell count	7.2 k/mm^3
Absolute neutrophil count	3.4 k/mm^3
Hemoglobin	4 g/dL
Mean corpuscular volume	104 fL
Mean corpuscular hemoglobin concentration	30.4 g/dL
Platelet count	415 k/mm^3
Reticulocyte count	0.2%

Physical examination is notable for the presence of triphalangeal thumbs. A bone marrow examination is performed and reveals a normocellular marrow with normal myeloid series and megakaryocytes. However, there is marked reduction in early erythroid precursors, and the few present appear to be immature proerythroblasts. Iron stain does not show iron deposits or ringed sideroblasts, and no multinucleated erythroblasts are seen.

Q Which of the following studies would be most helpful in establishing the diagnosis?

A Erythrocyte adenosine deaminase level
B Iron studies
C Direct antiglobulin (Coombs) test
D Osmotic fragility testing
E Heinz body preparation

Question 10

You are asked to see a 2-month-old girl with severe anemia since birth. She is suspected to have Diamond–Blackfan anemia. Her erythrocyte adenosine deaminase level comes back markedly elevated. Additional studies show elevated erythropoietin levels, negative parvovirus B19 polymerase chain reaction, and negative diepoxybutane testing. Over the next 6 months, she remains transfusion dependent, and her reticulocyte count never rises above 0.4%. She does not have an HLA-matched sibling.

Q Which of the following treatment options would be most appropriate to try at this point?

A Recombinant erythropoietin 200 U subcutaneously 3 times per week
B Vitamin B_{12} and folate supplementation
C Prednisone 2 mg/kg/d
D Intravenous immunoglobulin 1 g/kg
E Antithymocyte globulin and cyclosporine

Question 11

A 13-year-old boy is found to have moderate anemia on a screening complete blood cell count with a hemoglobin level of 9 g/dL. The mean corpuscular volume is 93 fl and the mean corpuscular hemoglobin concentration is 34 g/dL. Reticulocyte count is 4%. Leukocyte and platelet counts are within the normal range. There is slight jaundice and hepatosplenomegaly on physical examination. The bilirubin level is 4.1 total, 0.4 direct. The peripheral blood smear shows anisocytosis and poikilocytosis, with some basophilic stippling and teardrop forms. A bone marrow examination reveals 25% bi- and multinucleated erythroblasts. Cytogenetic studies are normal. Peripheral smear and marrow are shown (from ASH Image Bank #953, #1532).

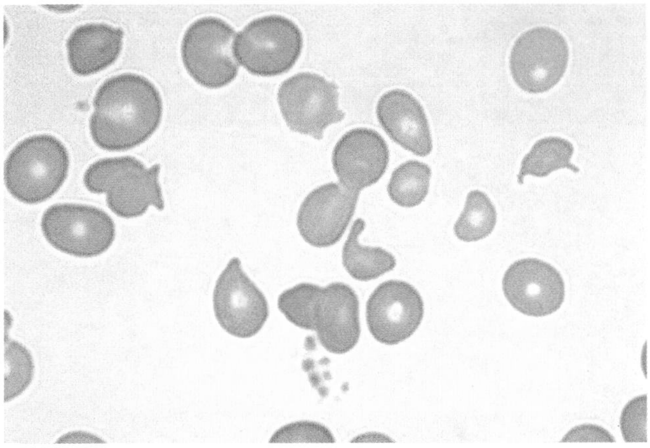
(a)

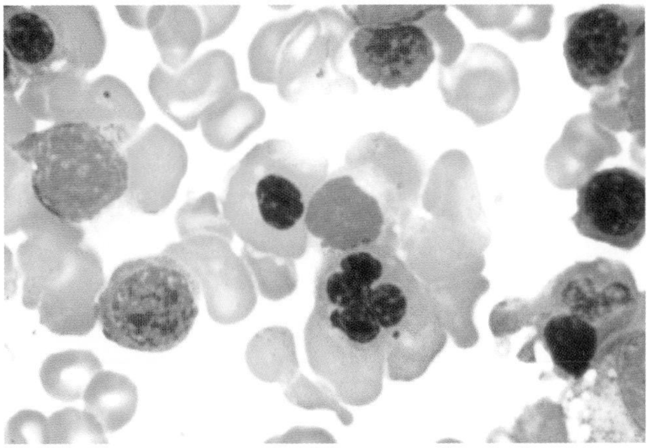
(b)

Q Which of the following diagnostic studies would be the most helpful in establishing the diagnosis?

A Osmotic fragility testing
B Direct antiglobulin test (Coombs)
C Hepatitis B serologies
D Serum transferrin saturation (Fe/total iron-binding capacity)
E Acid serum hemolysis test

Question 12

A 15-year-old boy is referred for consultation of worsening graft-versus-host disease despite initiation of immunosuppression. He had undergone an allogeneic bone marrow transplant from his HLA-matched sister for aplastic anemia at the age of 5. Physical examination is notable for a reticular rash, atrophic nails, and dry eyes. His blood counts are normal. Liver enzymes and bilirubin are normal. On his mother's side, he has a male cousin who died of aplastic anemia at the age of 6 and an uncle who died of an unspecified pulmonary disease.

Q What is the most appropriate next step in the management of this patient?

A Increase the immunosuppression for graft-versus-host disease
B Send a buccal swab for *DKC1* and *TERC* sequencing
C Refer to a rheumatologist

CHAPTER

03 Hematopoietic growth factors

Question 1

A 68-year-old man with a 2-year history of myelodysplasia presents to your clinic for his routine follow-up appointment. Over the past 2 weeks he has had brief episodes of chest pain while bicycling. On examination, his stool Hemoccult test is negative. His complete blood cell count shows a white blood cell count of 2,400/μL, a hematocrit 22%, and platelets 86,000/μL. His corrected reticulocyte count is 1%. A marrow performed 1 month ago shows dysplastic changes with <5% blasts.

Q Which of the following would be the most appropriate therapy for this patient?

A Epoetin alfa once per week
B Darbepoetin alfa once every 2 weeks
C Epoetin alfa once per week and daily filgrastim
D Transfusion of 2 U of packed erythrocytes
E Prednisone, 100 mg/d

Question 2

A 31-year-old human immunodeficiency virus-positive man with a CD4 count of 119/μL and a viral load of 200,000 copies/mL presents with easy bruising. He has had slight epistaxis and some gingival bleeding. His complete blood cell count shows a white blood cell (WBC) count of 3,500/μL, hematocrit 32%, and platelets 11,000/μL. His peripheral smear shows normal WBC and red blood cell morphology, and confirms fewer platelets.

Q Which of the following is the most appropriate management for this patient?

A Infuse fresh frozen plasma and begin plasma exchange
B Highly active antiretroviral therapy
C Splenectomy
D Platelet transfusion
E Thrombopoietin

Question 3

A 60-year-old man with multiple myeloma is referred for treatment with high-dose cyclophosphamide, etoposide, dexamethasone, and filgrastim followed by apheresis collection of $CD34^+$ progenitor cells in preparation for an autologous stem cell transplant. His HLA-matched brother also attends the interview in anticipation of serving as a donor for a subsequent nonmyeloablative allogeneic stem cell transplant.

Q Which of the following is the most likely effect of filgrastim therapy in this patient?

A More rapid engraftment when administered posttransplant
B Reduction of mortality risk and adverse effects
C Increased risk of graft-versus-host disease
D Rapid granulocyte recovery

Question 4

A 23-year-old man sustains an auto accident with major abdominal lacerations and contusions. He undergoes emergency exploratory surgery to identify and treat potential bleeding sites. With 15 U of packed red blood cells and 4 U of fresh frozen plasma, his condition is stable. Two days postoperatively, he develops high fevers and severe shortness of breath. Physical examination reveals a blood pressure of 90/60, heart rate of 140, and respiratory rate of 30 with diminished breath sounds and fine rales over the right base anteriorly. His oxygen saturation is 88% on room air. Initial blood cultures are positive for gram-negative rods. With increasing oxygen requirements, he is admitted to the intensive care unit and placed on 100% face mask with adequate oxygen saturation and is given broad spectrum antibiotics. A chest x-ray shows a dense consolidation in the right anterior lung base. His white blood cell count is 3,300/μL with 1500 neutrophils and a left-shifted differential; hematocrit is 32%, and the platelet count is 68,000/μL.

Q Which of the following is the most appropriate therapy for this patient?

A Epoetin alfa plus filgrastim plus imipenem
B Epoetin alfa plus ceftazadime/gentamicin
C Filgrastim and platelet transfusions plus granulocyte transfusions
D Filgrastim plus ceftazadime/gentamicin
E Ceftazadime/gentamicin

Question 5

A 22-year-old male serves as a normal stem cell donor for his HLA-identical sister with leukemia. He is in excellent health and asymptomatic. He begins granulocyte colony-stimulating factor (G-CSF) and notes mild abdominal pain. Gradually, his pain increases over the next 2 days. On the third day of treatment with G-CSF, he develops acute abdominal pain with a rigid abdomen on examination. His blood pressure is 90/60 with a heart rate of 140. His temperature is 36.6°C. His hematocrit has fallen from 45 to 34%. His white blood cell count is 19,000/μL with a left shift. His platelet count is 240,000/μL. The pain is localized to the left upper quadrant. His bowel sounds are absent, and he has rebound tenderness. Stools are guaiac negative. He has had no constipation, diarrhea, or other gastrointestinal symptoms.

Q Which of the following is the most likely diagnosis?

A Typhlitis
B Splenic rupture
C Appendicitis
D Filgrastim-related fever and muscular pain
E Filgrastim-induced peptic ulcer disease

Question 6

A 66-year-old diabetic man develops stage IVB large B-cell lymphoma with bone marrow involvement and central nervous system disease. His chest x-ray shows moderate mediastinal adenopathy, and a computed tomographic scan of his abdomen shows splenomegaly with slightly enlarged retrocrural lymph nodes. His white blood cell count is 3400/μL, platelet count is 356,000/μL, and hematocrit is 42%. His lactate dehydrogenase is 650 IU/L. His mother died of lymphoma in her 40s. He receives intrathecal methotrexate and begins brain irradiation simultaneously with rituximab, cyclophosphamide, doxorubicin, vincristine, and prednisone (R-CHOP) chemotherapy and granulocyte colony-stimulating factor (G-CSF). Shortly after completing his brain irradiation, his course is complicated by fever, neutropenia, and gram-negative sepsis with a 1-week hospitalization in the intensive care unit. His disease, however, responds nicely. His counts recover, and he improves sufficiently to begin his next cycle of chemotherapy.

Q Which of the following is the most appropriate chemotherapy at this time?

A R-CHOP at the same dose with G-CSF
B R-CHOP at a reduced dose with G-CSF
C R-CHOP at a reduced dose without G-CSF
D Etoposide, methylprednisolone, cytarabine, and cisplatin (ESHAP) with G-CSF
E Rituximab, ifosfamide, carboplatin, etoposide (R-ICE) with stem cell collection for autologous transplantation

Question 7

A 36-year-old man has developed fever and neutropenia 3 times despite dose adjustments while receiving CAE (cytoxan, adriamycin, etoposide) chemotherapy for extensive stage small cell lung cancer.

Q Which of the following would be the most likely result of adding a single dose of pegfilgastrim to the patient's next cycle of chemotherapy?

A The risk of mortality would be reduced
B The chance of remission increase
C The risk of fever and neutropenia would be reduced
D The adverse effects of therapy will be reduced
E No positive effect is likely

Question 8

A 76-year-old woman with hypertension and osteoarthritis is diagnosed with stage IIIA diffuse large B-cell lymphoma. Her bone marrow biopsy fails to show evidence of involvement by non-Hodgkin lymphoma, but it showed reduced stainable iron. A complete blood cell count obtained prior to the first cycle of rituximab, cyclophosphamide, doxorubicin, vincristine, and prednisone (R-CHOP) reveals mild anemia with hemoglobin (Hb) of 11.8 g/dL and a mean corpuscular volume of 79 fL. After 2 cycles of therapy, her Hb drops to 10.5. At that time, epoetin alfa is started; however, 8 weeks later her Hb is in fact lower at 9.5 g/dL. She is now complaining of fatigue and shortness of breath. Her physical examination is remarkable for alopecia, pallor, and notably smaller lymph nodes. The patient is to receive 2 U of blood in the clinic on that day.

Q Which of the following would be the most appropriate additional management for this patient?

A Measure iron studies including ferritin level
B Increase dose of epoetin alfa
C Reduce dose of R-CHOP for the next cycle
D Perform bone marrow biopsy to rule out progressive disease

Question 9

A 45-year-old woman presents to the clinic with complaints of fatigue and exercise intolerance. She had been recently diagnosed with stage III infiltrating ductal carcinoma of the breast. A lumpectomy and axillary lymph node dissection were performed, followed by adjuvant chemotherapy with Adriamycin/Cytoxan/Taxotere.

A complete blood cell count on day 1 of cycle 3 reveals hemoglobin (normal at base line) of 9.5 g/dL; white blood cell count and platelets are within normal limits.

Q Which of the following would be the most appropriate next step in the management of this patient?

A Reduce the dose of the next cycle of chemotherapy
B Begin therapy with epoetin alfa on a weekly basis
C Perform a bone marrow biopsy
D Measure erythropoietin level

Question 10

A 75-year-old otherwise healthy man is recently diagnosed with stage IV diffuse large B-cell lymphoma; his staging bone marrow biopsy is significant for involvement with lymphoma. His complete blood cell count at baseline reveals a white blood cell count of 3.0, absolute neutrophil count of 1,300 μL, hemoglobin of 11.2 g/dL, normal mean corpuscular volume at 98 fL, and a platelet count of 130 10^9/L.

Q Which of the following is the most appropriate therapy for this patient?

A Full-dose rituximab, cyclophosphamide, doxorubicin, vincristine, and prednisone (R-CHOP) and filgrastrim
B Full-dose R-CHOP
C R-CHOP at 25% reduced dose
D R-CHOP given at 6-week intervals

Question 11

A 65-year-old man presents with complaints of fatigue and exertional dyspnea. He was recently diagnosed with myelodysplastic syndrome, refractory anemia subtype. His complete blood cell count reveals hemoglobin of 8.9 g/dL, a mean corpuscular volume of 104 fL, and normal white blood cell and platelet counts. A ferritin level is high at 440 ng/dL. Cytogenetic studies show a normal male karyotype. His baseline erythropoietin level is elevated at 90 U/L. The patient requires red cell transfusion for the relief of symptomatic anemia once every 5–6 weeks.

Q Which of the following would be the most appropriate management for this patient?

A Therapeutic trial of epoetin alfa
B Iron chelation therapy
C Treatment with hypomethylating agents
D Nonmyeloablative allogeneic stem cell transplantation

CHAPTER
04
Iron metabolism, iron overload, and the porphyrias

Question 1

A 67-year-old woman with a 9-year history of myelodysplasia and >100 U of packed red blood cell transfusions presents with worsening fatigue and dyspnea. Physical examination reveals a bronzed woman with a liver edge palpable 3 cm below the right costal margin. She is found to have a ferritin of 4000 ng/mL. Her hemoglobin is 6.9 g/dL, and the hematocrit is 21%. Her transferrin saturation is 98%.

Which of the following is the most appropriate next step in the management of this patient?

A Phlebotomy
B Assay for HFE *C282Y* mutation
C Magnetic resonance imaging to assess liver iron stores
D Oral deferasirox therapy

Question 2

A 25-year-old woman with a history of thalassemia major and >100 U of packed red blood cell transfusions presents with fatigue and abdominal pain. Physical examination reveals a slender woman with palpable hepatosplenomegaly. She is found to have a ferritin of 4000 ng/mL. Her hemoglobin is 5.9 g/dL, and her hematocrit is 18%. Her transferrin saturation is 98%. She wishes to start chelation therapy.

Which of the following statements best reflects the counseling she should receive?

A Subcutaneous deferoxamine given for 12 hours nightly has proven superiority to any oral iron chelator
B She should undergo magnetic resonance imaging to evaluate hepatic iron stores before commencing therapy
C Oral deferasirox is safer than subcutaneous deferoxamine because it lacks ocular and ototoxicity
D Subcutaneous deferoxamine should be provided because oral deferasirox has not been approved by the Food and Drug Administration for treatment of patients with thalassemia major
E Oral deferasirox has been shown to be as effective as subcutaneous deferoxamine in reducing hepatic iron loads

Question 3

A 45-year-old man who is a professor at Tulane University in New Orleans with newly diagnosed hereditary hemochromatosis is undergoing a program of therapeutic phlebotomy. He does not drink alcohol or have other medical problems. He develops a fever and presents to the emergency room, where he is found to be hypotensive with numerous tense bullous skin lesions.

Which of the following infectious agents is the most likely cause of this patient's disorder?

A *Vibrio vulnificus*
B *Listeria monocytogenes*
C *Mycobacterium marinum*
D *Yersinia enterocolitica*
E *Sporothrix schenckii*

Question 4

A 35-year-old man with multidrug-resistant tuberculosis and acquired immunodeficiency syndrome presents with fever and hemoptysis. He is found to have multiple lung abscesses and requires intubation with mechanical ventilation. After 3 weeks in the intensive care unit, he develops pressure ulcers over his sacrum and a candidal infection of his groin and urine. He also develops anemia, for which hematology is consulted. His hemoglobin is 6.4 g/dL with a hematocrit of 22%. The mean corpuscular volume is 80 fL. The reticulocyte count is 1.1%.

Q Which of the following most likely explains the pathogenesis of the patient's anemia?

A Decreased hepcidin levels depress iron absorption from the gut and promote iron transport out of hepatocytes and macrophages
B Increased hepcidin levels depress iron absorption from the gut and promote iron transport out of hepatocytes and macrophages
C Increased hepcidin levels depress iron absorption from the gut and retard iron transport out of hepatocytes and macrophages
D Decreased hepcidin levels promote iron absorption from the gut and retard iron transport out of hepatocytes and macrophages

Question 5

A 45-year-old man presents for an initial visit. He has no current complaints but notes that his father was just diagnosed with cirrhosis and was found to be homozygous for the HFE *C282Y* mutation. The patient has no abnormalities found on physical examination. He has no siblings. He is married and neither drinks nor smokes. He and his wife have 3 sons, aged 21, 22, and 25, all of whom drink alcohol on a daily basis.

Q Which of the following is the most cost-effective next step in the evaluation of the risk for the family members?

A Screening of the patient and his children
B Screening of the children only, and not the patient
C Screening of the patient and his wife
D Screening of neither the patient nor his children
E Screening of the patient, his wife, and all his children

Question 6

A 45-year-old man presents for an initial visit. He has no current complaints but notes that his father was just diagnosed with cirrhosis and was found to be homozygous for the HFE *C282Y* mutation. The patient has no abnormalities found on physical. He is married and drinks 2 beers daily. He is also found to be homozygous for the HFE *C282Y* mutation. Current laboratory values show hemoglobin of 16.5 g/dL, hematocrit of 48%, transferrin saturation of 88%, and ferritin of 700 ng/mL. Weekly phlebotomy is begun.

Q Which of the following is the treatment goal of phlebotomy in this patient?

A Serum ferritin <100 ng/mL
B Until the patient is anemic
C Serum ferritin <50 ng/mL
D Serum ferritin <250 ng/mL

Question 7

A 16-year-old boy presents with shortness of breath and palpitations. Evaluation shows congestive heart failure, with an ejection fraction of 27%; absence of facial, genital, and underarm hair; small testes, consistent with hypogonadotropic hypogonadism; and glucose intolerance. His skin is slightly bronzed. Laboratory data show hemoglobin of 12.5 g/dL, hematocrit of 38%, transferrin saturation of 98%, and ferritin of 1700 ng/mL.

Q Which of the following is most likely to be mutated in this patient?

A HFE
B Ferroportin
C Hepcidin
D Hemojuvelin
E Hephaestin

Question 8

A 65-year-old man presents for an initial visit. He has complaints of fatique, lethargy, and weakness. He complains of some weight loss, with polyuria and polydipsia. His father died of cirrhosis. Physical examination reveals a bronzed-appearing man with pulmonary rales. He has tender hepatomegaly, and a palpable spleen is present. Testicles are atrophied. Current laboratory values show hemoglobin of 16.5 g/dL, hematocrit of 48%, transferrin saturation of 100%, and ferritin of 1800 ng/mL. Fasting glucose is 280. He is also found to be homozygous for the HFE *C282Y* mutation.

Q Which of the following is not expected to improve with phlebotomy?

A Cardiomyopathy
B Cirrhosis
C Hyperpigmentation
D Diabetes mellitus
E Hypogonadism

Question 9

A 25-year-old woman presents with abdominal pain, nausea, constipation, and confusion. She has had several episodes of similar pain over the past 6 years. Most of these were mild compared with her current pain. Last year she was hospitalized with severe abdominal pain and had an appendectomy. In follow up, she was told that the appendix was normal. On examination, she is confused and uncooperative. She has decreased muscle strength in her arms and legs and shallow respirations. Her blood pressure is 145/90, and her pulse is 110. She has a low-grade temperature. There is no rash. Her chest and cardiac exams are unremarkable. She has decreased bowel sounds and diffuse abdominal tenderness. There is no hepatosplenomegaly. The complete blood cell count shows a mild leukocytosis with no anemia or thrombocytopenia. Her serum sodium is 120 mEq/dL.

Q Which of the following is the most appropriate next step in the evaluation of this patient?

A Rapid screen of urine for porphobilinogen
B 24-hour stool collection for porphyrins
C 24-hour urine collection for porphyrins
D Plasma porphyrin determination
E Measurement of red blood cell PBG deaminase

Question 10

A 35-year-old man with a history of acute intermittent porphyria presents with severe abdominal pain and inability to walk following a period of heavy alcohol use.

Q Which one of the following is most likely to improve this patient's outcome?

A Intravenous 5% dextrose
B 3% normal saline infusion
C Hemin infusion
D Propranolol
E Surgical consult

Question 11

A young woman with known acute intermittent porphyria (AIP) was recently hospitalized for abdominal pain. After recovery, the patient asks your advice about preventing future episodes.

Q Which of the following is least likely to exacerbate AIP?

A Alcohol
B Stress
C Smoking
D Birth control pills
E Pregnancy

Question 12

A 50-year-old woman with a well-documented history of acute intermittent porphyria is referred to you by her primary care physician for management recommendations. She has no other medical problems at present. Her porphyria was discovered in her 20s after suffering multiple bouts of abdominal pain that led to 2 exploratory laparotomies. She has had several admissions over the past 20 years for abdominal pain treated with dextrose infusion and hemin. She does not smoke and avoids alcohol.

Q Which of the following yearly screening procedures is indicated in this patient?

A No additional recommendations
B Measurement of α-fetoprotein
C Peripheral nerve conduction tests
D Estrogen hormone replacement
E Measurement of urinary aminolevulinic acid and porphobilinogen

Question 13

A 23-year-old woman is referred after a hospitalization for abdominal pain. She was found to have 100× increased excretion of both aminolevulinic acid and porphobilinogen (PBG) in the urine. There were slightly increased levels of coproporphyrins and protoporphyrin in urine and stool collections. The pain resolved after treatment with hemin and dextrose. She has no history of photosensitivity. In retrospect, she has noticed increasing abdominal pain preceding her periods. Her red blood cell level of PBG deaminase was found to be normal.

Q Which one of the following is the most likely diagnosis?

A Acute intermittent porphyria
B Coproporphyria
C Variegate porphyria
D Plumbism

Question 14

A 48-year-old man with a long-standing history of hepatitis C presents with a 2-year history of blistering skin lesions on his hands and on sun-exposed areas, including his scalp. He finds that sun screens do not help. He wears gloves when working, and they seem to help reduce the number of lesions. There is no history of abdominal pain, and he is human immunodeficiency virus-negative. Despite advice from his physician, he continues to have "1 or 2" scotch and sodas per day and "maybe a third" on weekends.

Q Which of the following is the most likely diagnosis?

A Congenital erythropoietic porphyria
B Variegate porphyria
C Coproporphyria
D Protoporphyria
E Porphyria cutanea tarda

CHAPTER

05

Acquired underproduction anemias

Question 1

An 18-year-old otherwise healthy man is referred for evaluation of anemia. He reports frequent upper respiratory infections and cold symptoms. Although he denies taking any prescribed medications, he does take daily ascorbic acid (vitamin C), zinc lozenges, and selenium for cold prevention. His physical examination is unremarkable, and recent hematocrit values have ranged between 25% and 28% with normal white blood cell (WBC) and platelet counts. A complete blood count was normal at age 15. Blood and bone marrow studies reveal the following results:

Hematocrit	24%
WBC count	5700/μL
Platelet count	177,000/μL
Mean corpuscular volume	76 fL
Reticulocyte count	1.9%

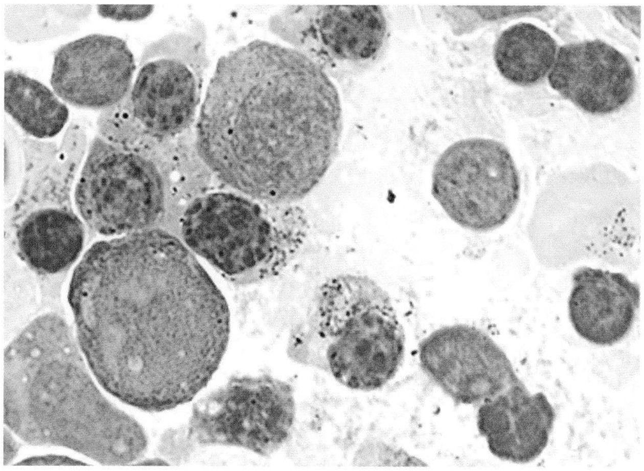

From ASH Image Bank #101383.

Q Which of the following is the most likely cause of this patient's anemia?

A Myelodysplasia
B Copper deficiency
C Selenium toxicity
D Vitamin C toxicity

Question 2

A 58-year-old man who presented to his primary care physician with progressive dyspnea and fatigue is referred to you when he is discovered to be anemic. His past medical history is significant for rheumatoid arthritis that is treated with 10 mg prednisone each day, diet-controlled diabetes mellitus, and hypertension (controlled with hydrochlorothiazide). He denies any other medications. His physical examination is remarkable for skin pallor and pale conjunctiva. Lymphadenopathy and hepatosplenomegaly are not appreciated on physical examination. Stool guaiac is negative. Initial laboratory evaluation is as follows:

Hematocrit	28%
White blood cell count	5700/μL
Platelet count	169,000/μL
Mean corpuscular volume	78 fL
Reticulocyte count	1.3%
Serum iron	18 μg/dL (normal range, 42–135 μg/dL)
Serum total iron-binding capacity	198 μg/dL (normal range, 225–430 μg/dL)
Transferrin saturation	9% (normal range, 20–50%)
Ferritin	337 ng/mL (normal range, 30–400 ng/mL)
Total bilirubin	1.0 mg/dL
Direct bilirubin	0.6 mg/dL
Lactate dehydrogenase	188 IU/L

Q Which of the following is the most likely diagnosis?

A Iron deficiency anemia
B Myelodysplasia
C α-Thalassemia
D Anemia of chronic inflammation/disease
E Autoimmune hemolytic anemia

Question 3

A 48-year-old woman is evaluated for progressive dyspnea and fatigue. The patient has a long-standing history of systemic lupus erythematosus, diabetes mellitus, and hypertension. Her medications include corticosteroids, metformin, ramipril, and aspirin. Initial evaluation reveals a microcytic anemia (mean corpuscular volume 77 fL), and anemia of chronic inflammation/disease is diagnosed after additional workup.

Q Which of the following would likely be found in this patient?

A Elevated hepcidin level
B Increased mobilization of iron from macrophages
C Increased sensitivity of erythrocyte precursors to endogenous erythropoietin
D Increased intestinal absorption of iron

Question 4

A 53-year-old African American man is referred for evaluation of anemia. He has recently become dialysis dependent secondary to hypertension leading to end-stage renal disease. When his hemoglobin was noted to be 9 g/dL, he was placed on a regimen of darbopoetin (60 μg/wk) and oral iron sulfate (325 mg twice daily). His hemoglobin subsequently improved to 12.7 g/dL. During the last 2 months, he has again become more fatigued and has experienced dyspnea on exertion. He was again noted to be anemic, with a hemoglobin level of 8.8 g/dL. His dose of darbopoetin was increased to 100 μg/wk without an adequate response. He has subsequently been referred to you for further evaluation. Current laboratory data include:

White blood cell count	6700/μL
Hemoglobin	8.3 g/dL
Mean corpuscular volume	80 fL
Platelets	424,000/μL
Reticulocyte count	1.2%
Serum iron	11 μg/dL (normal range, 42–135 μg/dL)
Serum total iron-binding capacity	98 μg/dL (normal range, 225–430 μg/dL)
Transferrin saturation	9% (normal range, 20–50%)
Ferritin	47 ng/mL (normal range, 30–400 ng/mL)

Review of the blood smear is unremarkable.

Q Which of the following would be the most appropriate therapy for this patient?

A Increase darbopoetin dose to 200 μg/wk
B Stop darbopoetin and begin erythropoietin 40,000 U/wk
C Increase oral iron sulfate intake to 325 mg orally 3 times daily
D Provide intravenous iron sucrose during dialysis

Question 5

A 53-year-old woman is referred for treatment recommendations concerning her anemia. She has recently been complaining of fatigue and shortness of breath when climbing stairs. She is otherwise well, is able to work 40 hours per week, and can easily perform all her activities of daily living. She has 5 healthy children. A recent screening colonoscopy was negative. She has entered menopause but describes a history of lifelong heavy menstrual periods. She has no other medical illnesses and takes no medications. She weighs 65 kg, is normotensive, and has a normal heart rate. The rest of her physical examination is also unremarkable. Laboratory studies include:

White blood cell count	7,400/μL
Hematocrit	27%
Platelet	234,000/μL
Mean corpuscular volume	73 fL
Reticulocyte count	1%
Serum creatinine	0.8 mg/dL
Serum iron	11 μg/dL (normal range, 42–135 μg/dL)
Serum total iron-binding capacity	498 μg/dL (normal range, 225–430 μg/dL)
Transferrin saturation	2% (normal range, 20–50%)
Ferritin	10 ng/mL (normal range, 30–400 ng/mL)

Q Which of the following would be the most appropriate therapy for this patient?

A Multivitamin with iron daily
B Iron dextran 1.5 g intravenously
C Ferrous sulfate 325 mg orally 3 times per day
D Transfusion of 2 units of packed red blood cells
E Iron sucrose 1.5 g intravenously

Question 6

A 15-year-old boy is referred for further evaluation of an anemia that has been unresponsive to oral iron therapy. The patient complains of abdominal bloating, intermittent diarrhea, and arthritis for the past 5 years. His past medical history is significant for type I diabetes mellitus and irritable bowel syndrome. He has been compliant taking oral iron sulfate 3 times per day. On examination he is thin and in the 25th percentile for height and weight. The rest of his physical examination, including the abdominal examination, is benign. Laboratory studies are as follows:

White blood cell count	5400/μL
Hematocrit	32%
Platelets	234,000/μL
Mean corpuscular volume	76 fL
Reticulocyte count	1.4%
Serum creatinine	0.8 mg/dL
Serum iron	20 μg/dL (normal range, 42–135 μg/dL)
Serum total iron-binding capacity	487 μg/dL (normal range, 225–430 μg/dL)
Transferrin saturation	4% (normal range, 20–50%)
Ferritin	12 ng/mL (normal range, 30–400 ng/mL)
Hemoglobin electrophoresis	Normal pattern

Review of the blood smear shows no target forms but a few cigar-shaped red blood cells.

Q Which of the following would be the most appropriate next step in the evaluation of this patient?

A Bone marrow aspirate and biopsy
B Measurement of serum vitamin B_{12}, folate, and thyroid-stimulating hormone levels
C Measurement of endomyseal and transglutaminase antibodies
D Globin gene synthesis studies

Question 7

A 53-year-old man with systemic lupus erythematosis and awaiting a renal transplant for end-stage renal disease secondary to lupus nephritis is transferred from a referring hospital where he was admitted with a 2-week history of chest pain, shortness of breath, and severe exertional dyspnea. The patient is otherwise healthy, and his lupus has been inactive over the last year. His medications at the time of initial admission include Nephrovite, calcium bicitra, prednisone 20 mg daily, Imuran 100 mg daily, and darbopoetin 60 μg weekly with dialysis. He denies any herbal remedies, over-the-counter medications, or recreational drug use. His grandchild was ill 1 month ago with a febrile illness and rash that resolved within 1 week without treatment. He denied any other sick contacts. On physical examination he appears weak and pale. He is afebrile, and his blood pressure is 87/40 and heart rate is 123 beats/min. There is no scleral icterus, lymphadenopathy, or hepatosplenomegaly. A 2-unit packed red blood cell transfusion has been ordered based upon his blood work. Recent blood counts are as follows:

	Current	6 months prior (routine)
Hematocrit	14%	34%
Mean corpuscular volume	98 fL	83 fL
Platelets	197,000/μL	268,000/μL
White blood cell count	4900/μL	5600/μL
Reticulocyte count	0.1%	2.8%

A bone marrow biopsy performed at the outside institution indicates that the most significant finding was a lack of red blood cell precursors. You are asked to see the patient for recommendations and further evaluation.

Q Which of the following is the most appropriate next step in the evaluation of this patient?

A Antiglobulin (Coombs) test
B Parvovirus DNA studies
C Anti-darbopoetin antibodies
D Antinuclear antibody (ANA) test

Question 8

A 39-year-old previously healthy African American man is admitted for fatigue, exertional dyspnea, and chest pain. He has had a transfusion-dependent anemia during the past 3 months. Previously blood counts had all been normal. White blood cell counts and platelet counts have been normal, and bone marrow aspirate and biopsy confirm the diagnosis of pure red cell aplasia. Flow cytometry and cytogenetic studies are unremarkable. Other evaluation including serologies for B_{12}, folate, thyrotropin, human immunodeficiency virus, LFTs, hepatitis, cytomegalovirus, and computed tomographic scan of the chest, abdomen, and pelvis have all been unremarkable. The patient appears reliable and denies taking any medications, herbal remedies, or recreational drugs. His only treatment has been red blood cell transfusion. Current blood counts include:

Hematocrit	18%
Platelets	167,000/μL
Reticulocyte count	0.1%
Direct antiglobulin test	Negative

Peripheral blood smear review reveals few red blood cells with normal morphology.

Q Which of the following is the most appropriate therapy for this patient?

A Thymectomy
B Splenectomy
C Erythropoietin
D Prednisone

Question 9

A 55-year-old woman with no previous medical problems and on no medications presents with increasing fatigue and weakness of several months' duration. Her review of systems is positive for a 40-lb weight gain over the last 2 years. A complete blood count (CBC) demonstrates a hemoglobin of 7 g/dL and a mean corpuscular volume of 108 fL. Serum B_{12} level is low, and the erythrocyte folate is borderline. A bone marrow examination reveals changes consistent with megaloblastic anemia. Iron stores are normal. She is diagnosed with B_{12} deficiency and begins daily vitamin B_{12} 1000 μg intramuscularly for 1 week followed by weekly administration for 1 month. She returns for a follow-up CBC after 1 month of therapy. On her return visit, her hemoglobin is 8 g/dL, with a corrected reticulocyte count of 2.0%.

Q What laboratory study is most likely to reveal the cause of the patient's persistent anemia?

A Ferritin
B Lactate dehydrogenase
C Direct Coombs test
D Thyrotropin

Questions 10/11

A 60-year-old woman presents with fatigue and dyspnea on exertion. Her past medical history is significant only for a deep venous thrombosis (DVT) and pulmonary embolism that occurred 2 years ago after a hip fracture. Following 6 months of Coumadin, anticoagulation was discontinued. One year later she experienced a recurrent DVT in the contralateral leg for which she remained on Coumadin up to the time of the current presentation. She is not on any other medications and has no other medical history. She has no family history of anemia or thrombosis. She denies any signs of bleeding such as hematemesis or melena.

A complete blood count reveals a hemoglobin of 6.6 g/dL, with a mean corpuscular volume of 106 fL. Her platelet count is 115,000/μL, and her absolute neutrophil count is 2200/μL. A peripheral smear shows ovalocytes and a rare hypersegmented neutrophil. Her international normalized ration is 2.1.

Q Which of the following is the most likely cause of this patient's anemia?

A Vitamin B_{12} deficiency
B Paroxysmal nocturnal hemoglobinuria
C Warm antibody hemolytic anemia
D Iron deficiency
E Anemia of chronic inflammation/disease

Q Her physician orders a laboratory evaluation for hypercoagulability. Which of the following laboratory abnormalities is most likely to be found in this patient?

A Antithrombin deficiency
B Protein C deficiency
C Hyperhomocysteinemia
D Deficiency of plasminogen activator inhibitor-1

Question 12

A 45-year-old woman with human immunodeficiency virus (HIV) presents for evaluation of fatigue, weakness, and increasing exercise intolerance. She is not taking any medications. In recent months, her CD4 count has fallen to 100 cells/μL, and her HIV viral load has been increasing. Laboratory studies show a hemoglobin of 10 g/dL, a mean corpuscular volume of 95 fL, a platelet count of 100,000/μL, and a normal white blood cell count and differential. A corrected reticulocyte count was 1.0%. Serum electrolytes, creatinine, lactate dehydrogenase, and haptoglobin are all normal. Ferritin is also normal at 287 ng/mL.

Q Which of the following therapies would be the most appropriate initial strategy for managing this patient's anemia?

A Epoetin alfa 40,000 units weekly
B Highly active antiretroviral therapy
C Epoetin alfa 100 U/kg 3 times weekly
D Epoetin alfa 100 U/kg 3 times weekly plus parenteral iron therapy

Question 13

A 76-year-old man presents for a routine physical examination. He is asymptomatic and leads an active lifestyle. He is on no medications. Routine laboratory studies show a hemoglobin of 10.5 g/dL, a mean corpuscular volume of 102 fL, platelets of 200,000/µL, and a white blood cell count of 7,500 uL with a normal differential. Urinalysis is normal, and stool guaiac does not reveal occult blood. Serum vitamin B_{12} level is 560 pg/L (normal range 243–894 pg/mL).

Q Which of the following is the next appropriate step in his evaluation?

A Obtain serum erythropoietin level
B Obtain erythrocyte sedimentation rate and C-reactive protein level
C Obtain a history of alcohol use
D Obtain iron studies

Question 14

A 35-year-old woman with known hemoglobin (Hb) S/β^+ thalassemia presents to the emergency room with complaints of severe weakness and dyspnea increasing over the previous week. The patient is on no medications. She has a recent history of substance abuse significant for both intravenous drugs and alcohol. Her appetite is poor, and she consumes only one meal each day. Her initial laboratory studies include an Hb of 4.5 g/dL, a mean corpuscular volume of 95 fL, platelets of 150,000/µL, a white blood cell count of 4,000/µL, and a corrected reticulocyte count of 1.0%.

Q Which of the following would be the most likely finding on examination of the patient's bone marrow?

A Hodgkin disease
B Megaloblastic changes
C End-stage myelofibrosis
D Disseminated candidiasis
E Myelodysplatic changes

Question 15

An 80-year-old female who lives alone presents with frequent falls and an unsteady gait. She has no other past medical history and is not on any medications. She has a normal complete blood count, creatinine, and liver function tests. A serum cobalamin level is 260 pg/L (normal range, 243–894 pg/mL). Serum folate is normal. Antiparietal cell antibodies are negative, and antiintrinsic factor antibodies are also negative. A gastrointestinal workup suggests atrophic gastritis. Serum homocysteine and methylmalonic acid levels return elevated.

Q Which of the following is the most appropriate therapeutic strategy at this point?

A Begin therapy with folic acid 1 mg orally each day
B Begin combination therapy with oral cobalamin, folate, and vitamin B_6
C Begin cobalamin 1000 µg intramuscularly each week for 4 weeks followed by monthly administration
D Begin oral cobalamin 250 µg orally each day

CHAPTER 06

Hemolytic anemias

Question 1

A 63-year-old man with chronic hepatitis C is being treated with pegylated interferon α (IFN-α) and ribavirin. He has had an excellent response to therapy with significant reduction of his viral load. He begins to notice darkening of his urine and decreased exercise tolerance. His physical examination is significant for slightly icteric sclera. His laboratory studies show hemoglobin of 7.7 g/dL and a reticulocyte count of 6%.

Q Which of the following is the most appropriate management for this patient?

A Reduce IFN-α dose by 25%
B Add high-dose vitamin E
C Discontinue IFN-α and ribavirin
D Add erythropoietin
E Reduce the dose of ribavirin

Question 2

A 29-year-old woman with persistent hemolytic anemia is found to have paroxysmal nocturnal hemoglobinuria. Flow cytometry shows that CD55 or CD59 are absent from approximately 60% of granulocytes. Her hemolysis is controlled with prednisone given every other day. She is not pregnant or taking oral contraceptives and has no history of thrombosis.

Q In addition to prednisone, which of the following would reduce the risk of thrombosis in this patient?

A No additional treatment necessary
B Aspirin
C Warfarin
D Aspirin and low-molecular-weight heparin

Question 3

A 22-year-old male soldier presents with shortness of breath. He has no significant past medical history. He returned from active duty in Afghanistan 5 months prior. His physical examination is significant for pallor with icteric sclera. He is febrile to 101ºF. His respiratory rate is 27, and he is tachycardic. His lung examination is unremarkable, and he has a 2/4 systolic murmur that does not radiate. The remainder of his examination is normal. His laboratory studies are significant for hemoglobin of 8 g/dL with a platelet count of 42,000/mm^3. His reticulocyte count is 17%. His peripheral smear stained with methylene blue is shown (from ASH Image Bank #100704).

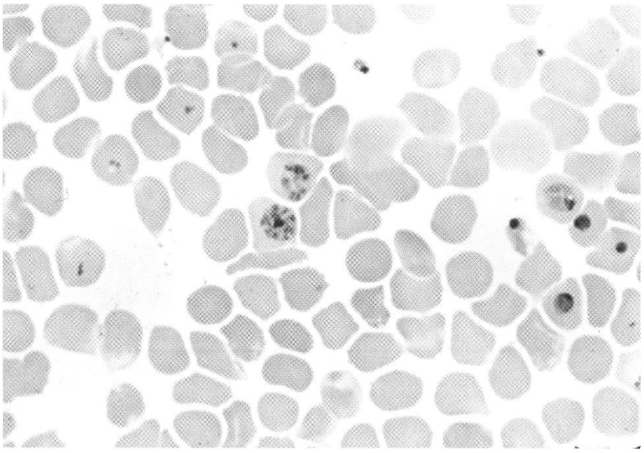

Q How should he be treated?

A Prednisone
B Intravenous immune globulin
C Plasmapheresis
D Chloroquine

Question 4

A 62-year-old African American man with chronic lymphocytic leukemia has undergone mechanical valve replacement. He now presents with anemia. He reports mild shortness of breath and dyspnea on exertion. He has recently been treated for a urinary tract infection with trimethoprim/sulfamethoxazole and phenazopyridine. His physical examination is significant for muffled mechanical valve sounds with a 2/4 diastolic murmur heard at the apex. His laboratory studies are significant for hemoglobin of 8.4 g/dL with a hematocrit of 25%. His reticulocyte count is 11%. His lactose dehydrogenase and indirect bilirubin are elevated. His peripheral smear (from ASH Image Bank #100249) is shown.

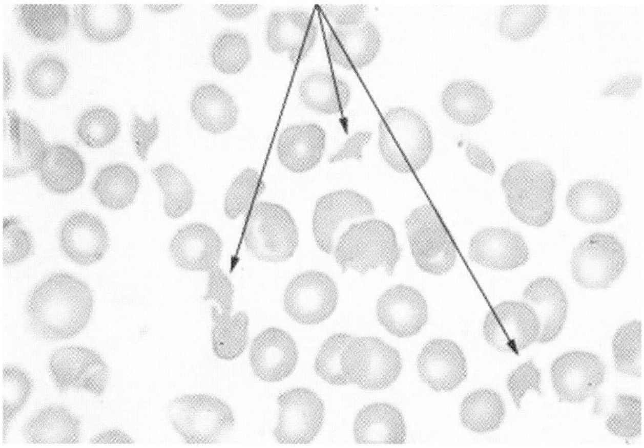

Q Which of the following is the most appropriate therapy for this patient's anemia?

A Prednisone
B Plasmapheresis
C Prosthetic valve replacement
D Discontinuation of phenazopyridine

Question 5

A 37-year-old woman who had undergone splenectomy as a teenager following a bicycle accident presents to the emergency department complaining of fevers, night sweats, headaches, dark urine, and myalgias of 2 weeks' duration. She had undergone a hysterectomy 1 month prior for uterine fibroids and menorrhagia and required a packed red blood cell transfusion prior to surgery. On physical examination, she is pale with icteric sclera. She is tachycardic, tachypneic, and has a 2/4 murmur heard best at the base without radiation. Her laboratory studies are significant for hemoglobin of 9.7 g/dL, a platelet count of 57,000/mm^3, and a normal white blood cell count and differential. Her peripheral smear is shown (ASH SAP. 2nd ed. Figure 6-19). Her creatinine is 4.6 mg/dL, her alanine aminotransferase is 220 IU/L, and her indirect bilirubin is 5.6 mg/dL.

Q Which of the following is the most appropriate therapy for this patient?

A Prednisone
B Quinine and chloroquine
C Clindamycin and ampicillin
D Azithromycin and atovaquone

Question 6

A 39-year-old man develops a delayed transfusion reaction following knee surgery. His serum, when incubated with a panel of red cells, reveals the agglutination pattern shown in

Question 6: Red cell panel

	D	C	E	c	e	K	k	Jk^a	Jk^b	Fy^a	Fy^b	Le^a	Le^b	S	s	M	N	P	Lu^a	Lu^b
1	+	+	0	0	+	0	+	+	0	0	+	0	+	0	+	+	+	+	0	+
2	+	+	0	0	+	0	+	0	+	+	0	0	+	+	+	+	+	+	0	+
3	+	0	+	+	0	0	+	+	+	+	+	0	+	0	+	0	+	+	0	+
4	+	0	0	+	+	0	+	0	+	0	0	0	0	0	+	+	+	+	0	+
5	0	+	0	+	+	0	+	+	0	0	+	0	+	+	+	+	0	0	0	+
6	0	0	+	+	+	0	+	+	+	0	+	+	0	+	+	+	+	+	0	+
7	0	0	0	+	+	+	+	0	+	0	+	0	+	+	+	0	+	+	0	+
8	0	0	0	+	+	0	+	+	0	+	0	0	+	0	+	+	+	0	0	+
9	0	0	0	+	+	0	+	0	0	0	+	0	0	+	0	+	0	+	0	+
10	0	0	0	+	+	0	+	+	+	0	+	+	0	+	0	+	+	+	0	+
11	+	+	0	0	+	+	+	+	+	0	+	0	+	+	+	+	0	+	0	+

the following when performed at 37°C. The red cell antigen panel is also shown.

Patient's agglutination pattern at 37°C

	37°C
1	+
2	+
3	–
4	–
5	+
6	–
7	–
8	–
9	–
10	–

Q To what antigen has this patient been sensitized?

A D
B C
C K
D JK[a]
E Lu[a]

Question 7

A venture capitalist consults you regarding potential therapies for paroxysmal nocturnal hemoglobinuria. He is interested in investing in strategies that have the most promise for future treatment of this disease.

Q Which one of the following treatment strategies is most likely to be effective?

A Monoclonal antibody therapy directed against C5
B Gene therapy to transfect hematopoietic stem cells with intact *PIG-A* genes
C Strategies to attach proteins artificially onto erythrocyte membranes using synthetic glycosyl phosphatidylinositol (GPI) anchors
D *Ex vivo* expansion of clonal hematopoietic stem cells expressing GPI-linked molecules followed by transplantation of these cells

Question 8

An 18-year-old woman with sickle cell anemia (SS) is admitted to the hospital with shortness of breath and pedal edema. She has 8 to 10 painful crisis per year. Her current oxygen saturation is 75% on room air. Her hemoglobin (Hb) is 8.3 g/dL. Her white count is 10.5×10^3 cells/μL. Review of her peripheral smear at the time of hospitalization reveals 30% nucleated red cells. Her hemoglobin electrophoresis reveals 94% Hb S and 6% Hb F.

Q Which of the following findings *most* increases this patient's risk for death from this hospitalization?

A Nucleated red blood cells on smear
B Her degree of anemia
C Elevated Hb F
D Peripheral edema

Question 9

A 66-year-old woman with a history of myelodysplasia, refractory anemia subtype, presents with a hemoglobin of 9.3 g/dL with a newly reduced mean corpuscular volume of 59 fL. Her iron studies are significant for a ferritin of 425 ng/mL, with an iron level of 245 μg/dL. A bone marrow aspirate shows increased erythroid precursors. Hemoglobin H inclusions are seen on her peripheral smear after staining with brilliant cresyl blue. The patient has no family history of anemia and has previous hemograms that have been unremarkable. Her peripheral smear stained with Wright–Giemsa is shown (from ASH Image Bank #100324).

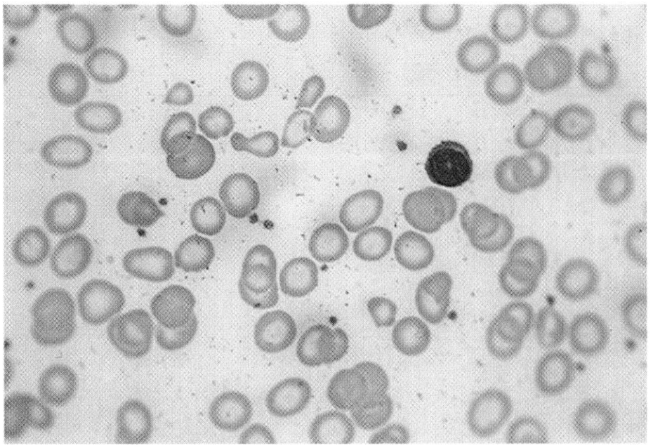

Q What is her most likely diagnosis?

A Cobalamin deficiency
B Myelofibrosis
C Hemoglobin C disease
D α Thalassemia

Question 10

A 7-year-old boy is noted to be lethargic following an episode of otitis media. His mother reports dark urine on the morning of his doctor's visit. On physical examination, he is noted to be pale with icteric sclera. He does not have splenomegaly. His laboratory studies are remarkable for a total bilirubin of 6.2 mg/dL of which 5.9 mg/dL is indirect. His complete blood cell count reveals hemoglobin of 8 g/dL with a hematocrit (Hct) of 23%. His reticulocyte count is 7%. He has a normal white count and platelet count. Further evaluation reveals a direct antibody test that is negative for immunoglobin G at room temperature but positive when run at 4°C.

Q The cause of this disorder is an immune-mediated reaction against which of the following?

A Rh antigen
B P antigen
C I/i antigens
D ABO antigens

Question 11

A 6-year-old girl with congenital cyanosis presents for evaluation. She was the product of a normal birth and delivery. Cardiopulmonary evaluation has been normal. Both of her parents are normal. She is on no medications. Evaluation reveals a normal hemogram. Her oxygen saturation on room air is 97%.

Q What is her most likely diagnosis?

A Sulfhemoglobinemia
B Low-oxygen-affinity hemoglobinopathy
C Nicotinamide-adenine-dinucleotide–diaphorase deficiency
D Hemoglobin M

CHAPTER 07

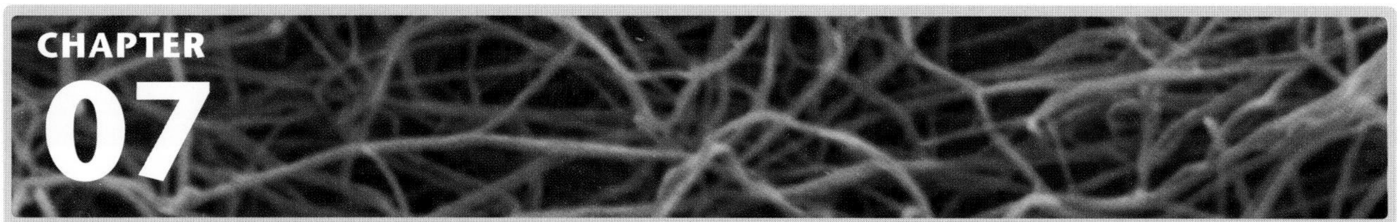

Myeloid disorders

Question 1

A 67-year-old female with Crohn disease for 10 years presents with fever, hypotension, and abdominal pain. Abdominal computed tomographic scan shows an intraabdominal abscess. The abscess is percutaneously drained, and broad-spectrum antibiotics are started. A complete blood cell count reveals an elevated white blood cell count of 28,000/μL.

Q Which of the following features would most warrant further investigation for a myeloproliferative disorder?

A Absolute neutrophil count of >15,000/μL
B Leukocyte differential with a preponderance of band neutrophils and occasional metamyelocytes
C Monocytosis
D Basophilia
E High leukocyte alkaline phosphatase score

Question 2

An 85-year-old male with a history of hypertension and benign prostatic hypertrophy presents with fever, fatigue, and sore throat. The patient reports starting trimethoprim-sulfamethoxazole 10 days ago for a urinary tract infection. A complete blood cell count and examination of the peripheral blood smear reveal normal white blood cell, red blood cell, and platelet counts but the absence of segmented or band neutrophils. Trimethoprim-sulfamethoxazole is stopped.

Q Which of the following is the most likely outcome for this patient's disorder?

A The neutropenia should resolve in 2–3 days
B The neutropenia should resolve within 2–3 weeks
C The neutropenia will persist, requiring indefinite granulocyte colony-stimulating factor therapy
D The neutropenia will progress to leukemia
E The neutropenia will progress to aplastic anemia

Question 3

A 37-year-old woman with recurrent bouts of anaphylactic shock is referred for evaluation. The patient has mild anemia, and bone marrow reveals multifocal aggregates of spindle-shaped mast cells with >25 cells per aggregate. There are no other obvious affected organs on physical examination or laboratory evaluation, and the serum tryptase on repeated measurement is within normal limits.

Q Which of the following would be the most appropriate next test in the evaluation of this patient?

A Flow cytometry of peripheral blood monocytes for CD2 and CD25
B Analysis of peripheral blood granulocytes for *c-kit* mutations
C Measurement of 24-hour specimen for histamine
D Measurement of red cell hexokinase
E Fluorescent *in situ* hybridization of bone marrow mast cells for 19q23 deletions

Question 4

A 30-year-old woman complains of headache and pressure behind her right eye, and radiograph reveals a lytic lesion in the temporal bone. Needle biopsy reveals histiocytic-appearing cells that are CD1a and S-100 positive. A complete blood cell count and octreotide scan are normal, but magnetic resonance imaging suggests pituitary stalk involvement, and serum sodium is 148 mEq/L.

Q In addition to desmopressin, which would be the most appropriate therapy for this patient?

A Radiation therapy
B Curettage of the lesion followed by radiation
C Systemic chemotherapy
D Interferon-α
E Concurrent cisplatin and radiation

Question 5

A 34-year-old woman presents with a macular skin rash, intermittent diarrhea, flushing, and hepatomegaly. Skin biopsy reveals spindle-shaped mast cells in large aggregates, and the bone marrow biopsy has similar findings. A serum tryptase is elevated, as is 24-hour urinary histamine excretion.

Q Which of the following is the most likely mutation to be found in the malignant cells?

A The *D816V c-kit* mutation
B The *bcr-abl* rearrangement
C The *AML-ETO* rearrangement
D The *C282Y* mutation
E Translocations involving the *MLL* gene

Question 6

A 48-year-old man presents with rash, flushing, diarrhea, and intermittent angiodema and bronchospasm. On examination, he has a macular skin rash with dermatographia, and hepatomegaly. Biopsy of the skin reveals dense aggregates of irregularly shaped mast cells, and a total serum tryptase level is markedly elevated. Molecular analysis reveals the *D816V* mutation in *c-kit*.

Q Which of the following therapies would not be effective in this patient?

A Cromolyn sodium
B Imatinib
C Antihistamines
D Corticosteroids
E H_2 antagonists

Question 7

An 8-year-old boy is brought to his pediatrician for a 10-day history of fever, nausea, vomiting, fatigue, and abdominal pain. On examination, his temperature is 39°C; there are 1–2-cm lymph nodes in anterior cervical, bilateral axillae, and bilateral inguinal areas and a spleen palpable 4 cm below the costal margin on the left. Laboratory data is remarkable for a hemoglobin of 8.5 g/dL, mean corpuscular volume of 75 fL, platelets of 68,000/μL, absolute reticulocyte count of 43,000/μL, triglycerides of 600 mg/dL, serum ferritin of 610 μg/L, and fibrinogen of 1.1 g/L. His bone marrow reveals marked hemophagocytosis.

Q Which of the following is the most likely diagnosis?

A Systemic lupus erythematosus
B Hemophagocytic lymphohistiocytosis
C Juvenile rheumatoid arthritis exacerbation
D Castleman disease
E Infectious mononucleosis

Question 8

A 5-year-old boy is diagnosed with hemophagocytic lymphohistiocytosis and is found to be homozygous for a mutation in the perforin (*PRF1*) gene. No other associated disorders or underlying malignancy is found.

Q Which of the following therapies would be most appropriate for this patient?

A High-dose corticosteroids
B Intravenous immunoglobulin, cyclosporine, and corticosteroids
C Concurrent high-dose corticosteroids, etoposide, and cyclosporine
D Allogeneic stem cell transplantation
E Cladarabine and CAMPATH-1H

Question 9

A 13-year-old boy presents with complaints of pain in the arms, legs, and hips for 3 months that has progressively worsened. Plain film radiographs of the affected areas show 1–3-cm lytic lesions with minimal sclerotic changes. Needle biopsy specimen of one of the lesions yields histiocytic cells positive for CD1a and S-100.

Q Which of the following is the most likely diagnosis?

A Langerhans cell histiocytosis
B Hodgkin disease

C Multiple myeloma
D Rosai–Dorfman disease
E Ewing sarcoma

Question 10

A 7-year-old boy presents with persistent pain in the left humerus for 2 months after a baseball injury. Plain film radiograph reveals a 2-cm lytic lesion. The rest of his plain film skeletal survey, bone scan, and laboratory evaluation are unremarkable. A needle biopsy reveals histiocytic cells positive for CD1a and S-100. He is treated with surgical curettage with good relief of symptoms.

Q Which of the following is the most likely prognosis for this patient's condition?

A High likelihood of local recurrence and progression
B High likelihood of systemic recurrence
C Low likelihood of recurrence
D High likelihood of pulmonary recurrence

Question 11

A 6-year-old boy presents with cellulitis and an absolute neutrophil count (ANC) of 200/uL. His history is notable for recurrent stomatitis and oral ulcers. His father had a similar history of stomatitis as a child but is now asymptomatic. The cellulitis clears with antibiotic therapy, and a repeat complete blood cell count 1 week later shows an ANC of 2,200/uL. Over the next few months, serial blood counts are obtained and show that the ANC fluctuates from normal to <200/uL.

Q What test would most likely establish the diagnosis?

A Antineutrophil antibodies
B Antinuclear antibody testing
C Empiric trial of granulocyte colony-stimulating factor
D Genetic testing for *ELA2* mutations
E Genetic testing for *BCR-ABL* mutations

Question 12

A 2-year-old boy with recurrent pneumonia and skin abscesses now presents with suppurative lymphadenitis. His neutrophil and other blood counts are normal. Neutrophil function testing shows reduced nitroblue tetrazolium reduction and impaired oxidation of dihydrorhodamine.

Q Which of the following is the most likely diagnosis?

A Cyclic neutropenia
B Chediak–Higashi syndrome
C Chronic granulomatous disease
D Myeloperoxidase deficiency
E Severe combined immunodeficiency

Question 13

A 10-month-old girl with recurrent otitis media presents with an absolute neutrophil count of 200/uL. Neutrophil morphology is normal. Her 2 siblings and parents have normal neutrophil counts. Bone marrow examination shows normocellularity with a mild reduction in the number of mature neutrophils. Antineutrophil antibodies against the HNA-1a (NA1) antigen are detected.

Q Which of the following is the most appropriate management for this patient?

A Genetic testing for *ELA2* mutations
B Serial bone marrow biopsy
C Indefinite granulocyte colony-stimulating factor therapy
D HLA typing of siblings
E Observation

Question 14

A 6-year-old girl presents with short stature (10%) and chronic diarrhea. Her complete blood cell count shows mild anemia (hemoglobin 10 g/dL), an absolute neutrophil count of 400/μL, and normal platelets. The blood smear is otherwise normal. Her serum trypsinogen is 5.9 μg/L (normal >16.7 μg/L). Fasting blood glucose is within normal limits. Magnetic resonance imaging of her abdomen shows a normal spleen size but fatty infiltration of the pancreas. The parents want to know if a 1-year-old sibling (or future siblings) might be affected.

Q Which of the following would be the most appropriate genetic testing for the patient and her sibling?

A No genetic testing because this syndrome is acquired
B Genetic testing for *ELA2*
C Genetic testing for *SBDS* mutation
D Genetic testing for *CXCR4* mutation

Question 15

A 2-year-old boy is brought in by his parents for a rash that has persisted over the last 3 weeks, and he has been unable to stop scratching. The rash involves the arms and legs but spares the palms, soles, and face. There is minimal involvement of the trunk with these brown macules. Urticaria and erythema occur when the affected area is rubbed. Physical examination is otherwise unremarkable, as are a complete blood count and chemistry panel, including alkaline phosphatase and bilirubin. A skin biopsy reveals increased irregular-appearing mast cells that are tryptase and chymase positive on immunohistochemical stains. Serum tryptase and urine histamine are normal; a bone marrow biopsy is also normal.

Q Which of the following would be the most appropriate treatment of this patient?

A Imatinib mesylate
B Interferon-α and prednisone
C Topical cromoglycate and an oral antihistamine
D Intravenous cladarabine
E Psoralen and ultraviolet A

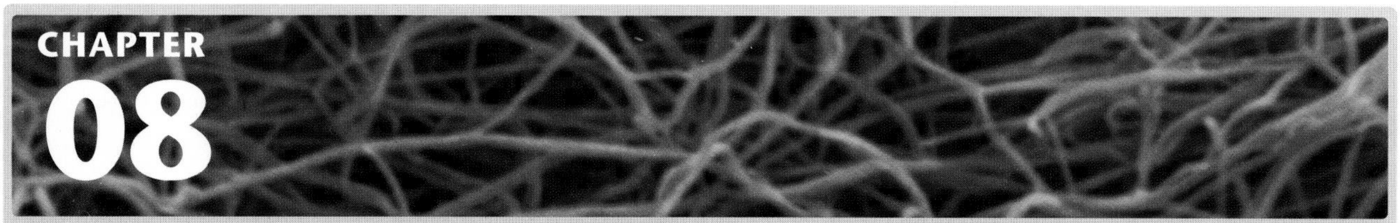

CHAPTER 08

Myeloproliferative disorders

Question 1

A previously healthy 67-year-old retired insurance salesman presents to his family doctor complaining of fatigue and vague abdominal discomfort. He is referred to the hematology clinic when physical examination reveals hepatosplenomegaly (the spleen tip was palpable 6 cm below the left costal margin on shallow inspiration), and blood tests demonstrate a hemoglobin of 8.7 g/dL, mean corpuscular volume of 96 fL, white count of 2200/μL with an absolute neutrophil count of 900/μL, and a platelet count of 74,000/μL. Transaminases (aspartate aminotransferase and alanine aminotransferase) and alkaline phosphatase are also moderately elevated above the normal range. Vitamin B_{12} and folate levels are normal. A bone marrow examination and liver biopsy are then performed. The bone marrow is hypercellular for age, with 9% undifferentiated blasts, trilineage myeloid dysplasia (including megakaryocyte clustering), and an abnormal increase in the number of mast cells, which are present in diffuse sheets with admixed myeloid progenitor cells. Eosinophilia is not present. The marrow karyotype shows del(5)(q13;q35) and trisomy 13 in all metaphases examined. Biopsy of the liver demonstrates atypical cells that express CD117, CD25, and CD2. Serum tryptase level is 35 ng/mL.

Q Which of the following is the most likely associated molecular lesion?

A FIP1L1-PDGFRA fusion
B JAK2 V617 mutation
C FLT3 D835 mutation
D C-KIT D816 mutation
E PDGFRB-EVI6 fusion

Question 2

A 66-year-old female homemaker is hospitalized for deep venous thrombosis of the right femoral vein. She is a smoker and underwent hysterectomy 4 years ago for irregular postmenopausal bleeding (no malignancy was identified). Her initial complete blood count shows a hemoglobin of 13.8 g/dL, white blood count of 6,500/μL with a normal differential, and a platelet count of 978,000/μL. At the time of her hysterectomy, her blood counts had been normal. Physical examination now discloses a palpable spleen tip and asymmetry in the diameter of her legs. There is no evidence of an inflammatory condition by history or examination, and her other laboratory tests (including erythrocyte sedimentation rate and C-reactive protein) are normal. Spiral computed tomography of the chest performed using a pulmonary embolism protocol is normal. Her bone marrow aspirate is slightly hypercellular, with scattered clusters of atypical megakaryocytes. Bone marrow cytogenetics, *BCR-ABL* reverse transcriptase polymerase chain reaction, and *JAK2* mutation testing results are all normal. Ristocetin cofactor assay is within normal limits. She is started on low-molecular-weight heparin in therapeutic doses for her thrombosis, instructed in the use and monitoring of oral warfarin, and encouraged to quit smoking.

Q Which of the following is the best initial management for this patient's thrombocytosis?

A Anagrelide
B Hydroxyurea
C Interferon-α
D High-dose aspirin
E Plateletpheresis

Question 3

A 75-year-old man is evaluated for lower extremity edema, dyspnea on exertion, fatigue, and increasing abdominal girth. He has a diagnosis of chronic idiopathic myelofibrosis and underwent splenectomy for mechanical symptoms 2 years ago. His current symptoms have made it challenging for him to work. Jugular venous pressure is elevated. Loop diuretic therapy does not help. Chest x-ray shows engorgement of pulmonary veins, whereas chest computed tomography shows ground-glass infiltrates in bilateral bases, but no evidence for thromboembolism. Echocardiography shows right-sided heart dilatation with severe tricuspid regurgitation, and the right ventricular systolic pressure is estimated at 90 mm Hg (systemic blood pressure is 140/100 mm Hg). Technetium-99m sulfur colloid nuclear medicine scanning shows diffuse bilateral lung uptake and a strong liver signal, as well as patchy bone marrow signal.

Q Which of the following is the most appropriate next step in the treatment of this patient?

A Pulmonary irradiation
B Epoprostenol
C Hydroxyurea
D Thrombolytic therapy
E Induction chemotherapy for acute myeloid leukemia

Question 4

A 55-year-old man is evaluated during a routine examination and found to have a hemoglobin of 19.2 g/dL, white blood count of 13,000/μL with neutrophilia, and a platelet count of 466,000/μL. He takes no medications and is a nonsmoker. Physical examination is unremarkable, and the spleen tip is just barely palpable with deep inspiration. Oxygen saturation is 96% on room air by pulse oximetry. He denies a family history of hematologic disorders. He exercises regularly and is a competitive cyclist. He denies using any performance-enhancing drugs. Endogenous erythropoietin level is 5 U/L, repeat erythropoietin testing reveals a level of 6 U/L, and endocrine testing is unremarkable. He refuses bone marrow examination.

Q Which of the following tests is most likely to establish a diagnosis?

A Red cell mass measurement with 51-chromium
B Sequencing of the *VHL* and *EPOR* genes
C Granulocyte expression of *PRV-1*
D Assay for JAK2 V617F
E Immunoassay for epoetin-alfa and darbepoetin-alfa

Question 5

A 28-year-old woman is evaluated in the emergency department for epistaxis. She mentions to the examining physician that her last menstrual period was heavier than usual. This concerns her because she has been trying to become pregnant. Physical examination reveals blood in the nares and in the pharynx, a spleen tip palpable 4 cm below the left costal margin, and a few ecchymoses on the patient's extremities that appear to be of varying ages. Pelvic examination is unremarkable, and a pregnancy test is negative. Her international normalized ratio is 1.1, and her activated partial thromboplastin time is 26 seconds. The erythrocyte sedimentation rate is 24 mm/h. Her complete blood count is as follows: hemoglobin 11.2 g/dL, mean corpuscular volume 83 fL, white blood count 9,000/μL, and platelet count 1,100,000/μL. Her ferritin is low. Peripheral smear shows occasional hypochromic cells, mild anisopoikilocytosis, scattered basophils, and numerous platelets of various sizes. Acute management of the epistaxis is undertaken. When she is stabilized, a bone marrow is performed. The final report of the marrow shows myeloid hyperplasia with megakaryocyte excess and 1+ fibrosis; there are 3% undifferentiated blasts. The karyotype is normal, but reverse transcriptase polymerase chain reaction (RT-PCR) demonstrates a strongly positive signal for the *BCR-ABL1* gene rearrangement.

Q Which of the following is the most appropriate next step in the management of this patient?

A Assay for JAK2 V617F mutation
B Repeat RT-PCR
C Start interferon-α therapy
D Start hydroxyurea therapy

Question 6

An 88-year-old man with a 13-year history of polycythemia vera is evaluated. His initial diagnosis was made at the time of hospitalization for a cerebrovascular accident, and he had 2 lower extremity thromboses in the 3 years prior to his stroke. His blood counts at present are as follows: hemoglobin 16.8 g/dL, hematocrit 50%, white blood count 12,000/μL, and platelet count 505,000/μL. His blood counts have always been difficult to control with hydroxyurea, and he has now developed nonhealing bilateral ankle ulcers, despite normal results from noninvasive lower extremity arterial studies. He tolerates phlebotomies poorly because of volume shifts leading to hypotension and near syncope. His spleen size has been stable, and the spleen tip is palpable about 4 cm below the left costal margin. At the time of his last marrow examination 15 months ago, the marrow findings were unchanged from diagnosis. His other medical problems include refractory heart failure, nonmelanomatous skin cancer, type 2 diabetes mellitus for which he is on an oral agent, and peripheral vascular disease. He quit smoking 6 months ago.

Q Which of the following is the most appropriate therapy for this patient?

A Anagrelide
B Radiophosphorous (^{32}P)
C Splenectomy
D Interferon-α

Question 7

A 55-year-old male prisoner develops unexplained fevers, fatigue, pruritus, cough, diarrhea, and insidious onset of lower extremity edema. Examination is remarkable for elevated jugular pressures, inspiratory basilar lung crackles, positive hepatojugular reflux, ascites, and 3+ pitting bilateral lower extremity edema. Chest x-ray shows cardiomegaly and patchy bibasilar lung infiltrates. Transthoracic echocardiography suggests endomyocardial thickening, a restrictive filling pattern, and also the possibility of a mural thrombus, though this is not well defined. Complete blood count is as follows: hemoglobin 12.2 g/dL, white blood count 17,000/μL with 6,500/μL eosinophils, and platelet count 334,000/μL. Viral serologies (human immunodeficiency virus, hepatitis) are negative, and studies for parasites (stool smears and *Giardia* and *Strongyloides* serologies) are also unremarkable. T-cell clonal rearrangement studies of peripheral blood are negative, and a serum tryptase level is normal. *C-Kit* mutation analysis is negative, and JAK2 V617F is absent, but a *FIP1L1-PDGFRA* fusion gene is present.

Q Which of the following is the best initial therapy for this patient?

A Hydroxyurea
B Chlorodeoxyadenosine (2-CDA, cladribine)
C Imatinib mesylate
D Interferon-α

Question 8

A 37-year-old woman who requires chronic oral corticosteroids for long-standing systemic lupus erythematosus is found to have anemia (hemoglobin 9.8 g/dL) and moderate thrombocytopenia (platelet count 96,000/μL). She complains of increased fatigue but otherwise notes no specific symptoms. Clot-based tests for lupus anticoagulant activity and antiphospholipid antibody assays are negative. The ferritin level is 540 ng/mL, iron 110 μg/dL, and total iron-binding capacity 220 μg/dL. An antinuclear antibody assay is positive in high titer in a speckled pattern. B^{12} and folate are normal. A Coombs test (direct antiglobulin test) is positive with the polyspecific (IgG and complement) reagent; a haptoglobin level is normal, as is the total bilirubin. Physical examination reveals cushingoid features and joint deformities, similar to previous examinations and consistent with her known treated lupus. The spleen is not palpable. Her blood smear shows occasional nucleated blood cells and anisopoikilocytosis with teardrop-shaped cells. No platelet clumping or agglutination is detected. A few variant lymphocytes are seen. The bone marrow is mildly hypercellular for age and demonstrates 3+ fibrosis without dysplasia. The marrow karyotype is 46,XX in all metaphases. Tests for *BCR-ABL* fusion and *JAK2* mutation are negative.

Q Which of the following is the most appropriate next step in the management of this patient?

A Hydroxyurea
B Interferon-α
C Low-dose thalidomide
D Referral to a marrow transplantation center
E Increase of corticosteroid dose

Question 9

A 44-year-old construction worker presents to his family doctor with fatigue, bloating, intermittent loose stools, and an involuntary 10-kg weight loss. His past medical history is unremarkable. Physical examination reveals mild pallor but is otherwise normal. The spleen tip is nonpalpable. The complete blood count shows a hemoglobin of 9.8 g/dL with a mean corpuscular volume of 77 fL, white blood count of 7,000/μL with an unremarkable differential, and a platelet count of 620,000/μL. Erythrocyte sedimentation rate is 22 mm/h, and a ferritin is 12 ng/mL. His stool is negative for occult blood, and upper and lower endoscopy are unremarkable. Despite 6 months of oral iron therapy with ferrous sulfate, his hemoglobin does not improve, and he continues to have thrombocytosis. He is then referred to the hematology clinic for further evaluation. He states that he has had no fevers, pruritus, or acral extremity symptoms. He has never had a surgery or major trauma. There is no family history of anemia. Hemoglobin electrophoresis shows no hemoglobin variant. Serum protein electrophoresis shows hypoalbuminemia but no monoclonal protein. Urine monoclonal protein studies are normal. Peripheral smear shows hypochromic microcytic erythrocytes, anisopoikilocytosis, and an increase in platelet count. Numerous red cells have small, single, rounded purple inclusions. Marrow is mildly hypercellular for age but is otherwise unremarkable. He continues to have fatigue and to feel generally unwell.

Q Which of the following is the most appropriate management for this patient?

A Start anagrelide
B Start hydroxyurea
C Start low-dose aspirin
D Refer to a dietician for gluten-free diet
E Refer for stem cell transplantation

Question 10

A 65-year-old woman presents with splenomegaly and an abnormal complete blood count on a routine examination. Her white blood count is 24,000/μL with 3% basophils, her hemoglobin is 11.6 g/dL, and her platelets are 580,000/μL. Peripheral blood is positive for the e13a2 *BCR-ABL* transcript by qualitative polymerase chain reaction (PCR). Her bone marrow does not demonstrate fibrosis, and a G-banded karyotype shows 20/20 metaphases with the Philadelphia chromosome, t(9;22)(q34;q11). After discussing treatment options, she decides to start imatinib mesylate at a dose of 400 mg/d.

Q Which of the following is the most appropriate method for monitoring this patient's response to therapy?

A Qualitative PCR of peripheral blood
B Bone marrow and G-banded karyotyping
C Fluorescence *in situ* hybridization of bone marrow
D Real-time quantitative reverse transcriptase PCR of peripheral blood

Question 11

A 42-year-old man presents to the emergency department with fever of 38.4°C, severe fatigue, and easy bruising. Laboratory studies are remarkable for a white blood count of 76,000/μL with 99% undifferentiated blasts. The hemoglobin is 7.1 g/dL, and the platelet count is 12,000/μL. He also has hyperuricemia and mild elevation in the creatinine level. He is admitted to the hospital and transfused with erythrocytes and platelets. He receives hydration, allopurinol, and broad-spectrum antibiotics after appropriate cultures are obtained. Flow cytometry demonstrates a primitive myeloid blast population that is CD19 negative and CD33, CD14, and CD34 positive. He is started on 12 mg/m^2/d of idarubicin for 3 days and 100 mg/m^2/d of cytarabine for 7 days. After 5 days of this, cytogenetic analysis results become available and demonstrate trisomy 8 and t(9;22)(q34;q11) translocation.

Q Which of the following choices is the most appropriate therapy?

A Continue induction therapy, followed by consolidation therapy
B Continue induction therapy, followed by consolidation therapy and autologous stem cell transplantation
C Add lenalidomide
D Add imatinib mesylate

Question 12

A 36-year-old woman complaining of early satiety presents for evaluation. Her primary care physician obtained a complete blood count that demonstrated a white blood count of 33,000/μL, a hemoglobin of 11.9 g/dL, and a platelet count of 550,000/μL. A complete blood count from 6 months ago showed a white blood count of 24,000/μL, which was attributed to sinusitis. She denies weakness, easy bruising, or bleeding; she has no history of thrombosis and is afebrile. On physical examination, her spleen is palpable 6 cm below the costal margin. Review of the peripheral blood smear shows abundant basophils, metamyelocytes, and myelocytes. Bone marrow cytogenetics is negative for t(9;22). Molecular analysis of peripheral blood cells found no JAK2 V617F mutation.

Q What is the most appropriate next step in the management of this patient?

A Perform polymerase chain reaction for the *BCR-ABL* fusion gene
B Determine leukocyte alkaline phosphatase (LAP) score
C Draw blood cultures and start empiric antibiotic
D Start an aspirin per day and hydroxyurea
E Send endogenous erythroid colony assays

Question 13

A 42-year-old man with chronic phase chronic myeloid leukemia was started on imatinib at 400 mg/d exactly 1 year ago. After 6 months, real-time quantitative polymerase chain reaction (PCR) for *BCR-ABL* rearrangement showed a decrease to an undetectable level. At the time of the patient's 9-month checkup, the laboratory reported the reappearance of a *BCR-ABL* PCR signal, and the test was repeated at both 10 and 11 months with a clear increase in the fusion signal (now at 0.8% relative to *BCR*). He has been compliant with imatinib therapy. He has 4 siblings.

Q Which of the following is the most appropriate next step in the management of this patient?

A Hold imatinib for 2 months and restart at 400 mg/d
B Increase imatinib to 800 mg/d and perform HLA typing of the patient and his siblings
C Discontinue imatinib
D Add hydroxyurea
E Continue imatinib at 400 mg/d and refer for experimental therapy

Question 14

A 72-year-old asymptomatic woman is diagnosed with chronic phase chronic myeloid leukemia as a result of a complete blood count obtained during a routine general examination. Her white blood count is 18,000/μL with a predominance of immature myeloid forms, her hemoglobin is 11.7 g/dL, and her platelet count is 540,000/μL. After confirmation of the presence of *BCR-ABL* fusion, she is started on imatinib at 400 mg/d. Six weeks later, she returns to the clinic complaining of severe fatigue and peripheral edema. Her repeat complete blood count shows a white blood count of 8,000/μL with a normal differential, her hemoglobin is now 8.8 g/dL, and her platelet count is 155,000/μL. She has a normal serum ferritin.

Q Which of the following treatment decisions would be most appropriate?

A Begin erythropoietin
B Discontinue imatinib until the hemoglobin increases to >10 g/dL
C Reduce the imatinib dose to 200 mg/d
D Begin transfusion to hemoglobin >10 g/dL

Question 15

A 42-year-old banker with chronic phase chronic myeloid leukemia has been treated with imatinib at a dose of 400 mg/d for 13 months. The patient achieved a hematologic remission within 3 months after beginning therapy and had a complete cytogenetic response by 6 months, but he continued to have *BCR-ABL* positivity using quantitative polymerase chain reaction (PCR; 2-log decrease in transcript) at each time point. The 12-month follow-up analysis demonstrated an increase in the PCR *BCR-ABL* transcript number, and 12 out of 200 metaphase nuclei were now positive for the *BCR-ABL* translocation by fluorescence *in situ* hybridization. He has been compliant with imatinib therapy. A research laboratory has detected the T315I *BCR-ABL* mutation in the patient's blood.

Q Which of the following treatment decisions would be appropriate?

A Initiate dasatinib
B Initiate hydroxyurea
C Increase the dose of imatinib to 800 mg/d
D Collect stem cells for an autologous stem cell transplant
E Recommend allogeneic transplant

CHAPTER 09

Myelodysplastic syndrome and overlap syndromes

Question 1

A 57-year-old woman who was diagnosed with myelodysplastic syndrome (MDS) 9 months ago now presents to the hematology clinic for a follow-up visit. At the time of initial diagnosis, she had complained to her physicians of fatigue and dyspnea and was ultimately found to have pancytopenia, 2% undifferentiated marrow blasts, 1+ reticulin fibrosis, and a marrow karyotype of 46,XX,del(20)(q11.2) in 18 of 20 metaphases examined. Epoetin alfa therapy was attempted, but failed. She has declined other therapies because she enjoys travel and does not want to be "tied down" by inconvenient drug regimens.

She has been receiving transfusions of 2 U of packed red blood cells every 2–3 weeks since her initial diagnosis. Last week, her bone marrow findings were found to be unchanged from the time of diagnosis. Iron studies now reveal a ferritin of 2126 μg/L and an iron saturation of 89%. Her creatinine and liver chemistries are normal.

Q In addition to continuing transfusion support, which of the following would be the most appropriate for this patient?

A Observation
B Parenteral deferoxamine by nocturnal infusion
C Parenteral deferoxamine by brief infusion after each transfusion
D Deferasirox orally once daily

Question 2

A 78-year-old previously healthy Scottish man is evaluated for progressive fatigue. Physical examination reveals moderate conjunctival pallor and a systolic flow murmur, and there is no splenomegaly. His hemoglobin is 9.8 g/dL, mean corpuscular volume is 77 fL, white blood count is 2800/μL with a reduced proportion of neutrophils (38%), and platelet count is 136,000/μL. The peripheral smear findings are remarkable for anisopoikilocytosis with frequent poorly hemoglobinized "ghost" red cells, rare giant platelets, and hypogranular pseudo-Pelger–Huet neutrophils. There are no circulating blasts. Iron studies are normal. Supravital staining with brilliant cresyl blue reveals that 38% of circulating red cells have multiple intracellular inclusions. Hemoglobin electrophoresis demonstrates 15% hemoglobin H (a β-globin tetramer) but is otherwise unremarkable, including normal levels of hemoglobin A_2 and fetal hemoglobin. There is no family history of thalassemia or another hemoglobinopathy, the patient has no Mediterranean or Asian ancestors, and α-globin gene cluster molecular analysis of a blood sample provided by the patient is normal. The bone marrow aspirate is hypercellular, with extensive erythroid dysplasia and hyperplasia, and milder dysplastic features in other lineages. The marrow blast proportion is normal, and ringed sideroblasts are not present. The karyotype is 46,XY.

Q Which one of the following genes is most likely to be mutated in this patient?

A *RUNX1/AML1* at chromosome 21q22.3
B *JAK2* at 9p24
C *ATRX* at Xq13.1-q21.1
D *TP53* at 17p13.1
E *NRAS* at 1p13.2

Question 3

A 66-year-old woman was recently diagnosed with refractory cytopenia with multilineage dysplasia, with a normal karyotype and normal marrow blast count. Her primary physician recommended a period of observation and blood count monitoring, and she comes now for a second opinion regarding therapy for her myelodysplastic syndrome (MDS). She has been receiving red blood cell transfusions every 2 weeks. Her white count and platelet count are normal, although hypogranular neutrophils and a few giant platelets can be seen on the peripheral blood smear. Her iron saturation is 41%, and her serum erythropoietin level is 615 U/L.

Q Which of the following would be the most appropriate recommendation regarding erythropoietic growth factors in MDS?

A Darbepoetin alfa at standard doses combined with filgrastim or sargramostim
B Increased-dose darbepoetin alfa alone (eg, 300 μg once weekly)
C Epoetin alfa alone for at least 18–24 weeks to determine response
D Epoetin alfa plus parenteral iron supplementation
E No erythropoietic growth factor indicated

Question 4

A 54-year-old woman is evaluated for fatigue of 6 months' duration. She is 3 years postmenopausal and had been previously healthy. Physical examination reveals only generalized pallor; the spleen is not palpable. She has a hemoglobin of 10.2 g/dL, mean corpuscular volume of 98 fL, white blood count of 6400/μL with an unremarkable differential, and a platelet count of 512,000/μL. Her ferritin is 205 μg/L, and her serum erythropoietin level is 666 U/L. B_{12} and folate levels are normal, as are the creatinine and liver tests. The bone marrow is hypercellular for age, with moderate dysplastic changes in erythroid precursors (megaloblastoid changes and a few binucleate cells), normal granulocytic series, and clusters of atypical monolobated megakaryocytes. The blast proportion is 1%, and the karyotype is 46,XX,del(5)(q13q35) in 16 of 20 metaphases examined.

Q Which of the following is the most appropriate initial treatment of this patient?

A Lenalidomide
B Antithymocyte globulin
C Epoetin alfa
D Hematopoietic stem cell transplantation
E Decitabine

Question 5

A 75-year-old woman presents to her primary care physician with complaints of fatigue and decreased exercise tolerance of several months' duration. Her physical examination is unremarkable with the exception of pale mucous membranes and sinus tachycardia. A complete blood cell count reveals the following:

White blood cell count	3.1×10^9/L
Absolute neutrophil count	1600/μL
Hemoglobin	8.9 g/dL
Mean corpuscular volume	104 fL
Platelet count	489,000/μL

Full hematologic workup is inconclusive as to the exact cause of her anemia. A bone marrow biopsy is performed, showing a hypercellular marrow with mild dyserythropoiesis and clusters of micromegakaryocytes. Cytogenetic examination results are not yet available.

Q Which of the following represents a false statement about his disease?

A Disease is likely to respond to vitamin B_{12} supplements
B The risk of leukemic transformation is low
C This clinical entity will result in a transfusion-dependent state
D She should be treated with an immunomodulatory drug

Question 6

A 50-year-old painter is recently diagnosed with myelodysplastic syndrome (MDS). He had been complaining of fatigue for about a year and eventually went for a blood test, which revealed severe anemia with a hemoglobin of 6.7 g/dL. His white cell count and platelets were within normal limits. His bone marrow biopsy demonstrated dyserythropoiesis and <5% blasts. His cytogenetic examination revealed a normal male karyotype.

Q Which of the following represents a true statement about his disease?

A His International Prognostic Scoring System score is 2
B He has high-risk MDS
C He should receive a packed red blood cell transfusion
D He should undergo allogeneic bone marrow transplantation

Question 7

A 19-month-old boy is brought to his pediatrician for evaluation of a progressive skin rash and a protuberant abdomen. His parents also describe decreased activity over the past 2–3 weeks without fever or other systemic signs. Physical examination reveals multiple café au lait macules on the trunk and extremities and a diffuse erythematous rash without petechiae. The liver edge is palpated 4 cm below the right costal margin, and the spleen is massively enlarged with extension into the pelvis and across the midline. A complete blood cell count shows a white blood cell count of 22,600/μL with an absolute monocyte count of 5000/μL, hemoglobin of 8.1 g/dL, and a platelet count of 49,000/μL. The bone marrow is hypercellular with <5% blasts and an expanded number of myelomonocytic cells.

Q What is the most likely diagnosis?

A Refractory anemia with excess blasts (RAEB) in a child with Fanconi anemia
B RAEB in a child with neurofibromatosis, type 1
C RAEB in a child with Noonan syndrome
E Juvenile myelomonocytic leukemia (JMML) in a child with Fanconi anemia
E JMML in a child with neurofibromatosis, type 1

Question 8

A healthy 9-year-old girl has a routine yearly complete blood cell count performed in the cancer follow-up clinic. This shows a white blood cell count of 2400/μL, hemoglobin of 8.6 g/dL, and platelets of 109,000/μL. The history is remarkable for successful treatment of an embryonal rhabdomyosarcoma of the jaw between ages 3 and 5. Her therapy included surgery, involved field radiation, and combination chemotherapy with high-dose alkylating agents and other drugs. Her physical examination today is unremarkable. The bone marrow is mildly hypocellular with <5% blasts and moderate trilineage dysplasia.

Q What is the most likely diagnosis?

A Acquired bone marrow failure (aplastic anemia) that is unrelated to her previous treatment
B Acquired bone marrow failure (aplastic anemia) due to her previous treatment
C Myelodysplastic syndrome (MDS) secondary to treatment with alkylating agents and/or radiation
D MDS secondary to treatment with a topoisomerase inhibitor
E Acute myeloid leukemia secondary to treatment with alkylating agents and/or radiation

Question 9

Q Which of the following signaling proteins do genetic and biochemical studies of children with inherited predispositions to myelodysplastic/myeloproliferative overlap disorders strongly implicate in leukomogenesis?

A Jak/STAT
B Ras
C c-kit
D PI3 kinase/Akt

CHAPTER

10

Acute myeloid leukemia

Question 1

A 22-year-old man is diagnosed with acute myelogenous leukemia of French-American-British classification M4Eo, and cytogenetics show inv(16). He has no siblings. After one course of induction therapy, bone marrow is in morphologic remission and inv(16) no longer detected.

Q Which of the following would be the most appropriate therapy for this patient?

A One more course of chemotherapy followed by unrelated allogeneic stem cell transplantation (SCT)
B Three more courses of chemotherapy followed by unrelated allogeneic SCT
C Three more courses of chemotherapy that include high-dose cytarabine
D Three more courses of chemotherapy followed by low-dose cytarabine maintenance
E At least 5 more courses of intensive chemotherapy

Question 2

An 18-year-old man with diploid acute myelogenous leukemia promptly achieves complete remission following induction therapy and subsequently receives 3 postremission intensive chemotherapy courses. He relapses 6 months after completing therapy. His white blood cell count is 40,000/μL. He has no siblings.

Q What is the most appropriate treatment of this patient?

A Phase I agent
B Immediate stem cell transplantation (SCT) from an unrelated donor
C Five courses of intensive chemotherapy
D Cytarabine-containing regimen followed by SCT from an unrelated donor
E Cytarabine-containing regimen followed by autologous transplant

Question 3

A previously healthy 34-year-old woman presents with a 1-week history of increased bruisability. On physical examination, she is pale and has several bruises over upper and lower extremities. A complete blood cell count shows a hemoglobin of 9 g/dL, platelet count of 40,000/μL, and white blood cell count of 8,600/μL with circulating blasts. Bone marrow shows dysplastic features with 46% blasts, and cytogenetics show t(8;21)(q22;q22).

Q Which of the following statements is true?

A This patient has myelodysplastic syndrome (MDS) and a poor prognosis
B MDS with t(8;21) has a better prognosis than MDS with other translocations
C This patient has no MDS but is a candidate for stem cell transplantation
D This patient has favorable acute myelogenous leukemia that responds well to cytarabine
E This patient has acute promyelocytic leukemia and a good prognosis if treated with all-*trans* retinoic acid

Question 4

A 24-year-old man is referred to you with a 10-month history of progressive thrombocytopenia and anemia. He received cyclophosphamide, vincristine, prednisone, procarbazine (COPP) and mantle-field radiotherapy for Hodgkin disease when he was 14 years old. He had been doing well until he developed easy bruisability that has worsened over the past few months. He has no other symptoms. Physical examination is otherwise unremarkable. Scans are negative.

Q Which of the following is the most likely finding on bone marrow examination?

A Translocation involving 11q23
B t(12;22)
C Relapsed Hodgkin disease
D Monosomy 7

Question 5

A 45-year-old woman presents to the emergency room with a 2-week history of fatigue that has worsened over the past 2 days with development of rapidly progressive breathing difficulty and drowsiness. A complete blood cell count reveals a white blood cell count of 120,000/μL, with blasts; a platelet count of 69,000/μL; and hemoglobin of 9.2 g/dL. Chest x-ray shows bilateral diffuse infiltrate. You have the patient on oxygen.

Q Which of the following would be the most appropriate next step in the management of this patient?

A Perform blood cultures and begin antimicrobial therapy
B Transfuse with red blood cells to improve oxygenation
C Start leukapheresis and repeat daily until patient is stable for evaluation
D Establish diagnosis and initiate therapy
E Start leukapheresis, while establishing the diagnosis to initiate therapy

Question 6

A 33-year-old man is diagnosed with acute promyelocytic leukemia t(15;17) and started on treatment with all-*trans* retinoic acid (ATRA). A few days later, his white blood cell count is up from 4,600/μL to 36,240/μL. He has a low-grade fever and a mild cough and is retaining fluid.

Q Which of the following would be the most appropriate next step in the management of this patient?

A Start high-dose cytarabine
B Discontinue ATRA
C Discontinue ATRA and start high-dose dexamethasone
D Continue current therapy
E Start antibiotics

Question 7

A 72-year-old man is diagnosed with diploid acute myelogenous leukemia (AML). He has no other health problems, is in good physical condition, and voices that he would like to receive treatment for his leukemia.

Q Which of the following would be the most appropriate therapy for this patient?

A High-dose cytarabine-based standard AML regimen
B Palliative care
C Adjusted-dose standard AML therapy
D All-*trans* retinoic acid

Question 8

A 5-months-pregnant woman is experiencing bruising and epistaxis. She is more fatigued than usual. A complete blood cell count reveals a hemoglobin of 8.2 g/dL, a white blood cell count of 24,000/μL with 8% blasts, and a platelet count of 20,000/μL. She is diagnosed with t(8;21) acute myelogenous leukemia (AML).

Q Which of the following would be the most appropriate therapy for this patient?

A Terminate the pregnancy and initiate AML therapy
B Hold therapy until early delivery is induced
C Start standard AML therapy
D Start a low-dose chemotherapy to control disease progression until delivery

Question 9

A 67-year-old presents with a recent history of progressive fatigue and increased bruisability. A complete blood cell count documents anemia and thrombocytopenia. Bone marrow aspirates shows 46% blasts; myeloperoxidase 1%; positive terminal deoxynucleotidyl transferase, CD19, CD117, CD34, and CD33; and negative CD41, CD61, and CD22. Two Auer rods are noted.

Q Which of the following is the most likely diagnosis?

A Acute lymphoblastic leukemia
B Acute myeloid leukemia, French-American-British (FAB) classification M0
C Acute promyelocytic leukemia, FAB M3
D Acute myeloid leukemia, FAB M1
E Acute megakaryocytic leukemia, FAB M7

Question 10

Q Which of the following is the oncologic emergency most commonly associated with acute myeloid leukemia?

A Tumor lysis syndrome
B Superior vena cava syndrome
C Leukostasis
D Splenic rupture
E Central nervous system involvement

Question 11

Heavy granularity differentiates this acute myelogenous leukemia French-American-British classification subtype from others (from ASH Image Bank #101126, Figure 3).

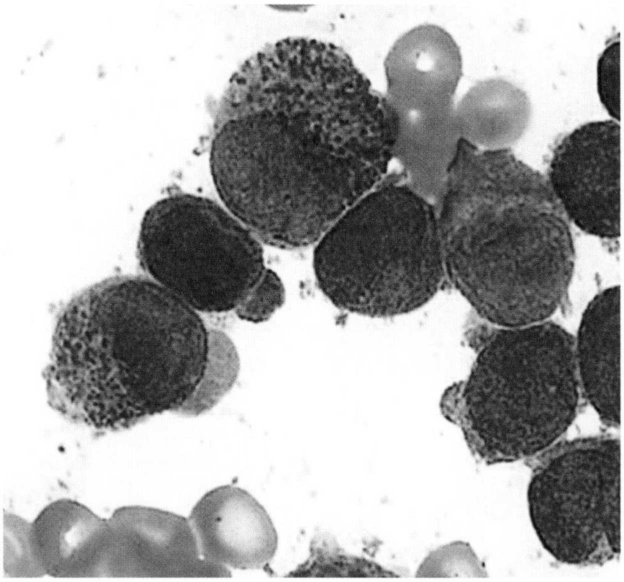

Q What differentiates it in terms of therapy?

A It responds to maintenance with high-dose cytarabine
B It is not sensitive to anthracyclines
C It does not require postremission therapy
D Remission can be achieved without cytotoxic chemotherapy

Question 12

A newborn with Down syndrome has a white blood cell count of 80,000/μL, with French-American-British classification M7 morphology and trisomy 21. The baby is stable with an Apgar score of 9 and adequate platelet and hemoglobin levels.

Q Which of the following would be the most appropriate therapy for this patient at this time?

A Acute myelogenous leukemia chemotherapy
B Exchange transfusion
C Observation
D Low-dose cytarabine

Question 13

A 6-year-old girl is diagnosed with acute myelogenous leukemia with a translocation involving 11q23. Her mother reports that the patient was treated for acute lymphoblastic leukemia at the age of 3. You ask for prior medical records.

Q Which of the following findings do you expect?

A The patient has received prior alkylating agents
B The patient has received prior topoisomerase inhibitors
C The patient has received prior cranial irradiation

Question 14

A 9-year-old boy with history of seizure disorder presents to the emergency room with extensive gingival hypertrophy, bilateral pulmonary infiltrates, and a white blood cell count of 90,000/μL. Morphologically, the majority of the cells are of monocytic lineage, mostly promonocytes. Myeloperoxidase is negative.

Q Which is the most likely cause of this patient's symptoms?

A Infectious mononucleosis
B Acute myelogenous leukemia (AML), t(9;11)
C AML, inv(16)
D Reaction to phenytoin
E AML, t(8;21)

Question 15

A 2-year-old girl presents with a 6-week history of diffuse progressive bone pain. She has required several red blood cell and platelet transfusions over the past month. Two attempts at a bone marrow aspirate were reported as "dry tap" and nondiagnostic. You repeat a bone marrow aspirate and biopsy. The aspirate proves very difficult to perform, with very little marrow obtained. Pathology shows extensive fibrosis and small blue round blasts negative for myeloperoxidase. Some blasts manifest cytoplasmic blebbing. CD41 and CD61 are positive.

Q Which of the following is the most likely translocation in this patient?

A t(12;21)
B t(8;21)
C t(9;22)
D t(1;22)
E t(1;19)

CHAPTER

11

Acute lymphoblastic leukemia and lymphoblastic lymphoma

Question 1

All of the following patients with acute lymphoblastic leukemia (ALL) are in first remission.

Q In which of these patients has allogeneic stem cell transplantation been shown to improve disease-free survival?

A A 3-year-old girl with precursor B-cell ALL and a *TEL-AML1* fusion gene
B A 10-year-old boy who presents with precursor B-cell ALL and a hyperdiploid karyotype
C A 30-year-old woman with precursor B-cell ALL and a t(9;22) resulting in a *BCR-ABL* fusion gene
D A 19-year-old man who presents with precursor T-cell ALL and a large mediastinal mass

Question 2

A 25-year-old woman presents with complaints of fever and increasing fatigue. Further workup reveals bulky retroperitoneal adenopathy, an elevated lactate dehydrogenase of 5000 U/L, and a markedly hypercellular bone marrow replaced by basophilic lymphoblasts with prominent vacuoles. Cytogenetic analysis reveals the following karyotype: t(8;14)(q23;q32).

Q Which of the following is the most appropriate management for this patient?

A The immunophenotype in this case is characterized by the presence of strong CD20 expression and surface immunoglobulin
B The optimal treatment of this patient should include the incorporation of the targeted tyrosine kinase inhibitor imatinib mesylate
C The risk of central nervous system involvement is very low
D Survival for this patient has improved as a result of increasing the duration of postremission therapy with use of prolonged maintenance therapy

Question 3

A 54-year-old man with newly diagnosed precursor B-cell acute lymphoblastic leukemia in remission is completing his seventh month of long-term maintenance therapy. Over the last few months, he has noticed that he has had increasing difficulty holding small objects, including a pen. He also has been asking his wife for help in buttoning his shirts and complains of burning in his fingers.

Q Which of the following is the most likely cause of this patient's symptoms?

A Corticosteroid-induced myopathy
B Central nervous system relapse
C L-Asparaginase-induced central nervous system toxicity
D Vincristine-induced peripheral neuropathy

Question 4

A 63-year-old woman undergoing treatment of a precursor B-cell acute lymphoblastic leukemia comes to the clinic complaining of nausea, vomiting, light-headedness, and recent dysuria and urinary urgency. Two days prior to this presentation, she received a consolidation course of chemotherapy that contained high-dose methotrexate. Leucovorin was administered per routine, but the patient vomited shortly after her most recent dose. She is now orthostatic on examination, with dry mucous membranes. A chemistry profile reveals a serum creatinine of 3.2 mg/dL.

Urinalysis has many white blood cells and is positive for nitrite and leukocyte esterase. A methotrexate level is drawn and is 3 μmol/L. The patient is admitted to the hospital.

Q Which of the following therapeutic options will delay clearance of the methotrexate?

A Intravenous hydration with sodium bicarbonate to achieve urinary pH > 7
B Treatment of the urinary tract infection with trimethoprim sulfa
C Increasing the leucovorin dose with intravenous administration
D Hemodialysis using a high-flux membrane
E Administration of carboxypeptidase

Question 5

A 64-year-old man is diagnosed with precursor B-cell acute lymphoblastic leukemia.

Q Which of the following would have the greatest effect on survival in this patient?

A Addition of a targeted *FLT3* inhibitor to combination chemotherapy
B Incorporation of nelarabine into consolidation therapy
C Inclusion of imatinib mesylate as frontline therapy
D Consolidation with a myeloablative allogeneic transplant in first remission

Question 6

Both clinical and molecular genetic features of acute lymphoblastic leukemia (ALL) have been demonstrated to have prognostic relevance.

Q Which of the following features of ALL in a 5-year-old patient is most associated with a good prognosis?

A Significant residual disease after first remission
B Philadelphia chromosome-positive disease
C Abnormalities of the *MLL* gene
D Age <10 years

Question 7

A 2-month-old infant presents to the pediatrician with a history of irritability, rash, and abdominal distention. Physical examination reveals a fussy infant covered with a petechial rash on the trunk and extremities and a liver palpated 3 cm below the right costal margin and the spleen palpated 6 cm below the left costal margin. The complete blood cell count reveals a white blood cell count of 400,000/μL, hemoglobin of 6.5 g/dL, and platelets of 43,000/μL. The differential shows 79% blasts. Bone marrow is completely replaced with cells that are $CD10^-$, CD 19^+, $CD3^-$, $CD4^-$, and $CD7^-$. Cytogenetics show t(4;11).

Q Which of the following is the most likely finding/prognosis for this patient?

A Development of central nervous system disease
B Good response to therapy
C Lack of CD10 expression
D Hyperdiploidy and a poor prognosis

Question 8

All of the following patients have a matched-related donor.

Q In which patient would a stem cell transplant be the treatment of choice?

A A 7-year-old girl with B-cell acute lymphoblastic leukemia (ALL), white blood cell count (WBC) at presentation of 9800/μL, and a t(12;21)
B A 9-year-old girl with B-cell ALL, WBC of 12,000/μL, and balanced t(1;19)
C A 15-year-old boy with B-cell ALL, WBC of 87,000/μL, and t(9;22)
D A 16-year-old boy with T-cell ALL and WBC of 250,000/μL

Question 9

A 13-year-old boy with acute lymphoblastic leukemia is in maintenance therapy including corticosteroids. There is no history of trauma. Plain x-ray of the knee is normal.

Q Which of the following would be the most appropriate management for this patient?

A Analgesia
B Bone marrow biopsy
C Magnetic resonance imaging and bone scan
D Reassurance

Question 10

All of the following patients have relapsed acute lymphoblastic leukemia (ALL).

Q Which patient has the best chance of long-term survival with further chemotherapy?

A A 15-year-old boy with B-cell precursor ALL who experiences a central nervous system relapse in maintenance therapy
B A 12-year-old girl with B-cell precursor ALL who has been off therapy for 4 years and develops a central nervous system relapse

C A 14-year-old boy with T-cell ALL who experiences a bone marrow relapse during interim maintenance

D A 7-year-old boy with B-cell ALL and a white blood cell count of 125,000/μL at initial diagnosis who develops a bone marrow and testicular relapse 14 months after completion of therapy

Question 11

A 9-year-old previously healthy boy with a history of cough for several days presents to the emergency room. A chest x-ray is obtained (see below). A complete blood cell count shows a white blood cell count of 25,000/μL with platelets of 95,000/μL.

Q Which of the following is the most appropriate management for this patient?

A Bone marrow biopsy

B Immunophenotyping of cells in pleural fluid

C Biopsy of the mediastinal mass

D Cytogenetics of the mediastinal mass

CHAPTER 12

Lymphoproliferative disorders

Question 1

A 65-year-old man is evaluated for lower gastrointestinal bleeding. Biopsy of multiple masses in the colon that were seen during colonoscopy shows dense infiltration by intermediate-sized lymphocytes which are CD5$^+$, CD10$^-$, sIg$^+$, CD20$^+$, cyclin D1$^+$, and FMC7$^+$.

Q Which of the following is the most likely diagnosis?

A Follicular lymphoma, grade 2
B Mantle cell lymphoma
C Marginal zone lymphoma
D Diffuse large B cell lymphoma

Question 2

Q Which of the following patients with a lymphoid malignancy would benefit from prophylactic therapy for the central nervous system?

A A 56-year-old man with peripheral T cell lymphoma involving lymph nodes above and below the diaphragm as well as the right lung
B A 60-year-old man with isolated left testicular large B-cell lymphoma
C A 46-year-old woman with diffuse large cell lymphoma involving the lymph nodes in the neck, axilla, and retroperitoneum
D A 39-year-old man with stage IV chronic lymphocytic leukemia with bulky lymphadenopathy
E A 65-year-old woman with follicular grade 3 lymphoma with involvement of mediastinal and retroperitoneal lymph nodes

Question 3

A 29-year-old man presents to his internist with facial swelling and headache of 3 weeks' duration. A chest x-ray reveals a large mediastinal mass. The radiologist reports that this is most likely Hodgkin lymphoma. Physical examination is significant for facial swelling but no bleeding or palpable lymphadenopathy or organomegaly. Blood counts, serum chemistry, and lactate dehydrogenase are within normal limits.

Q Which of the following would be the most appropriate management for this patient?

A High-dose corticosteroids
B Emergent radiation therapy to mediastinum
C Surgical biopsy
D ABVD (doxorubicin, bleomycin, vinblastine, and dacarbazine) chemotherapy
E Placement of a stent

Question 4

A 50-year-old man presents with history of headache and impaired vision. Computed tomographic (CT) scan of the head reveals a 4-cm mass in the right occipital region. A human immunodeficiency virus test is negative. A stereotactic biopsy of the cerebral mass reveals diffuse large B cell lymphoma. CT scan, positron emission tomographic scan, bone marrow, and cerebrospinal fluid studies are negative for evidence of disease elsewhere.

Q Which of the following would be the most appropriate initial therapy for this patient?

A Whole brain radiation therapy
B High-dose methotrexate with leucovorin rescue
C Hyper-CVAD (hyperfractionated cyclophosphamide, vincristine, adriamycin, doxorubicin) + rituximab therapy
D CHOP (cyclophosphamide, doxorubicin, vincristine, and prednisone) + rituximab therapy
E High-dose cytarabine

Question 5

A 62-year-old woman is evaluated for swelling over the left side of her neck. Biopsy reveals an Epstein–Barr virus–positive lymphoproliferative disorder with a mixture of small and large monoclonal B cells. She has no other symptoms. She has a 3-year history of polymyositis well controlled with methotrexate therapy. Her blood counts and serum chemistry are within normal limits.

Q Which of the following is the most appropriate next step in the management of this patient?

A Discontinue methotrexate therapy
B Rituximab weekly × 4 doses
C CVP (cyclophosphamide, vincristine, and prednisone) every 3 weeks × 6 cycles
D CHOP (cyclophosphamide, doxorubicin, vincristine, and prednisone) + rituximab every 3 weeks × 6 cycles
E Observation

Question 6

A 34-year-old woman presents with relapsed diffuse large B cell lymphoma with lymphadenopathy in the neck and mediastinum. Six months ago, she completed 6 cycles of CHOP + R (cyclophosphamide, doxorubicin, vincristine, and prednisone plus rituximab) and had achieved complete remission. A positron emission tomographic scan shows uptake in both sides of the neck and mediastinum. Bone marrow biopsy is negative for lymphoma. She has an HLA-matched brother who is 25 years old.

Q Which of the following is the most appropriate therapy for this patient?

A Autologous stem cell transplantation (SCT)
B Allogeneic SCT from her HLA-matched brother
C CHOP + R
D Radioimmunotherapy

Question 7

A 57-year-old woman with no significant past medical history presents to her primary physician with complaints of fatigue, increasing dyspnea on exertion, and abdominal discomfort. Physical examination reveals pallor and a spleen palpable 10 cm below the costal margin. A complete blood cell count reveals hemoglobin of 7.0 g/dL, white blood cell count of 2400/μL (neutrophils 48%, lymphocytes 44%, eosinophils 6%, and monocytes 2%), and platelets of 110,000/μL. A computed tomographic scan confirms splenomegaly with no lymphadenopathy or other abnormalities. Bone marrow biopsy reveals 5% involvement with $CD20^{+}$ small lymphocytes consistent with marginal zone lymphoma. After 2 U of packed red blood cell transfusions, her fatigue and dyspnea improve but abdominal symptoms persist.

Q Which of the following would be the most appropriate management for this patient?

A Observation without therapy
B CVP (cyclophosphamide, vincristine, and prednisone) × 8 cycles
C CHOP (cyclophosphamide, doxorubicin, vincristine, and prednisone) + rituximab × 6 cycles
D Rituximab weekly × 4 cycles
E Splenectomy

Question 8

A 48-year-old truck driver presents with lymphadenopathy over the left side of the neck. Biopsy reveals non-Hodgkin lymphoma, follicular, grade IIIB. Computed tomographic scan shows lymphadenopathy in the neck, axilla, and retroperitoneum. Bone marrow biopsy is negative for lymphoma. Lactate dehydrogenase is >2 × the upper limit of normal.

Q Which of the following is the most appropriate management for this patient?

A CHOP (cyclophosphamide, doxorubicin, vincristine, and prednisone) + rituximab × 6–8 cycles
B CVP (cyclophosphamide, vincristine, and prednisone) + rituximab × 6–8 cycles
C Rituximab weekly × 4 cycles
D Autologous stem cell transplantation
E Observation

Question 9

An 82-year-old woman with a history of congestive heart failure and atrial fibrillation (left ventricular ejection fraction of 25%) was diagnosed with stage IV small lymphocytic lymphoma 2 years ago. She achieved partial remission with chlorambucil and prednisone and remained asymptomatic until 3 weeks ago when she started complaining of night sweats, fatigue, and weight loss. Physical examination during the current clinic visit reveals significant lymphadenopathy (largest 3 cm) in the neck, axilla, and inguinal region. Her spleen is palpable 6 cm below the costal margin. Bone marrow biopsy reveals 40% involvement with small lymphocytic lymphoma. Her blood counts and chemistry including lactate dehydrogenase are within normal limits.

Q Which of the following is the most appropriate management for this patient?

A Chlorambucil and prednisone
B Radioimmunotherapy
C CHOP (cyclophosphamide, doxorubicin, vincristine, and prednisone) + rituximab × 6–8 cycles
D Observation

Question 10

You are seeing a 32-year-old female patient who has recurrent Hodgkin lymphoma. A bone marrow analysis at the time of relapse revealed no evidence of Hodgkin lymphoma, but cytogenetic analysis revealed deletion of chromosome 7 in 40% of the cells. Physical examination, blood counts, and chemistry are within normal limits. She has 7 siblings, among whom 2 are HLA matched to the patient and 1 is the patient's identical twin. You have recommended that she proceed to stem cell transplantation.

Q Which of the following is the most appropriate type of stem cell transplantation for this patient?

A Autologous stem cell transplantation
B Allogeneic stem cell transplantation from an HLA-matched sibling
C Syngeneic stem cell transplantation from the identical twin
D Matched unrelated stem cell transplantation
E Umbilical cord stem cell transplantation

Question 11

A 65-year-old woman is evaluated for dyspepsia and abdominal bloating. An upper gastrointestinal endoscopy shows an ulcerative lesion in the gastric fundus. Biopsy reveals low-grade mucosa-associated lymphoid tissue lymphoma. *Helicobacter pylori* is identified in the specimen, and cytogenetic studies reveal t(11;18). Computed tomographic scans of the chest, abdomen, and pelvis as well as bilateral bone marrow biopsies do not reveal any evidence of disease elsewhere.

Q Which of the following is the most appropriate therapy for this patient?

A A course of amoxicillin, clarithromycin, and lansoprazole
B Local radiotherapy
C CVP (cyclophosphamide, vincristine, and prednisone) chemotherapy × 6–8 cycles
D Rituximab every week × 4 doses
E CHOP (cyclophosphamide, doxorubicin, vincristine, and prednisone) + rituximab × 6–8 cycles

Question 12

A 68-year-old previously healthy man is admitted for management of rectal abscess. He is found to have pancytopenia. Physical examination reveals palpable spleen 6 cm below the costal margin. A bone marrow biopsy reveals classic morphologic immunophenotypic features of hairy cell leukemia. Tartrate-resistant acid phosphatase staining is positive.

Q Which of the following is the most appropriate therapy for this patient?

A Cladribine
B Rituximab
C Fludarabine
D CHOP (cyclophosphamide, doxorubicin, vincristine, and prednisone) + rituximab
E Splenectomy

Question 13

A 32-year-old man is evaluated for fatigue and swelling on the left side of his face. Physical examination reveals significant lymphadenopathy over both sides of the neck, axilla, and groin. Computed tomographic scan shows an enlarged spleen. Biopsy of a lymph node from the left side of the neck is reported as nodular lymphocyte-predominant Hodgkin disease. Blood counts and chemistry are normal. Bone marrow biopsy is negative for lymphoma.

Q Which of the following would be the most appropriate management for this patient?

A ABVD (doxorubicin, bleomycin, vinblastine, and dacarbazine) × 6–8 cycles
B Autologous stem cell transplantation
C Rituximab weekly × 4 cycles
D Total nodal irradiation
E Observation

Question 14

An 85-year-old man presents to you for consultation regarding worsening pancytopenia. Hairy cell leukemia was diagnosed 10 months ago, and he was treated with a 5-day course of cladribine and attained a complete remission. Three months ago, he developed dyspnea and fatigue. Physical examination during this clinic visit reveals palpable spleen 5 cm below the costal margin. A complete blood cell count shows hemoglobin of 7.6 g/dL, white blood cell count of 1800/μL with 300 neutrophils, and platelets of 55,000/μL. A bone marrow biopsy reveals massive infiltration with cells that are morphologically and immunophenotypically consistent with hairy cell leukemia. He is given 2 U of packed red blood cells, following which his symptoms improved.

Q Which of the following is the most appropriate therapy for this patient?

A Repeat a 5-day course of cladribine
B 2-Chlorodeoxyadenosine as a continuous infusion over 7 days
C Rituximab weekly for 4 weeks
D Chlorambucil and prednisone
E Chemotherapy with CVP (cyclophosphamide, vincristine, and prednisone)

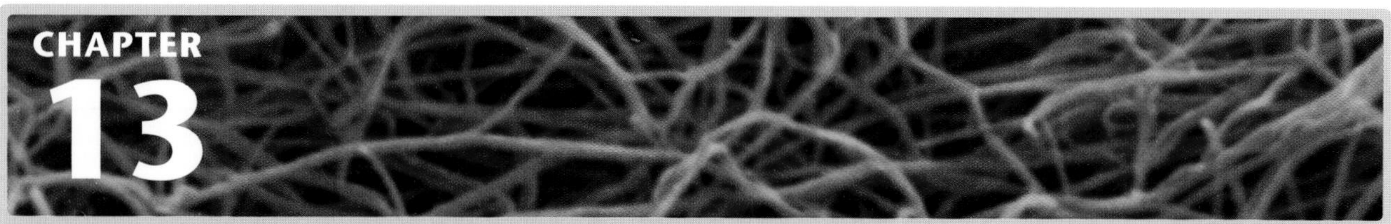

CHAPTER 13

Plasma cell dyscrasias

Question 1

A 54-year-old schoolteacher presents to her internist with progressive dyspnea on exercise and worsening pain in her right hip over 2 months' duration. Her physical examination is unrevealing except for pallor, and her initial laboratory values are notable for a hemoglobin of 9.8 g/dL. Hip films reveal at least 2 lytic lesions in the right femur, and skeletal survey reveals multiple lesions scattered throughout the axial and appendicular skeleton. Serum protein electrophoresis reveals a 3.6-g monoclonal spike, IgA-κ on immunofixation. A posterior iliac crest bone marrow biopsy shows 30% monoclonal plasma cells, with a plasma cell labeling index of 0.2%. Cytogenetics and fluorescence *in situ* hybridization for deletion 13 are both normal. The serum calcium and creatinine are normal. Serum β_2-microglobulin is 2.4 μg/mL; C-reactive protein, lactate dehydrogenase, and serum albumin are normal. Magnetic resonance imaging of the hips reveals a pathologic fracture of the right hip requiring surgical fixation.

The patient is recovering from surgical repair of the right hip and has begun erythropoietin. Left ventricular ejection fraction is normal.

Q Which of the following is the most appropriate treatment of this patient?

A Melphalan and prednisone
B Thalidomide + dexamethasone
C Dexamethasone
D Bortezomib + dexamethasone
E VAD (vincristine, doxorubicin, dexamethasone)

Question 2

Genetic instabilities are frequently identified in multiple myeloma (MM) cells.

Q Which of the following chromosomes is the most frequent translocation partner to 14q32 (IgH) in MM cells?

A 8q24 (*c-myc*)
B 11q13 (*cyclin D1*)
C 16q23 (*c-maf*)
D 4p16 (*FGFR3, MMSET*)

Question 3

A 78-year-old retired electrician develops severe back pain. He consults an orthopedic surgeon, who orders plain x-rays of the lumbosacral spine, which show collapse of the second and fourth lumbar vertebrae. A skeletal survey reveals diffuse osteoporosis and multiple lytic lesions involving the ribs and pelvis. His hemoglobin is 10.1 g/dL; renal function and serum calcium are normal, serum β_2-microglobulin is 6.2 μg/mL, and serum albumin is 3.5 g/dL. A bone marrow examination reveals 30% plasma cells in sheets. Serum immunoglobulins show an elevated IgG of 5.3 g/dL that on immunoelectrophoresis reveals an IgG-λ monoclonal spike.

Past medical history is notable for hypertension, coronary artery disease, noninsulin dependent diabetes mellitus, and mild chronic obstructive pulmonary disease. Left ventricular ejection fraction is moderately suppressed at 45%.

Q What is the most appropriate next step in the management of this patient?

A Melphalan and prednisone
B Thalidomide + dexamethasone
C Dexamethasone
D Bortezomib + dexamethasone
E MPT (melphalan, prednisone, thalidomide)

Question 4

A 56-year-old landscape engineer presents with bone pain and anemia. He is diagnosed with IgG-κ multiple myeloma. Otherwise, his prior health has been excellent, and physical examination is unremarkable. Laboratory studies show hemoglobin of 9.3 g/dL, white blood cell count of 6200/μL, and platelet count of 178,000/μL. Serum protein electrophoresis reveals a 5.2 g/dL IgG-κ monoclonal protein and 24-hour urine total protein of 1200 mg/24 hours with monoclonal IgG-κ protein of 800 mg/24 hours. Serum creatinine is 1.3 mg/dL, and albumin is 3.8 g/dL. Workup reveals lytic lesions in the skull and right femur. Bone marrow biopsy shows 55% plasma cells with normal cytogenetic analysis including fluorescence *in situ* hybridization analysis. Eastern Cooperative Oncology Group performance status is 1.

He is treated with thalidomide and dexamethasone and, after 3 months of therapy, reevaluation shows a 50% reduction in paraprotein with 15% residual marrow plasma cells and urine IgG-κ 400 mg/24 hours. Hemoglobin has increased to 11 g/dL.

Q What is the most appropriate next step in the management of this patient?

A Thalidomide and dexamethasone at current dose
B Autologous stem cell transplant
C Bortezomib-based regimen
D VAD (vincristine, doxorubicin, dexamethasone)

Question 5

A 59-year-old insurance broker is diagnosed with multiple myeloma after presenting with progressive back pain and anemia. Initial presenting labs are notable for hemoglobin of 8.9 g/dL, white blood cell count of 4.8 with normal differential, and platelet count of 243,000/μL. Serum chemistries including creatinine, calcium, and liver function tests are normal. He has an IgG-κ monoclonal (M) spike of 4.1 g/dL. Serum β_2-microglobulin is elevated at 5.3 μg/mL, and his bone marrow reveals a 60% plasmacytosis. Cytogenetic analysis for deletion 13 is normal. Initial skeletal survey reveals diffuse osteolytic disease, with at least 2 vertebral compression fractures. Magnetic resonance imaging of the spine confirms skeletal survey findings and reveals no cord compression.

His initial therapy consists of thalidomide and dexamethasone (Thal/Dex), as well as pamidronate and erythropoietin. Aside from moderate somnolence in the first month of therapy, he tolerates the thalidomide well. After 4 months of Thal/Dex (200 mg of thalidomide), his complete blood count is normal, and his IgG is 1.2 g/dL. After peripheral stem cell harvesting, he is treated with high-dose melphalan and autologous stem cell support. He has an uneventful recovery from the transplant, is off of growth factors, and is back to work within 2 months of his transplant. His routine labs are now normal, but his serum immunoglobulins and immunoelectrophoresis are noteworthy for a residual M-protein of 0.3 g/dL of IgG-κ.

Q What is the most appropriate next step in the management of this patient?

A Observation
B Prednisone or dexamethasone maintenance
C Low-dose α interferon
D Thalidomide

Question 6

Bone marrow microenvironment plays a crucial role in multiple myeloma (MM) cell pathogenesis. Upon cytokine stimulation, 3 major signaling cascades including extracellular signal-regulated kinases, signal transducers and activators of transcription 3, and phosphatidylinositol 3-kinase/Akt are activated, which mediate proliferation, survival, and drug resistance in MM cells.

Q Which of the following cytokines secreted from bone marrow stromal cells stimulates all 3 of these signaling cascades in MM cells?

A Interleukin-6
B Insulin-like growth factor 1
C Vascular endothelial growth factor
D Stromal cell-derived factor 1α
E B-cell activating factor

Question 7

The first-in-class proteasome inhibitor bortezomib has significant anti–multiple myeloma (MM) activity in preclinical studies and is effective in patients. Besides direct cytotoxicity against MM cells, bortezomib down-regulates adhesion molecules and inhibits interleukin 6 secretion in bone marrow stromal cells.

Q Which of the following transcriptional factors has been shown to mediate these effects in bone marrow stromal cells after bortezomib treatment?

A Signal transducers and activators of transcription 3 (STAT3)
B STAT5
C Nuclear factor-κB
D c-Jun
E PU.1

Question 8

A 49-year-old woman develops progressive anemia and bone pain and is diagnosed with stage IIIa IgG-κ multiple myeloma (multiple bone lesions, high paraprotein level). She is treated with thalidomide and dexamethasone for 4 months and obtains a near-complete remission. This is followed by high-dose melphalan and autologous stem cell transplantation. She remains progression free off all therapy except for monthly pamidronate.

Two years later, she is found to have a rising paraprotein level, progressive anemia, and worsening renal function with a creatinine of 2.7 mg/dL; 24-hour urine immunoelectrophoresis confirms significant κ light-chain secretion at 2000 mg/24 hours. Her hemoglobin is 10.8 g/dL, white blood cell count is 3.8, and platelet count is 198,000/μL. Chemistry profile, including renal and liver function, is otherwise normal. Skeletal survey reveals 2 new lytic lesions but otherwise is unchanged. Repeat bone marrow reveals 35% plasmacytosis. She is now 52 years old, and her Eastern Cooperative Oncology Group performance status is 0.

Q Which of the following would be the most appropriate therapy for this patient?

A Dexamethasone
B Thalidomide + dexamethasone
C Bortezomib ± dexamethasone
D VAD (vincristine, doxorubicin, dexamethasone)
E Lenalidomide + dexamethasone

Question 9

A 61-year-old beautician is diagnosed with IgG-λ multiple myeloma following evaluation of anemia and bone pain. Her prior health has been excellent, and physical examination is unremarkable. Laboratory studies show hemoglobin of 8.8 g/dL, white blood cell count of 5400/μL, and platelet count of 135,000/μL. Laboratory evaluation confirms the diagnosis, with serum protein electrophoresis that reveals a 4.4 g/dL IgG-λ monoclonal protein and 24-hour urine total protein of 900 mg/24 hours with monoclonal IgG-λ protein of 600 mg/24 hours. Serum creatinine is 1.7 mg/dL, β_2-microglobulin is 6.4 μg/mL (normal <4), and albumin is 3.6 g/dL. Skeletal survey reveals multiple lytic lesions in the skull and left humerus without cortical erosion. Bone marrow biopsy shows 45% plasma cells. Conventional cytogenetic studies show a normal karyotype 46,XX, with normal fluorescence *in situ* hybridization analysis for del(13) and t(11;14). Eastern Cooperative Oncology Group performance status is 1. The patient is started on monthly zoledronic acid at 4 mg and erythropoietin weekly. She prefers an oral regimen if at all possible. She has no prior history of thrombosis, and her family history is similarly unrevealing. You prescribe thalidomide and dexamethasone as initial therapy.

Q Which of the following is the most appropriate therapy for this patient?

A Low-dose aspirin
B Full-dose aspirin
C Low-dose coumadin
D Enoxaparin

Question 10

A 56-year-old landscape engineer presents with bone pain and anemia. He is diagnosed with IgG-κ multiple myeloma. Otherwise, his prior health has been excellent, and physical examination is unremarkable. Laboratory studies show hemoglobin of 9.3 g/dL, white blood cell count of 6200/μL, and platelet count of 178,000/μL. Serum protein electrophoresis reveals a 5.2 g/dL IgG-κ monoclonal protein and 24-hour urine total protein of 1200 mg/24 hours with monoclonal IgG-κ protein of 800 mg/24 hours. Serum creatinine is 1.3 mg/dL, and albumin is 3.8 g/dL.

Workup reveals lytic lesions in the skull and right femur. Bone marrow biopsy shows 55% plasma cells with normal cytogenetic analysis including fluorescence *in situ* hybridization analysis. Eastern Cooperative Oncology Group performance status is 1.

He is treated with thalidomide and dexamethasone and, after 6 months of therapy, reevaluation shows a 50% reduction in paraprotein with 15% residual marrow plasma cells and urine IgG-κ 400 mg/24 hours. Hemoglobin has increased to 11 g/dL.

He undergoes an autologous stem cell transplant and achieves a complete remission following the transplant. Eighteen months later, his paraprotein level increases 40%, with recurrence of 20% plasma cells in the marrow, and he has new back pain. He is otherwise well but troubled by residual peripheral neuropathy (grade 2) from his prior thalidomide exposure. Magnetic resonance imaging of his thoracolumbar spine shows diffuse disease involvement but no spinal cord compression or compression fracture.

Q Which of the following is the most appropriate therapy for this patient?

A Bortezomib with dexamethasone
B Lenalidomide with dexamethasone
C Thalidomide with dexamethasone
D VAD (vincristine, doxorubicin, dexamethasone)
E Melphalan and prednisone

CHAPTER

14

Stem cell transplantation

Question 1

A 26-year-old male patient was diagnosed with chronic myelogenous leukemia 12 months ago. He has been treated with imatinib at 400 mg per os daily since diagnosis. His blood counts have been controlled, but a bone marrow performed 2 weeks prior to the clinic showed persistence of the Philadelphia chromosome in 17 of 20 metaphases. He has a twin brother and 4 other siblings. The twin and 1 other brother are HLA-identical to the patient.

Q Which of the following would be the most appropriate therapy for this patient?

A Increase imatinib to a dose of 800 mg. Repeat marrow in 6 months

B Initiate treatment with a novel tyrosine kinase/SRC inhibitor. Transplant is no longer indicated in CML

C Proceed to transplant using the HLA-identical sibling. Avoid using the twin brother as donor

D Confirm monozygosity of twin by DNA-fingerprinting. Recommend transplant. Discuss pros and cons of syngeneic transplantation versus HLA-identical sibling transplantation

Question 2

A 45-year-old patient underwent a matched unrelated donor transplantation 1 year ago. He has developed extensive chronic graft-versus-host disease (GVHD), which is partially controlled with steroid therapy. He is considering taking out a mortgage for a new house but wants to discuss his prognosis.

He was originally diagnosed 16 months ago with acute myelogenous leukemia with an unfavorable karyotype. He obtained remission after induction with standard-dose cytarabine and daunorubicin and received one cycle of consolidation with high-dose cytarabine prior to the allogeneic transplant. He has been able to do his job as an accountant for the past 6 months.

Physical examination is nearly unremarkable, except for the presence of mild lichenoid changes on the buccal mucosa and mild erythema of the conjunctivae. Labs show a hemoglobin of 12 g/dL, white blood cell count of 5×10^9/L, and platelet count of 250×10^9/L. Differential shows approximately 10% eosinophils. Bilirubin is mildly elevated at 1.3 mg/dL, and alkaline phosphatase is 288 IU/mL. Transaminases are normal, and serum urea nitrogen and creatinine are within normal limits. His medications include prednisone 20 mg per os every other day, bactrim DS on weekends, and fluconazole 200 mg/d.

Q Which of the following best characterizes this patient's extent of GVHD and his prognosis?

A Extensive GVHD; low risk with 2-year survival approximately 80%

B Limited GVHD; low risk but with lifelong corticosteroid dependence

C Extensive GVHD; high risk with 2-year survival approximately 20%

D Limited GVHD; high risk as a result of eosinophilia

Question 3

A 65-year-old man was diagnosed with follicular lymphoma grade I, stage IV (bone marrow involvement) 3 years ago. He was initially followed without treatment, but worsening anemia, increasing adenopathy, and fatigue led his oncologist to recommend treatment about 18 months ago. He received 6 cycles of CVP (cyclophosphamide, vincristine, and prednisone)-rituximab and obtained a complete remission.

Now, 12 months after completing treatment, he presents with fatigue and new lymphadenopathy. He is pale and has palpable lymph nodes in the neck, axilla, and groins. The largest lymph node, in the right axilla, measures approximately 4 cm. Laboratory examination shows a hemoglobin of 9 g/dL, a platelet count of 130 × 10^9/L, and a slightly increased lactate dehydrogenase at 258 (normal < 245). All other labs are normal. A lymph node biopsy shows follicular lymphoma grade I. Bone marrow shows 40% involvement by small cleaved cells. The patient's only sibling died last year from a heart attack.

Q Which of the following is the most appropriate management of this patient?

A ESHAP (etoposide, methylprednisolone, cytarabine, cisplatin) chemotherapy followed by autologous stem cell transplantation
B Rituximab therapy
C Unrelated donor stem cell transplantation
D Observation

Question 4

A 69-year-old patient was diagnosed with immunoglobulin G (IgG) myeloma approximately 3 years ago. He was initially treated with melphalan and prednisone and obtained a partial response. Recently, he was found to have progressive disease as indicated by a rapidly rising paraprotein and increasing bone pain. He now receives treatment with thalidomide and decadron and appears to be responding again. He comes to discuss the possibility of an autologous transplantation. He is a healthy appearing man. His only past medical history is mild hypertension treated with a beta-blocker. He also underwent transurethral resection of the prostate 5 years ago for benign prostatic hyperplasia. Labs are normal except for a hemoglobin of 11 g/dL and an IgG-κ paraprotein of 2.5 g/dL with suppression of IgA and IgM. Creatinine is normal.

Q Which of the following is the most appropriate therapy for this patient?

A Autologous stem cell transplantation after total body irradiation
B Allogeneic transplantation
C Continued therapy with thalidomide and decadron
D Autologous stem cell transplantation with high-dose melphalan conditioning

Question 5

A 35-year-old woman with Philadelphia-positive acute lymphoblastic leukemia underwent an allogeneic bone marrow transplantation from a one-allele mismatched unrelated donor after conditioning with cyclophosphamide and total body irradiation. Graft-versus-host disease prophylaxis consisted of tacrolimus and short-course methotrexate. Her initial posttransplant course was uneventful, except for severe mucositis requiring treatment with narcotic analgesics. Her white blood cell count recovered to 1.0 × 10^9/L by day 16. She was discharged on day 20 after transplant.

On day 24 after transplant, she comes for her first clinic visit. She feels quite well and has a reasonable appetite with no nausea or diarrhea. Medications include tacrolimus 1 mg per os twice daily and Diflucan 400 mg per os daily. Physical

Blood pressure	110/60
Heart rate	60/min
Respiratory rate	18/min
Hemoglobin	10 g/dL
White blood cell count	3.0
Platelet count	50 × 10^9/L

examination is completely unremarkable. Her temperature is slightly elevated at 38.0°C, and physical examination reveals the following:
The next day, the result of a cytomegalovirus (CMV) polymerase chain reaction (PCR) test shows a level of 5000/μL (normal undetectable).

Q Which of the following is the most appropriate management for this patient?

A Oral valacyclovir
B PCR in 1 week
C Chest radiograph
D CMV immune globulin
E Intravenous ganciclovir

Question 6

A 53-year-old female had follicular lymphoma in second complete remission. She underwent an allogeneic stem cell transplant from her 50-year-old HLA-identical brother. The conditioning regimen consisted of the combination of total body irradiation and cyclophosphamide. Graft-versus-host disease prophylaxis included cyclosporine and short methotrexate (15 mg/m^2 on day 1 and 10 mg/m^2 days 3, 6, and 11).

She is 28 days posttransplant with excellent graft function. However, she complains of persistent nausea since transplant, and her appetite remains poor. She has vomited 1–2 times per day, and has loose stool 2 times per day (<500 mL). Physical examination reveals minimal tenderness over the epigastrium. There is no new skin rash. Stool for *Clostridium difficile* is negative × 3.

Q What is the most appropriate next step in the management of this patient?

A Total parenteral nutrition
B Methylprednisolone
C Upper endoscopy and biopsy
D Ganciclovir therapy
E Caspofungin therapy

Question 7

A 20-year-old man has acute myelogenous leukemia in first complete remission. He is herpes simplex virus $(HSV)^{+ve}$, cytomegalovirus $(CMV)^{+ve}$, and varicella-zoster virus $(VZV)^{+ve}$. He has an 18-year-old HLA-identical sister who is HSV^{-ve}, CMV^{+ve}, and VZV^{+ve}.

Q What is the most appropriate CMV prophylaxis and monitoring strategy?

A CMV-negative blood products and weekly CMV blood culture
B Leukocyte-reduced blood products and weekly CMV blood culture
C Leukocyte-reduced blood products and weekly CMV DNA polymerase chain reaction (PCR) assay
D CMV-negative blood products and weekly CMV DNA PCR assay

Question 8

A 32-year-old man is day 18 status post matched unrelated donor stem cell transplantation for Philadelphia $chromosome^{+ve}$ acute lymphocytic leukemia in first complete remission. The conditioning regimen consisted of the combination of total body irradiation and cyclophosphamide. Graft-versus-host disease prophylaxis consisted of the combination of cyclosporine, sirolimus, and minimethotrexate (10 mg/m^2 on day, 1 and 5 mg/m^2 on days 3 and 6). He developed neutropenic fever on day 15 posttransplant, and on day 18 because of persistent fever and a new pulmonary infiltrate in the right lower lobe, infectious disease (ID) service is consulted. The ID consultant recommends initiation of voriconazole and a pulmonary consult for bronchoalveolar lavage. You decide to defer bronchoscopy and agree to treat the patient empirically with voriconazole.

Q How will you adjust the immunosuppressive therapy?

A Decrease cyclosporine by 50%; no change in sirolimus
B Decrease cyclosporine by 50%; decrease sirolimus by 50%
C Decrease cyclosporine by 50%; discontinue sirolimus
D Discontinue cyclosporine; decrease sirolimus by 50%
E Replace cyclosporine and sirolimus with tacrolimus and mycophenolate mofetil

Question 9

A 29-year-old female is status post allogeneic stem cell transplant (SCT) from a matched unrelated donor for Philadelphia $chromosome^{+ve}$ acute lymphocytic leukemia in first complete remission. Her conditioning regimen consisted of the combination of busulfan and fludarabine. Graft-versus-host disease prophylaxis consisted of the combination of tacrolimus and short methotrexate. She received all the prescribed doses of methotrexate. On day 13 post-SCT, she develops a generalized seizure. Physical examination fails to reveal any focal neurologic deficit: Noncontrast computed tomography scan is unremarkable. Phenytoin therapy is started.

Temperature	37.7°C
Blood pressure	160/95
Pulse	105/min
Respiratory rate	22/min
Hemoglobin	8.5 g/dL
White blood cell count	0.1 × 10^9/L
Platelet count	15 × 10^9/L
Electrolytes, glucose	Normal
FK506 trough level	10 mg/L

Q What is the most appropriate next therapeutic intervention?

A Add ceftriaxone
B Add phenobarbitrone
C Discontinue tacrolimus
D Start decadron
E Start high-dose acyclovir

Question 10

A 55-year-old man with acute myeloid leukemia is in second complete remission. His blood group is O^{+ve} and cytomegalovirus $(CMV)^{+ve}$. The patient does not have a histocompatible sibling. Unrelated donor search identified 4 HLA-ABCDRDQ allele-matched donors.

Q Which of the following unrelated HLA-matched donors would be appropriate for this patient?

A A 55-year-old male, O^{+ve}, CMV^{-ve}
B A 20-year-old male, A^{+ve}, CMV^{+ve}

C A 48-year-old female, G3P3, O^{+ve}, CMV^{+ve}
D A 55-year-old female, G0P0, O^{+ve}, CMV^{-ve}

Question 11

A 19-year-old woman is referred to you for evaluation of pancytopenia after she notes increased bruising and fatigue. She was diagnosed as a child with Fanconi anemia after being noted as small for her age. She has 3 siblings, including her identical twin. A bone marrow biopsy reveals a relatively acellular marrow.

Q Which of the following is the most appropriate management for this patient?

A High-dose cyclophosphamide
B Cyclosporine and antithymocyte globulin
C Syngeneic stem cell transplantation with her identical twin as the donor
D Allogeneic stem cell transplantation with her matched sibling as the donor

Question 12

A 13-year-old boy presents with a history of mixed cellularity Hodgkin disease that was treated with standard therapy including chemotherapy and radiation. He has been referred to the transplant center after the diagnosis of relapse was confirmed by biopsy immediately following the completion of his radiation. His bone marrow is not involved. The family wishes to understand the options for his continued care. The family is African American with some Native American background. He has 1 sister who is HLA identical.

Q Which of the following would be the most appropriate management for this patient?

A Allogeneic transplantation from his sister
B Cord blood transplantation
C Autologous transplantation
D Chemotherapy only

Question 13

A 6-year-old boy presents to his primary pediatrician with paleness and has been tiring faster with activity than in the past. On review of systems, his parents do think that he has been bruising more than his siblings despite decreasing activity and increasing quiet play. The pediatrician requests that the child have a complete blood cell count (CBC) and a monospot test performed. The CBC demonstrates a white blood cell count of 150,000/μL and a platelet count of 9×10^9/L. The patient is sent to the local emergency room for evaluation. The peripheral smear reveals the presence of blasts, and flow cytometry confirms the presence of acute myeloid leukemia. The family asks what the treatment plan is.

Q Which of the following would be the most appropriate therapy for this patient?

A Cord blood transplantation
B There is no indication for a transplant unless there is a relapse.
C Chemotherapy and HLA typing of the patient's family
D Stem cell transplantation with an HLA-matched unrelated donor

Question 14

A 16-year-old girl is diagnosed with acute lymphoblastic leukemia and begins therapy. She develops a bone marrow relapse 15 months after achieving a remission.

Q Which of the following is the most appropriate therapy for this patient?

A Proceed immediately to cord blood transplantation
B Chemotherapy and search for an HLA-matched donor for stem cell transplantation
C Chemotherapy followed by autologous stem cell transplantation
D Chemotherapy only

Question 15

An adolescent presents to your clinic 5 years after undergoing stem cell transplant for acute myeloid leukemia (AML). She wants to know what she should expect and what medical follow-up she needs now that her leukemia is "cured."

Q Which of the following is the most likely complication of this patient's treatment?

A She will be noticeably shorter then her siblings
B She is likely to have no long-term effects if they have not manifested themselves within the first 5 years posttransplant
C A 20-point drop in IQ from high dose
D Amenorrhea and possible lack of sexual characteristics
E Significantly increased risk of secondary AML but not other cancers

CHAPTER

15

Hemostasis and thrombosis

Question 1

A 35-year-old woman presents with acute left leg deep venous thrombosis (DVT), which occurred in the setting of plaster cast immobilization as a result of a fibular fracture requiring open reduction and internal fixation. Her mother died of pulmonary embolism after hip replacement surgery, and a maternal aunt is on long-term "blood thinning therapy" for "blood clots in her legs." She wishes advice on the optimal duration of anticoagulant therapy and wonders whether she should be screened for hypercoagulable states.

Q Which is the most appropriate response to her questions?

A Her DVT is clearly secondary to the immobilization and surgery; therefore, 3 months of anticoagulants are sufficient. Her family history is not significant because her mother's DVT was also secondary, and the history from the aunt is not useful given its lack of detail. As a result, hypercoagulable screening is not indicated.

B Her DVT is clearly secondary to immobilization and surgery; however, her family history is of sufficient concern that extended-duration anticoagulants (>1 year) are indicated. Screening for a hypercoagulable state is not indicated because such a disorder must exist and delineating the specific state is unnecessary.

C The history of surgery-associated DVT is irrelevant; her family history mandates long-term anticoagulants.

D Her DVT is clearly secondary to immobilization and surgery, and her family history is of sufficient concern that hypercoagulable testing is indicated.

Question 2

A 75-year-old man presents to the emergency department with arterial ischemia to the right leg. Emergency surgical intervention and embolectomy are required; during surgery, unanticipated bleeding occurs, and it is noted that the patient had a coagulopathy prior to arriving in the operating room (international normalized ratio of 5.6, activated partial thromboplastin time of 84 seconds, fibrinogen of <1 g/L, and platelet count of 40×10^9/L). He is not known to be taking anticoagulants but does report increased bruising for approximately 6 months. He is afebrile and normotensive, and he has not seen a physician or required hospital care in >10 years.

Q Which of the following is the most likely cause of this patient's coagulopathy?

A Accidental administration of heparin during the surgical procedure

B Unanticipated gram-negative septicemia with associated disseminated intravascular coagulation

C Surreptitious ingestion of warfarin prior to hospital admission

D Prostate carcinoma

Question 3

A 45-year-old woman presents to the emergency department complaining of 4 days of left-sided chest pain that is pleuritic in nature. She denies fevers and chills but does have a mild cough that is not productive of sputum. The pain is described as being worse with inspiration, absent during rest, and located predominantly over the anterior left lower chest. She has not identified any factors that make the pain better or worse, and there are no associated symptoms such as dyspnea, syncope, or a sensation of tachycardia. Past medical history reveals that she has recently completed chemotherapy for breast cancer after primary lumpectomy and local radiation. She currently takes no medications on a day-to-day basis. On examination, the oxygen saturation on room air is 92%, the heart rate is 86, and the temperature is 37.5°C. Physical examination reveals possible reduced air entry over the right lower chest. There is no physical examination evidence of acute deep vein thrombosis. Chest x-ray reveals a possible infiltrate in the right lower lobe; electrocardiogram is normal. D-dimer is elevated.

Q Which of the following strategies are most likely to yield a definite diagnosis in this case?

A Ventilation perfusion lung scan
B Ultrasonography of the leg
C Computed tomographic pulmonary angiogram
D Direct pulmonary angiogram

Question 4

A 36-year-old man presents to the emergency department with a 36-hour history of headache and intermittent episodes of aphasia. He has no significant past medical history and takes no medications. Other symptoms include intermittent low-grade fevers with temperatures to 38.5°C. On examination, he has mild left-sided weakness without other abnormalities. Initial laboratory examination reveals moderate renal insufficiency, a hemoglobin of 9.2 g/dL, and a platelet count of $42 \times 10^9/L$. Coagulation tests are normal. Examination of the peripheral blood smear reveals frequent red cell fragments. The lactate dehydrogenase level is approximately 4 times the upper limit of normal.

Q Which of the following is the most likely cause of this patient's disorder?

A Disseminated intravascular coagulation
B Drug-associated toxic reaction
C A hereditary form of thrombotic thrombocytopenic purpura
D An acquired antibody-mediated microangiopathic disorder

Question 5

A full-term well male infant is born without complications after a normal pregnancy and initial nursery stay. The baby is noted to have prolonged oozing from the heelstick metabolic screen. To assess a potential coagulopathy, a complete blood cell count with platelet count, prothrombin time, partial thromboplastin time, and fibrinogen are sent, and the results are all normal. Family history is negative for any bleeding disorder. He returns for the 2-week check, and the mother states that the umbilical cord has been oozing blood for 4 days. A screening test for factor XIII deficiency is ordered, and this test shows that the baby's clot does not dissolve in 5 M urea. The euglobulin lysis time is very short (<1 hour).

Q Which of the following is the most likely diagnosis?

A Antiplasmin deficiency
B Severe hemophilia B (factor IX deficiency)
C von Willebrand disease
D Tissue plasminogen activator excess

Question 6

A 5-year-old girl has recurrent strep pharyngitis and enlarged tonsils. Her pediatrician consults with an ear, nose, and throat surgeon, who recommends a tonsillectomy and adenoidectomy. She comes to see you for a preoperative assessment. History reveals a recent strep infection 1 week ago, and she is still on penicillin. Family history confirms maternal menses lasting 5 days (changing pads that are partially soaked, 4 times daily) and a brother with a few scattered (1 cm) bruises on the lower extremity. The patient has nosebleeds 1–2 times per month during the winter season, associated with upper respiratory infections, which last <1 minute and stop with pressure. Laboratory findings on this patient reveal normal complete blood cell and platelet counts, a prothrombin time of 12 seconds, a partial thromboplastin time (PTT) of 48 seconds (10 seconds prolonged), and fibrinogen of 200 mg/dL. Also, 1:1 mixing studies of the prolonged activated PTT (APTT) show a correction (immediately) of only 3 seconds and a similarly prolonged APTT at 1 hour.

Q Which would be the best test to order to confirm the suspected diagnosis?

A Obtain a more detailed family bleeding history
B Repeat the APTT
C Perform a phospholipid neutralization of the APTT
D Perform factor VIII, IX, and XI assays

Question 7

A term, appropriate-weight female infant is born after uncomplicated pregnancy and delivery. The mother is a vegetarian and is breast-feeding her child. The mother argues, against your advice, to not administer the usual 0.5-mg vitamin K shot prior to her baby's discharge, and the medication is not given. The baby appears to be thriving until, at 2 months of age, she has what appears to be a viral infection with 3 days of watery diarrhea. She presents to the emergency room 2 days later with an intracranial hemorrhage. Laboratory shows normal complete blood cell and platelet counts but an extremely elevated prothrombin time and activated partial thromboplastin time, both of which are >100 seconds.

Q What is the most likely cause for this condition?

A The mother is a vegetarian
B Undiagnosed cystic fibrosis
C Breast-feeding
D Vitamin K deficiency

Question 8

A 4-year-old boy presents to the emergency room with petechiae and bruising. He is a normally active 4-year-old boy and was ill with an upper respiratory infection and low-grade fever 3 weeks ago. He recovered from this infection and was well until today when the mother noticed his new symptoms. His vital signs are normal, and he appears well without complaints except for some petechiae on his face and groin region and scattered bruising (1 × 1 cm in size) on his lower extremity and arms. He has no bleeding from his nose or mouth or in his stool. A complete blood cell count reveals a white blood cell count of 10,800/μL, hemoglobin of 12.5 g/dL, mean corpuscular volume of 82 fL, and platelet count of 15,000/μL. Review of the peripheral smear is normal with the exception of few platelets, and the ones observed appear larger than normal.

Q Which of the following is the most appropriate next step in the evaluation of this patient?

A Bone marrow biopsy
B Admit for observation
C Corticosteroids and intravenous γ globulin
D Reassurance and follow-up in 1 week

Question 9

A 9-year-old male Greek child with homozygous β thalassemia is receiving his regular every-3-week red blood cell transfusion. His trough hemoglobin prior to the transfusion is usually 10 g/dL. Midway through the transfusion, he develops fever, chills, hypotension, gross hematuria, and extensive bleeding from his mouth. Initial laboratory results reveal the following:

White blood cell count	21,000 (60% phagocytes, 15% basophils, 29% lymphocytes)
Hemoglobin	4.5 g/dL
Platelets	75,000/μL
Prothrombin time	30 seconds
Activated partial thromboplastin time	55 seconds
Fibrinogen	70 mg/dL
D-Dimer	4500 ng/mL

You presume a hemolytic transfusion reaction and secondary disseminated intravascular coagulation.

Q Which of the following is the most appropriate choice for initial therapy?

A Normal saline, antibiotics, red blood cells, and fresh frozen plasma
B Normal saline, antithrombin III concentrates, red blood cells, and platelet transfusion
C Aminocaproic acid, red blood cells, and platelet transfusion
D Low-dose heparin, normal saline bolus, red cell transfusion, and cryoprecipitate

Question 10

A 9-month-old female infant presents to your office with a several-month history of bruising on the extremities and trunk, some quite extensive (3 × 3 cm) and not associated with trauma. Additionally, the girl has been oozing for several hours from a tooth eruption. A complete blood cell count is normal (including the platelet count and peripheral morphology) as is the prothrombin time, activated partial thromboplastin time, and fibrinogen. You order von Willebrand disease and factor XIII screens as well as an antiplasmin level, all of which are normal. The moderately severe bleeding seems out of proportion to the normal laboratory testing, and you suspect a moderately severe platelet function defect such as Glanzmann thrombasthenia.

Q Which of the following platelet aggregation patterns would be most indicative of this diagnosis?

A Absent aggregation to adenosine diphosphate (ADP) and collagen but normal aggregation to ristocetin
B Absent aggregation to ristocetin and normal aggregation to ADP and collagen
C Normal platelet aggregation to all agonists (ADP, collagen, and ristocetin)

D Decreased aggregation and adenosine triphosphate (ATP) release to arachidonic acid and normal aggregation and ATP release to other agonists (ADP, collagen, and ristocetin)

Question 11

An 18-month-old boy with a known diagnosis of hemophilia A (factor VIII deficiency) presents to the Hemophilia Treatment Center with a new right knee bleed that does not appear to be responding to his usual FVIII dosing schedule. The father has been treating this bleed for 3 days now (50 IU/kg of recombinant (r) FVIII per day). The boy has received 12 exposure doses to rFVIII in the past. You suspect an inhibitor to FVIII and send a Bethesda titer, which is 25 BU.

Q Which of the following is the most appropriate next step in the management of this patient?

A High-dose rFVIII
B Low-dose immune tolerance therapy
C Continue current dose of rFVIII
D No therapy until the Bethesda titer is <10 BU

CHAPTER

16

Transfusion medicine

Question 1

A 57-year-old Hispanic man is admitted to an inner-city teaching hospital emergency department with subacute dyspnea. Physical examination reveals a normal cardiopulmonary examination but black heme-positive stool on rectal examination. Laboratory examination reveals hemoglobin of 6.8 g/dL but is otherwise normal. Five minutes into infusion of the first unit, the patient begins to complain of dyspnea. Examination reveals temperature 38.3°C, pulse 120/min, blood pressure 85/60 mm Hg, and respirations 32/min.

Q What is the most likely cause of the patient's acute decompensation?

A Acute febrile transfusion reaction
B Acute hemolytic transfusion reaction
C Volume overload
D Allergic transfusion reaction
E Transfusion-induced acute lung injury

Question 2

A 59-year-old woman with recently diagnosed nonmetastatic breast cancer receives her first cycle of adjuvant chemotherapy and is brought to the emergency room 10 days later complaining of inability to move her left leg. Physical examination is normal except for marked left leg weakness, and an emergency magnetic resonance imaging scan of the brain reveals a 3-cm hemorrhage in the right frontoparietal region. The patient's level of consciousness significantly declines over the first hour in the emergency department. Complete blood count reveals white blood count 200/μL, hemoglobin 9.9 g/dL, and platelet count 3,000/μL. The patient's blood type is O Rh-negative.

Q Which of the following is the most appropriate platelet product for the initial management of her bleeding diathesis?

A Type O Rh-negative single-donor apheresis platelet product expected to be available the next day
B Type A Rh-negative random-donor 6-pack expected to be available in 2 hours
C Type O Rh-positive single-donor apheresis product expected to be available in 1 hour
D Type A Rh-positive random-donor 6-pack expected to be available in 20 minutes

Question 3

A 36-year-old man with acute myelogenous leukemia in second relapse receives high-dose myeloablative chemotherapy followed by an infusion of human leukocyte antigen (HLA)-identical hematopoietic stem cells from his 32-year-old sister. The recipient's pretransplant blood specimen typed as O Rh-negative, whereas the donor's blood is type A Rh-positive. The patient's neutrophil count recovers promptly at day 12 following the transplant, and his platelet count recovers a few days thereafter, but at day 100 the patient still requires red cell transfusions on a regular basis. His peripheral blood reticulocyte count remains at 0.1%, and the peripheral blood lactate dehydrogenase level is normal.

Q What is the most likely explanation for the failure of the patient's erythroid recovery?

A Pure red cell aplasia due to donor–recipient gender mismatch
B Pure red cell aplasia due to donor–recipient Rh mismatch
C Alloimmune hemolytic anemia due to donor–recipient ABO mismatch

D Pure red cell aplasia due to donor–recipient ABO mismatch
E Pure red cell aplasia due to undetected non-HLA ("minor") histocompatibility antigen mismatches

Question 4

A 25-year-old woman with metastatic breast cancer receives high-dose myeloablative chemotherapy followed by infusion of autologous hematopoietic stem cells according to an institutional review board–approved clinical research protocol. At day 5 following the transplant, she develops painless facial and upper extremity swelling. Magnetic resonance angiography demonstrates near-complete thrombotic occlusion of the superior vena cava. The peripheral blood platelet count is 5,000/μL.

Q What is the best short-term management strategy for this patient?

A Do nothing, ie, allow the platelet count to remain at 5,000/μL or below
B Administer therapeutic-dose unfractionated heparin
C Administer therapeutic-dose unfractionated heparin in addition to platelet transfusions to keep the peripheral blood platelet count at 50,000/μL or higher
D Administer low-molecular-weight heparin in addition to platelet transfusions to keep the peripheral blood platelet count at 50,000/μL or higher
E Administer streptokinase

Question 5

A 55-year-old multiparous woman requires repeated platelet transfusions after receiving induction chemotherapy for acute myelogenous leukemia. On each day that her daily 6:00 AM peripheral blood platelet count is $<$10,000/μL, her attending physician orders platelets, which typically arrive and are transfused before noon on the day they are ordered. After each of the first 4 transfusions, the next morning's 6:00 AM platelet count is $>$20,000/μL, but after the fifth and sixth transfusions, the next morning's platelet counts remain $<$10,000/μL.

Q Which diagnostic strategy is most likely to yield the correct explanation for her platelet transfusion refractoriness?

A Order a lymphocytotoxic antibody screen
B Order an assay for platelet-specific antibodies
C Order a computed tomographic scan to quantitate the size of the spleen
D Order a screen for disseminated intravascular coagulation
E Order an assay for von Willebrand factor multimers

Question 6

A 40-year-old man with chronic myelogenous leukemia that has progressed to myeloid blast crisis on imatinib is referred to your center for consideration of bone marrow transplantation. Standard acute leukemia induction therapy is administered while a bone marrow donor search is initiated, and the patient becomes severely pancytopenic. The patient's blood type is A Rh-negative, and a serologic antibody screen for cytomegalovirus (CMV) is negative.

Q Which of the following red cell products would you select for this patient?

A γ-Irradiated, leukoreduced, directed-donor red cells obtained from the patient's type A Rh-negative, CMV-negative brother
B γ-Irradiated, leukoreduced red cells obtained from a type O Rh-positive, CMV-positive volunteer donor
C γ-Irradiated, leukoreduced red cells obtained from a type A Rh-negative, CMV-negative volunteer donor
D γ-Irradiated, leukoreduced red cells obtained from a type A Rh-negative, CMV-positive volunteer donor

Question 7

A 90-year-old Caucasian woman who is healthy other than a history of multiple urinary tract infections is admitted to the hospital with mental status changes, temperature 39.4°C, pulse 145/min, respiratory rate 42/min, and blood pressure 80/60. Appropriate intravenous fluid resuscitation and broad-spectrum antibiotics are initiated, and multiple blood cultures grow out gram-negative rods within hours of admission. The patient's vital signs have stabilized 12 hours after admission, but the physical examination now reveals blood oozing from the patient's nose, gums, and line insertion sites. In addition, the tips of 3 separate toes on the patient's left foot are now found to be cold and black. Examination of the blood reveals mild to moderate schistocytosis. Laboratory evaluation reveals markedly reduced plasma fibrinogen but markedly elevated fibrin degradation products, D-dimer levels, and prothrombin time. The platelet count is 30,000/μL.

Q Which of the following is the most appropriate therapy for this patient?

A Steroids and plasma exchange
B Cryoprecipitate, fresh frozen plasma, and platelets
C Cryoprecipitate and platelets
D Fresh frozen plasma and platelets

Question 8

A 28-year-old woman has just learned that she is 5 weeks pregnant and is having her first prenatal obstetrical visit. The physician sends off a blood sample for type and screen and receives a report from the blood bank that the patient is Rh(D)-negative and has a positive antibody screen for anti-Rh(D). The blood bank also reports that the Rh(D) titer is 1:16. The patient is an excellent historian and denies having been given Rh(D) immune globulin in the past 3 months, or ever, for that matter.

Q Given these laboratory results, how many vials of Rh(D) immune globulin should the obstetrician administer to the patient (each vial contains 300 μg)?

A One vial, immediately
B Two vials, given the titer of anti-Rh(D) present in the patient's serum
C One vial, when she is at 28-weeks gestation
D None

Question 9

The following table presents forward and reverse ABO typing reaction results for 4 patients and should be used to answer questions 9 and 10.

Patient	Forward typing reaction of patient's RBCs with:		Reverse typing reaction of patient's serum with:	
	anti-A	anti-B	A RBCs*	B RBCs
1	0	0	+	+
2	+	0	0	+
3	0	+	+	+
4	+	+	0	0

*RBC = red blood cell.

Q If the need for transfusion of fresh frozen plasma (FFP) should arise, which patient can receive only FFP collected from a blood donor who is blood group AB?

A 1
B 2
C 3
D 4

Question 10

Patient 3 from the table in question 9 was recently diagnosed with a B-cell lymphoma and was found to have a drop in hemoglobin over the past few weeks from 14.5 g/dL to 9.5 g/dL. The blood bank reports that the patient has a direct antiglobulin test (DAT) that is negative for immunoglobulin G (IgG) but positive for complement 3 and that the patient's serum displayed evidence of marked hemolysis. The blood bank also reports that the patient's red blood cells had to be washed with warm saline before forward ABO typing and the DAT could be performed. The blood bank requests a transfusion history from this patient and is told that he has never been transfused with red blood cells but had received a platelet transfusion earlier in the week as an outpatient at another facility.

Q What is the most likely cause of this patient's anemia?

A Cold-reactive IgM red cell autoantibodies
B Red cell alloantibodies to a high-frequency alloantigen
C ABO blood group isohemagglutinins
D Complement-fixing IgG autoantibodies

Question 11

A 78-year-old woman with a history of chronic renal disease on dialysis has symptomatic anemia and hemoglobin of 9.0 g/dL. In the dialysis unit, 2 U of packed red blood cells (RBCs) are ordered from the blood bank. The blood bank director pages the ordering physician and reports that the patient's antibody screen was positive for anti-K1, anti-E, anti-Fy^a and anti-S alloantibodies, and consequently there will be a delay of at least a couple of hours while the blood bank screens a number of ABO/Rh-compatible units to find ones that lack those 4 alloantigens. After screening approximately 2 dozen units, a pair of units that were K1-, E-, Fy^a-, and S-negative are identified. A full Coombs crossmatch is performed for each unit, and both are found to be crossmatch compatible. The units are transfused to the patient uneventfully, and a posttransfusion hemoglobin of 11.8 g/dL is obtained. Though the patient's anemia-related symptoms appear to resolve shortly thereafter, over the following week the patient develops some shortness of breath and returns to the emergency department. She is noted to be mildly jaundiced, and her hemoglobin is now 10.5 g/dL. The ER physician reviews her recent history of transfusion and suspects that there was some incompatibility with at least one of the transfused units she had received a week earlier and contacts the blood bank director. The blood bank director informs the physician that the blood bank still has some of the patient's pretransfusion blood sample and also has a policy of saving aliquots of blood from transfused units (tubing segments). The blood bank director requests that a fresh sample of blood from the patient be sent to the blood bank right away.

Q Which of the following serologic tests performed by the blood bank would be most informative?

A Retype RBCs in the retained tubing segments (the transfused units) for K1, E, Fy^a, and S
B Repeat the crossmatches of the RBCs in the retained tubing segments (the transfused units) with the patient's pretransfusion specimen
C Perform an antibody screen and panel on a fresh sample of the patient's blood
D Retype the patient's RBCs in the pretransfusion sample for K1, E, Fy^a, and S

Question 12

A 65-year-old woman with a 10-year history of warm autoimmune hemolytic anemia (ie, immunoglobulin G [IgG]-type AIHA) is transferred from an outside community hospital for further management of her underlying disease. She has had a long history of red cell transfusions in the past, most recently receiving 2 U of packed red blood cells (RBCs) earlier in the week in the setting of chest pain and hemoglobin of 7.5 g/dL. Currently, her hemoglobin is 7.0 g/dL, and 3 U of RBCs are ordered. Initial blood bank workup reveals a B Rh-positive patient with an antibody screen strongly positive on both screening cells. An antibody identification panel was run and, as expected for a patient with AIHA, pan-reactivity was observed across the 11 RBCs in the panel. The patient's direct antiglobulin test was positive for IgG and negative for complement 3. The blood bank calls the ordering physician to inquire about the patient's recent transfusion history and to alert the physician that it will take at least several hours to complete the workup before blood will be available. From past experience with patients with AIHA, the physician knows that any units of blood for this patient will be crossmatch incompatible and does not understand why further workup is required, much less a workup that may take hours.

Q Which of the following serologic procedures does the blood bank want to perform prior to selecting RBC units for crossmatch?

A Extended antibody identification panel of selected reagent RBCs to identify the specificity of the autoantigen
B Absorption of the patient's serum with autologous cells
C Extended phenotyping of the patient's RBCs so RBC units can be selected that match for more than just the A, B, and Rh(D) antigens
D Differential absorption of the patient's serum with a set of allogeneic reagent red cells

Question 13

A 13-year-old boy with newly diagnosed acute lymphoblastic leukemia accompanied by marked anemia develops laryngospasm, abdominal pain, and marked hypotension shortly after his nurse begins an infusion of packed red blood cells. The transfusion is stopped immediately, and workup reveals complete absence of immunoglobulin A (IgA) in his plasma along with anti-IgA antibodies.

Q What is the most appropriate way to prevent further reactions of this type when administering subsequent red cell transfusions?

A Leukoreduced red cells
B Washed red cells
C Red blood cells from IgA-deficient individuals
D Irradiated red cells
E Cytomegalovirus-negative red cells

Question 14

A 6-year-old girl with moderately severe T-cell-restricted congenital immunodeficiency syndrome is a passenger in a high-speed motor vehicle accident and arrives in a local emergency room severely hypotensive and tachycardic with bilateral pelvic fractures, bilateral hip fractures, and a peripheral blood hemoglobin level of 4.8 g/dL. She is successfully resuscitated with emergency surgery, crystalloid, and type O Rh-negative blood obtained from the hospital's blood bank. The surgical wounds become infected, and broad-spectrum antibiotics are administered. While making preparations for hospital discharge 14 days after admission, the girl begins to complain of skin itching and diarrhea, and the attending physician notices that her peripheral blood hemoglobin, white cell count, and platelet count are all falling rapidly and that her bilirubin, alkaline phosphatase, and aspartate aminotransferase levels are all rising.

Q What is the most likely explanation for this constellation of findings?

A Viral hepatitis
B Delayed transfusion reaction due to the development of antibodies against Kidd (Jk[a]) antigens
C Antibiotic-induced marrow suppression
D Transfusion-induced graft-versus-host disease
E Cytomegalovirus infection

Question 15

A newborn was delivered at term from a 35-year-old woman after an uneventful pregnancy. Records indicate that this is her first pregnancy, she has never received a transfusion in the past, her blood type is blood group O Rh-negative, and her negative antibody screen was negative at the outset of her pregnancy. She received the standard 1-vial dose of Rh(D)-immune globulin at 28-weeks gestation. Shortly after birth, the infant is noted to be jaundiced with a total bilirubin of 6.5 mg/dL (direct bilirubin of 0.9 mg/dL) and a hematocrit of 29.5%. The baby is followed over the course of the day, and her bilirubin continues to rise with a concomitant fall in hemoglobin. After ruling out nonimmune causes of hyperbilirubinemia and hemolysis, the neonatologist asks the blood bank if there might be an immune basis for this newborn's apparent hemolytic anemia. At this point in time, the blood bank has determined that the baby's blood type was A Rh-negative and her direct antiglobulin test was positive for immunoglobulin G (IgG). Hearing this, the neonatologist requests that that the blood bank identify the specificity of the IgG bound to the baby's cells, which are presumably responsible for the baby's hemolysis and hyperbilirubinemia. In response, the blood bank elutes the IgG off of the newborn's red blood cells (RBCs) and runs the eluate against antibody screening cells. The eluate was unreactive with the screening cells.

Q Which of the following serologic tests would be most helpful at this point in time?

A Performing an antibody screen on the baby's serum
B Performing an antibody identification panel with the baby's eluate and a select panel of RBCs expressing low-frequency antigens
C Reacting the baby's serum against maternal RBCs
D Testing the baby's red cell eluate using the A and B cells usually reserved for reverse typing

CHAPTER 17

Laboratory hematology

Question 1

You are called during hospital rounds about the following values obtained on an EDTA blood sample drawn from a female outpatient and run on an automated cell counter in your office. Your office staff tells you the instrument has "flagged" the results as suspect. The white blood cell and platelet counts are normal and "unflagged."

Red blood cell count	2.8 T/L (normal range, 4.1–5.1)
Hemoglobin	14.0 g/dL (normal range, 12.3–15.3)
Hematocrit	32.7% (normal range, 36–45)
Mean corpuscular volume	117 fL (normal range, 80–96)
Mean corpuscular hemoglobin concentration	38.5 g/dL (normal range, 33.4–35.5)

Q What is the most likely diagnosis of the patient?

A Hereditary spherocytosis
B Pernicious anemia
C Myelodysplastic syndrome
D Lymphoplasmacytic lymphoma
E Renal anemia

Question 2

The platelet function laboratory asks you to interpret the following aggregation results from a patient with a platelet count of 350,000.

Adenine diphosphate (ADP) low dose	Normal
ADP standard dose	Normal
Collagen low dose	Normal
Collagen standard dose	Normal
Ristocetin high dose	Markedly reduced
Epinephrine	Normal

Resuspending the platelets in normal plasma improved response to ristocetin to normal.

Q Which of the following is the most likely cause of these findings?

A Bernard–Soulier syndrome
B Glanzmann thrombasthenia
C Storage pool defect
D Aspirin effect
E von Willebrand disorder

Question 3

A 67-year-old woman with diabetes, hypertension, and chronic obstructive pulmonary disease complains of increasing exertional fatigue and intermittent pain in her hips, but denies other symptoms. Her physical examination is essentially normal, with no direct bony tenderness or arthritis findings. Her white blood cell count is normal, with a normal differential; hemoglobin 11.3 g/dL; mean corpuscular volume 94 fL; and platelets 245,000/μL. Absolute reticulocyte count is 103,000/μL (normal range, 25,000–76,000). A picture of her smear is shown below (from ASH Image Bank 2004 #101153).

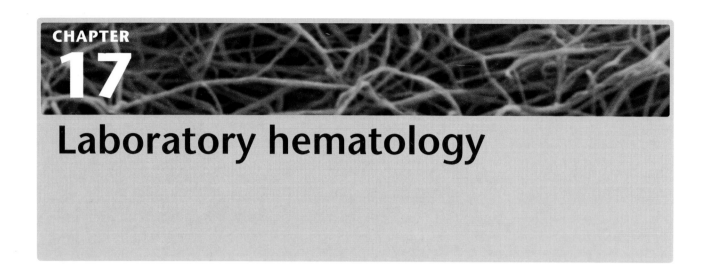

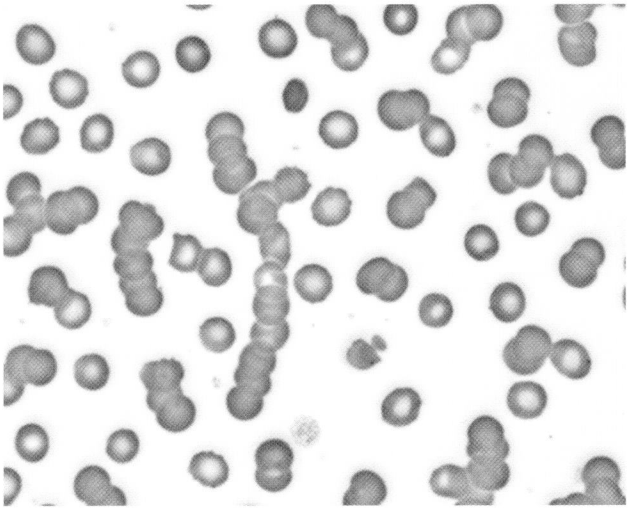

Q **Which diagnostic test would be most helpful in determining the cause of her anemia?**

A Direct antiglobulin test
B Serum protein electrophoresis
C Fibrinogen level
D Skeletal survey
E Computed tomography of chest, abdomen, and pelvis

Question 4

A 63-year-old female with diabetes, hyperlipidemia, obesity, and renal insufficiency has her left lower leg amputated for osteomyelitis. She is on clopidogrel for a history of transient ischemic attack. Daily low-molecular-weight heparin is started on day 1, but a deep venous thrombosis develops in her unaffected leg on day 5. Her preadmission complete blood cell count showed a white blood cell count of $8.2 \times 10^9/L$ with a normal differential, hemoglobin of 8.9 g/dL, and platelet count of 148,000/μL. The platelet count drops to 48,000. Examination of her blood smear reveals the following (from ASH Image Bank 2005 #101285).

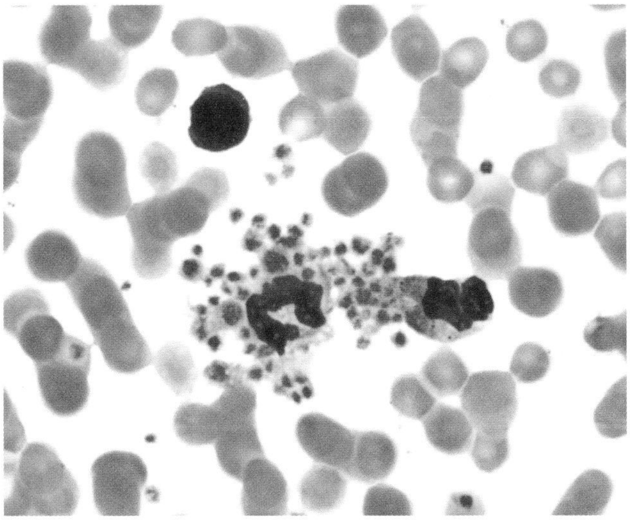

Q **Which of the following is the most likely cause of this patient's reduced platelet count?**

A Sepsis
B Heparin-induced thrombocytopenia
C Platelet agglutinin
D Antiphospholipid antibody
E Thrombotic microangiopathy

Question 5

A 77-year-old female Vietnamese immigrant notes heavy vaginal bleeding over the past week, requiring transfusion to maintain her hemoglobin above 8.0 mg/dL. Dilation and curettage did not help the bleeding. She denies a past history of excessive bleeding, jaundice, or melena, but has had constipation alternating with diarrhea intermittently for the past year. Prior to this episode, she had not seen a physician for 15 years. She lives with her son, who is on warfarin for atrial fibrillation. Laboratory testing reveals a prothrombin time of 12.7 seconds, an international normalized ratio of 0.98, and a partial thromboplastin time (PTT) of 78 seconds. The PTT was 62 seconds after mixing with normal plasma.

Q **What is the most likely cause of her vaginal bleeding?**

A Warfarin ingestion
B Factor inhibitor
C Lupus anticoagulant
D Factor XI deficiency
E Vitamin K deficiency

Question 6

A 33-year-old African American female has had mild anemia for years, unresponsive to oral iron supplementation. She was diagnosed with irritable bowel syndrome in her teens, which she manages by diet. Her menses are regular but self-described as heavy. She is on no medication other than oral iron. Laboratory data are as follows:

White blood cell count	$4.3 \times 10^9/L$
Hemoglobin (Hb)	11.9 g/dL
Hematocrit	31.9%
Red blood cell count	5.9 million cells/mm^3
Mean corpuscular volume	63 fL
Mean corpuscular hemoglobin	20.4 pg
Red blood cell distribution width	14.9%
Platelets	280,000/μL
Reticulocyte count	37,000/μL

Analysis by high-performance liquid chromatography revealed Hb A, 70%, Hb S, 26%, Hb A_2, 3.4%, and Hb F, <1%.

Q What is the most likely explanation for her anemia?

A Anemia of chronic disease
B α Thalassemia
C β Thalassemia
D Iron deficiency
E Sickle hemoglobinopathy

Question 7

A 55-year-old male with active hepatitis C virus is admitted for fever and increasing ascites. He has lost 15 pounds in the past 4 months. He is dialysis dependent from renal failure secondary to cryoglobulinemia. Coagulation testing shows the following:

Prothrombin time	21.2 seconds
Partial thromboplastin time	43 seconds
Fibrinogen	206 mg/dL
Thrombin time	44.3 seconds
Reptilase time	23 seconds

These tests were performed using coagulometric assays.

Q What is the most likely cause of his abnormal coagulation tests?

A Heparin effect
B Vitamin K deficiency
C Disseminated intravascular coagulation
D Dysfibrinogenemia
E Cryoglobulinemia

CHAPTER

18

Consultative hematology

Question 1

A 60-year-old female undergoes cardiac catheterization for exercise-induced chest pain and is found to have 3-vessel coronary artery disease not amenable to stent placement. Seven days later she is admitted for coronary artery bypass grafting using heparin anticoagulation. Her platelet count preoperatively is 220,000/µL. Though the platelet count falls to 110,000/µL 12 hours after surgery, by day 4 it has increased to 175,000/µL, and the patient is discharged on postoperative day 5. Three weeks after discharge, the patient is admitted with shortness of breath and malaise. The chest x-ray reveals a small, wedge-shaped opacity in the right mid lung area. Ventilation–perfusion is interpreted as high probability for pulmonary embolism, and the patient is treated with unfractionated heparin. The platelet count on admission is 95,000/µL and falls to 60,000/µL the morning after admission, at which time the patient notes increased shortness of breath.

Q Which of the following would the best course of management include at this time?

A Increase the infusion rate of unfractionated heparin
B Stop unfractionated heparin, begin low-molecular-weight heparin
C Stop heparin
D Stop unfractionated heparin, begin therapy with a direct thrombin inhibitor
E Begin corticosteroid therapy for presumed immune thrombocytopenia

Question 2

A 32-year-old female presents in the 30th week of pregnancy with a 2-week history of malaise, difficulty concentrating, and easy bruisability. Physical examination reveals an oral temperature of 38.2°C, a blood pressure of 126/78 mm Hg, and several purpuric lesions over the tibia bilaterally. The complete blood cell count demonstrates a hemoglobin of 8.7 g/dL, hematocrit of 26%, and a platelet count of 27,000/µL, and the urinalysis reveals 3–4 red blood cells per high-power field but only trace proteinuria. The creatinine, alanine aminotransferase, and aspartate aminotransferase levels are normal, though the lactose dehydrogenase is 1800 U/dL. The peripheral blood film is depicted below (from ASH Image Bank 2001 #100174, Figure 2).

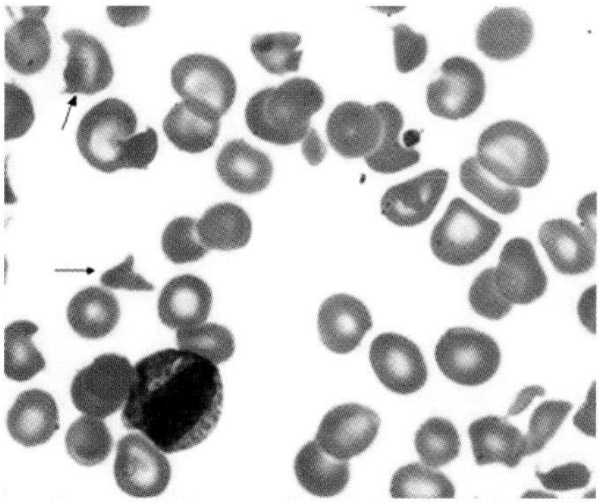

Q Which of the following is the most appropriate management strategy for this patient?

A Initiate bethamethasone therapy to promote fetal lung maturity with plans to deliver the fetus expeditiously
B Initiate therapy with pulse dexamethasone
C Initiate therapy with rituximab
D Obtain a fetal platelet count by percutaneous umbilical cord blood sampling
E Initiate daily plasma exchange

Question 3

A 26-year-old female is self-referred for recommendations concerning anticoagulation during pregnancy. She is not yet pregnant, but contemplating becoming so. Her past medical history is notable for a deep venous thrombosis at age 22 following an ankle fracture that required immobilization in a cast. She was subsequently evaluated for thrombophilia but was found to be negative for factor V Leiden, prothrombin G20210A, an elevated homocysteine level, antithrombin, protein C and S deficiencies, and antiphospholipid antibodies. She has not had any further thrombotic events. Her family history is notable for a 28-year-old sister who was found to have factor V Leiden upon thrombophilia screening following a fetal loss at 6 weeks. One other sister is 32 years old and has had one successful pregnancy and no fetal losses. She does not know the factor V Leiden status of her parents, but neither one of them has had thrombotic events.

Q Which of the following would be the most appropriate management for this patient?

A Follow with close clinical surveillance and initiate coumadin in the postpartum period
B Repeat screening for factor V Leiden
C Repeat antiphospholipid antibody testing
D Initiate therapy with low-molecular-weight heparin coincident with attempts to conceive, and continue throughout pregnancy and the postpartum period
E Initiate coumadin therapy coincident with attempts to conceive, and continue throughout pregnancy and the postpartum period

Question 4

A 29-year-old female who is 36 weeks pregnant presents with generalized malaise, right upper quadrant pain, and vomiting. On physical examination, the patient is afebrile with a blood pressure of 144/92 and significant right upper quadrant tenderness to deep palpation. The hemoglobin is 8.6 g/dL, hematocrit 27 g/dL, and the platelet count 40,000/μL. The creatinine is 1.1 g/dL, the serum urea nitrogen 23 mg/dL, the alanine aminotransferase 96 U/dL, and the aspartate aminotransferase 108 U/dL. The urinalysis reveals 4–6 red blood cells per high-power field, and 3+ proteinuria. The prothrombin time and activated partial thromboplastin time are normal, though the D-dimer level is slightly elevated at 2 μg/mL. A left upper quadrant ultrasound reveals a small subcapsular hemorrhage surrounding the right lobe of the liver. The peripheral blood film is depicted below (from ASH Image Bank 2001 #100249, Figure 1).

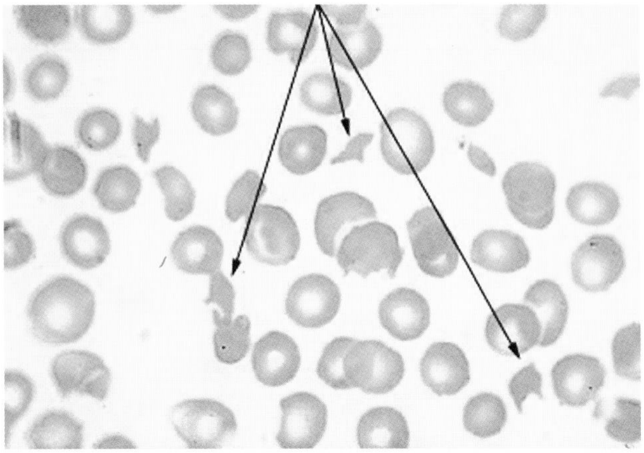

Q What is the most appropriate management strategy for this patient?

A Initiate daily plasma exchange
B Manage hypertension, ensure fetal lung maturity, and initiate expeditious delivery
C Initiate rituximab therapy
D Infuse fresh frozen plasma
E Refer for laparoscopic cholecystectomy

Question 5

A 24-year-old nullipara is referred to you in her 16th week of pregnancy for isolated thrombocytopenia. She was first noted to have a platelet count of 30,000/μL during her eighth week, and treated with a 3-week course of corticosteroids for presumed idiopathic thrombocytopenic purpura (ITP) with no improvement. One course of intravenous immunoglobulin was subsequently given, with an increment in the platelet count of only 10,000/μL that persisted for only 1 week. She has no record of previous platelet counts. Likewise, the patient has no bleeding history, though she has not undergone surgery. The family history is notable for an older sister with ITP who had previously had 2 successful pregnancies, during one of which she may have received corticosteroids.

On presentation to your office, the platelet count is 42,000/μL, the hemoglobin 12.3 g/dL, and the hematocrit 37.1%. The leukocyte count is 6100/μL with normal differential (from McArthur, ASH Education Program Book 2000;1:457):

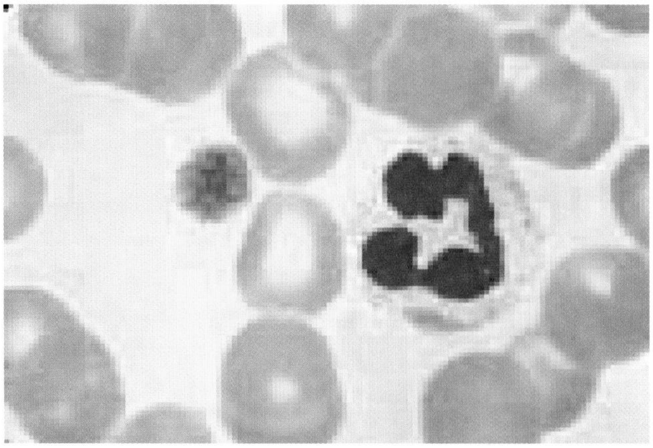

Q Which of the following is the most appropriate intervention for this patient?

A Bone marrow aspirate and biopsy
B Initiation of a trial of high-dose dexamethasone
C Rituximab
D Splenectomy
E Careful monitoring of the platelet count and review of the blood smears from other family members

Question 6

You are asked to evaluate a 58-year-old woman who was found on preoperative evaluation for elective total abdominal hysterectomy to have an abnormal coagulation test. She is postmenopausal and has had progressive problems with pelvic pain and relaxation secondary to large uterine leiomyomata. She denies a previous or recent history of menorrhagia or vaginal bleeding, bleeding after prior dental procedures, after tonsillectomy, or after 2 vaginal deliveries. She has no family history of unusual bleeding or easy bruising. Her past medical history is unremarkable except for obesity and cholecystitis. She is currently taking acetaminophen with oxycodone, iron supplement, and mutivitamins. Her weight is 100 kg, and her blood pressure is 154/90. Examination is unremarkable except for obesity and mild suprapubic tenderness on palpation. No petechiae, purpura, or ecchymoses are visible on the skin. Laboratory studies are as follows:

Hematocrit	38%
Leukocyte count	9800/μL
Platelet count	380,000/μL
Prothrombin time	12 seconds (normal range, 11–16 seconds)
International normalized ratio	1.1 (normal range, 0.8–1.3)
Activated partial thromboplastin time (APTT)	55 seconds (normal range, 22–35 seconds)
Thrombin time	22 seconds (normal range, 16–25 seconds)

Q Which of the following is the most likely cause of the prolonged APTT in this patient?

A von Willebrand disease
B Factor XI deficiency
C Lupus anticoagulant
D Acquired inhibitor to factor VIII

Question 7

You are asked to consult on a 52-year-old man in the surgical intensive care unit who underwent a cadaveric donor orthotopic liver transplant 2 hours ago and now has persistent bleeding. The patient was not bleeding preoperatively; the baseline prothrombin time/international normalized ratio was 20 seconds/1.8, and the platelet count was 85,000/μL. He received prophylactic aprotinin in the operating room. A vascular leak developed during initial reperfusion of the donor liver, and massive intraoperative hemorrhage ensued. He was stabilized with 8 U of packed red blood cells, 6 U of fresh frozen plasma, and 2 single-donor apheresis platelet products. He has been hemodynamically stable postoperatively and is currently receiving intravenous crystalloid and 1 U of packed red blood cells. Examination reveals a heavily sedated patient on a mechanical ventilator. Blood is slowly oozing from the abdominal wound incision site and from the exit sites of the central venous catheter and arterial catheter. A drain from the abdominal wound has yielded 80 mL of blood since arriving in the intensive care unit.

Postoperative hematology studies reveal the following:

Hematocrit	25%
Leukocyte count	3800/μL
Platelet count	65,000/μL
Prothrombin time	25 seconds (normal range, 12–16 seconds)
International normalized ratio	2.2 (normal range, 0.8–1.3)
Activated partial thromboplastin time	55 seconds (normal range, 22–35 seconds)
Thrombin time	40 seconds (normal range, 16–25 seconds)
Fibrinogen	0.7 g/L (normal range, 1.5–4 g/L)
D-dimer	8.8 mcg/mL (normal range, 0–0.59 mcg/mL)

Q What is the most appropriate next step in the management of this patient?

A Cryoprecipitate infusion
B Infusion of recombinant factor VIIa
C Platelet transfusion
D Infusion of aminocaproic acid

Question 8

A 22-year-old woman who is 18 months status-post a double lung transplant for cystic fibrosis is referred for evaluation of anemia and mild thrombocytopenia. Past medical history is notable for recurrent pneumonias and pancreatic insufficiency related to cystic fibrosis. She has not had major pulmonary or opportunistic infections since the transplant. She required anti-T-cell antibody therapy for acute rejection at 1-month posttransplant and has been on various immunosuppressive agents to control chronic rejection over the last year. Recent pulmonary function tests are stable. Current medications include azathioprine, low-dose prednisone, and tacrolimus. Her primary provider started levofloxacin 5 days ago for fever and presumed bronchitis. Chest x-ray at that time revealed increased bronchial markings and new left hilar fullness. She reports intermittent fevers and involuntary 5-lb weight loss over the last month. Examination is notable for a 3-cm nontender, firm lymph node in the left supraclavicular region. Lung examination reveals bilateral course breath sounds. No hepatosplenomegaly is appreciated on abdominal palpation. Laboratory studies reveal the following:

Hematocrit	29%
Hemoglobin	9.4 g/dL
Reticulocyte count	65,000/μL
Mean corpuscular volume	102 fL
Leukocyte count	3800/μL
Platelet count	110,000/μL
Peripheral smear	Mild erythrocyte anisocytosis and macrocytosis with a rare schistocyte; normal leukocyte and platelet morphology

Q What is the most appropriate next step in the evaluation of this patient?

A Assay peripheral blood ADAMTS13 activity
B Bone marrow aspirate and biopsy
C Assay peripheral blood Epstein–Barr virus DNA copy number
D Supraclavicular lymph node biopsy
E Bronchoscopy with bronchoalveolar lavage

Question 9

You are asked to manage a 62-year-old man who developed a left lower extremity deep venous thrombosis on the second postoperative day following a partial colectomy for acute large bowel obstruction. At surgery, he was found to have metastatic adenocarcinoma of the colon with involvement of the liver and omentum. Prior to hospitalization, he was healthy and active with no past history of venous thromboembolism or other medical problems. He has no family history of thrombosis. His postoperative course has been otherwise stable. There has been minimal drainage from the wound, and the hematocrit and platelet count have been stable. He had been receiving twice-daily low-molecular-weight heparin for thromboprophylaxis. He complains of pain at the surgical site and new pain in the left calf. He is hemodynamically stable, and oxygen saturation is 98% on room air. Examination is notable for a clean and dry abdominal surgical wound and colostomy with hypoactive bowel sounds and mild abdominal tenderness on palpation. The left lower leg is swollen, erythematous, and tender to palpation. Peripheral pulses and capillary refill are normal. Duplex ultrasound reveals occlusive thrombi involving the popliteal and superficial femoral veins of the left leg. No abnormalities are found in the right leg.

Q Which of the following is the safest and most effective therapeutic plan for this patient's venous thromboembolism?

A Acute placement of an inferior vena cava filter and long-term therapy with low-molecular-weight heparin
B Acute infusion of tissue plasminogen activator and long-term therapy with low-molecular-weight heparin
C Acute and long-term therapy with low-molecular-weight heparin
D Acute therapy with continuous-infusion unfractionated heparin and long-term therapy with low-molecular-weight heparin
E Acute therapy with low-molecular-weight heparin and long-term therapy with warfarin

Question 10

A 24-year-old woman in the 30th week of pregnancy is referred for management of Hodgkin disease. She noted progressive painless swelling in the neck over the past 4 months. Excisional biopsy of a 3-cm cervical lymph node revealed nodular sclerosing Hodgkin disease. Magnetic resonance imaging of the chest, abdomen, and pelvis noted a 6-cm mediastinal mass but no other adenopathy, splenomegaly, or evidence of parenchymal disease. She denies weight loss, fever, or night sweats. Prenatal evaluations revealed normal fetal growth and development for gestational age and no abnormalities involving the placenta. Examination is notable for a healing surgical wound in the lower neck with some residual adenopathy in both lower cervical chains. There is no palpable lymphadenopathy elsewhere and no palpable hepatosplenomegaly. The peripheral blood counts are appropriate for third-trimester pregnancy, including a hematocrit of 34%. Blood chemistries, erythrocyte sedimentation rate, and liver function tests are normal. Bilateral bone marrow biopsies found no involvement with disease.

Q What is the most appropriate management of this patient?

A Involved field radiotherapy with abdominal shielding
B Delay antitumor therapy until after the fetus can be safely delivered

C Doxorubicin, bleomycin, vinblastine, and dacarbazine every 3 weeks
D Doxorubicin and vinblastine every 3 weeks plus involved field radiotherapy with abdominal shielding

Question 11

Parents desire that their newborn son be circumcised, but they mention that there is a distant family history of "some kind of hemophilia." Screening coagulation testing on the infant included a prothrombin time of 17.3 seconds and a partial thromboplastin time of 46 seconds. Additional factor activity levels reveal the following:

Factor VIII activity	83%
Factor IX activity	19%
Factor VII activity	45%
Factor XI activity	73%

Q What is the most appropriate interpretation of these results?

A It is not safe to circumcise their infant
B The infant has mild hemophilia B
C The infant must not have received vitamin K injection at birth
D The factor levels are within normal limits
E The infant has probably inherited one abnormal gene for factor VII

Question 12

A 4-year-old boy is about to undergo tonsillectomy and adenoidectomy after experiencing frequent episodes of otitis media and pharyngitis. He has no history of excess bruising, epistaxis, or other bleeding, and family history is negative for known bleeding disorders. Preoperative screening reveals a normal complete blood cell count and platelet count, prothrombin time of 11.9 seconds (international normalized ratio 1.0), and partial thromboplastin time (PTT) of 47 seconds. A PTT 1:1 mix is 42 seconds, and a lupus anticoagulant screen is positive.

Q What is the most appropriate next step in the management of this patient?

A Proceed with surgery
B Perform assays for factors VIII and IX
C Infuse fresh frozen plasma
D Administer intravenous desmopressin
E Administer prednisone

Question 13

A 3.8-kg male infant is delivered vaginally following an uncomplicated 40-week pregnancy. Apgars are 8 and 9 at 1 and 5 minutes. This is the first pregnancy for this mother. On rechecking vital signs at 2 hours, the nurse notices striking ecchymoses on the arms, trunk, and forehead, and scattered petechiae. Additionally, a few small streaks of blood are noted in his stool. On examination, vital signs are normal for age. The infant is well formed and vigorous, with an active suck reflex. There is no mucosal bleeding noted, no adenopathy, and no hepatosplenomegaly. Other than multiple ecchymoses as noted, some of which are palpable, and petechiae most notable on face and scalp, the examination is normal. The following laboratory values are obtained:

Hematocrit	58%
Hemoglobin	19 g/dL
White blood cell count	11,200/μL with normal differential
Platelets	9000/μL
Prothrombin time	16 seconds
International normalized ratio	1.3
Partial thromboplastin time	43 seconds

Peripheral smear is consistent with the calculated platelet count, with both normal-appearing and large platelets present.

Mother herself has been healthy, both prior to and during the pregnancy, and has no history of excess bleeding. Her complete blood cell count is normal with a platelet count of 272,000/μL.

Q Which of the following interventions would be optimal?

A Administer intravenous immunoglobulin 1 g/kg/d for 2 days
B Administer prednisone 2 mg/kg/d divided every 8 hours
C Transfuse I U of irradiated full-volume random-donor platelets
D Transfuse I U of irradiated full-volume maternal platelets
E Transfuse I U of irradiated washed maternal platelets

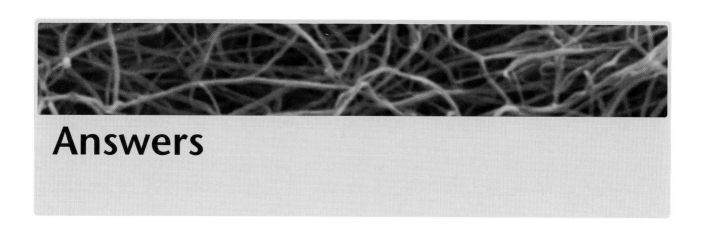

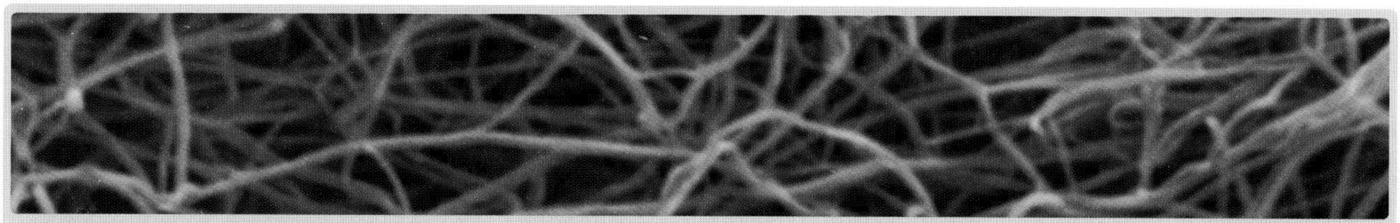

Answers

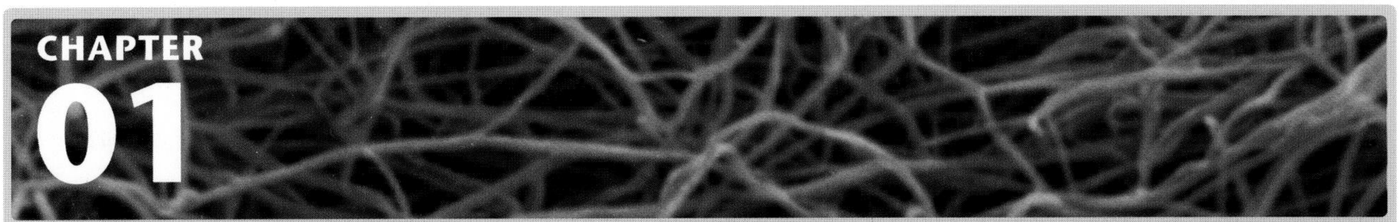

CHAPTER 01

Molecular basis of hematology

Answer to question 1: B

Educational objective

To recognize that gene expression is a complex process regulated by a number of factors including the transcriptional level, the translational level, and the protein level

Critique

All of the therapies mentioned have been used to treat myelodysplastic syndrome; however, only 5-azacytidine acts at the level of gene expression. A significant step in understanding epigenetic gene regulation was the discovery of gene inactivation by hypermethylation of cytosine-phosphate-guanosine (CpG) islands located in the promoter region. Methylation of CpG islands plays a role in the control of gene transcription. Fully methylated sites are associated with suppression of gene expression, whereas hypo- or unmethylated CpG islands are associated with active transcription. Hypermethylation can lead to silencing of important genes including tumor suppressor genes and other genes critical in regulation of the cell cycle and cell differentiation. In myelodysplasia, this mechanism may interfere with regulation of normal hematopoiesis. 5-Azacitidine may also inhibit DNA histone acetylation. Histone acetylation plays a critical role in chromatin structure, which when modified can affect access to genes and represent another regulatory mechanism in silencing genes.

References

Jain PK. Epigenetics: the role of methylation in the mechanism of action of tumor suppressor genes. Ann NY Acad Sci. 2003;983:71.

Kuykendall JR. 5-Azacytidine and decitabine monotherapies of myelodysplastic disorders. Ann Pharmacother. 2005;39:1700.

Answer to question 2: C

Educational objective

To recognize that alternative splicing is a mechanism by which a few genes can code for many proteins

Critique

The total number of human genes is estimated at 30,000—much lower than previous estimates of 80,000 to 140,000 that had been based on extrapolations from gene-rich areas as opposed to a composite of gene-rich and gene-poor areas. The number of human genes is only 2 to 3 times larger than the genomes of *Drosophila* (~13,500 genes) and *Caenorhabditis elegans* (~19,000 genes) and represents only 1–2% of the total DNA in the cell. Many human protein-encoding genes produce more than one protein product by alternative splicing of the primary transcript of the gene. On average, each human open reading frame produces 2 to 3 different proteins. Thus, the human proteome may actually be 10 times larger than that of the *Drosophila* or *C. elegans*.

References

Black D. Protein diversity from alternative splicing: a challenge for bioinformatics and post-genome biology. Cell. 2000;103:367.

Graveley BR. Alternative splicing: increasing diversity in the proteomic world. Trends Genet. 2001;17:100.

Answer to question 3: B

Educational objective

To recognize that a single nucleotide substitution in an exon can have a number of potential consequences including phenotypic silence, change in phenotype, creation of a new stop codon or splice site, and abrogation of a wild-type splice site

Critique

A single nucleotide substitution in an exon may have a number of potential consequences. If the substitution is in the first or second nucleotide of the codon, the consequence may be a change in the coded-for amino acid (missense mutation) or a creation of a stop codon (nonsense mutation). A change in the third nucleotide of the codon is often, but not always, silent (wobble), and there is no change in the coded-for amino acid. A single nucleotide substitution in an exon can also result in the creation of a new splice site or obliteration of the normal splice site at the ends of the exon. Splice site mutations are observed in many hematologic disorders, including hemoglobin E disease where a new splice site is created in the middle of β globin exon 1. Individuals with this mutation make only around 60% of the normal amount of β globin protein because the mutation creates a cryptic splice site such that 40% of the hemoglobin E messenger RNA is shorter by 16 nucleotides and does not give rise to detectable β globin protein. Substitution of one nucleotide for another cannot create a frameshift mutation—this requires insertion or deletion of a number of base pairs that is not a multiple of three and consequently disrupts the triplet reading frame.

References

Chasman D, Adams RM. Predicting the functional consequences of non-synonymous single nucleotide polymorphisms: structure-based assessment of amino acid variation. J Mol Biol. 2001;307:683.

Orkin SH, Kazazian HH, Antonarakis SE, et al. Abnormal RNA processing due to the exon mutation of beta E-globin gene. Nature. 1982;300:768.

Answer to question 4: B

Educational objective

To recognize that restriction fragment length polymorphism analysis can be used to map genetic linkage even if the disease-causing mutation is not known

Critique

In evaluating genetic linkage, often one relies on the use of a polymorphism that is not the disease-causing mutation but is closely linked to the gene of interest. If one is interested in mapping the disease in a family using a linked polymorphism, there must be proof that the polymorphism is found only in individuals who have the disease (ie, a particular polymorphism is in linkage disequilibrium with the disease-causing mutation). In the case presented here, at a minimum, one must show that only the patient's mother carries the polymorphism and that it is passed, along with the mutated factor VIII gene, to the brother. This requires testing both maternal and paternal sides of the patient's family for the polymorphism. Thus, at a minimum, one must document the genotypes of the patient's parents.

Reference

Laird NM, Lange C. Family-based designs in the age of large-scale gene-association studies. Nat Rev Genet. 2006;7:385–94.

Answer to question 5: D

Educational objective

To recognize the limitations of conventional cytogenetics

Critique

The patient presented here has acute myeloid leukemia with no cytogenetic abnormalities detectable by conventional techniques. Conventional cytogenetics has a number of limitations including sensitivity, the requirement for dividing cells, and the inability to detect cryptic translocations or microdeletions. In the case presented here, conventional cytogenetics would be sensitive enough to detect a significant translocation (such as 15;17) or a large deletion if it existed as adequate dividing cells were evaluated (100). Conventional cytogenetics could not, however, detect a microdeletion. This would require the use of more sensitive techniques such as fluorescence *in situ* hybridization or polymerase chain reaction.

References

Casas S, Aventin A, Fuentes F, et al. Genetic diagnosis by comparative genomic hybridization in adult de novo acute myelocytic leukemia. Cancer Genet Cytogenet. 2004;153:16.

Wang N. Methodologies in cancer cytogenetics and molecular cytogenetics. Am J Med Genet. 2002;115:118.

Answer to question 6: A

Educational objective

To recognize that real time polymerase chain reaction (PCR) permits quantitation of specific RNA species and is thus useful in detection of minimal residual disease

Critique

Criteria based on evaluation of marrow and peripheral blood smears as well as conventional cytogenetics have been helpful in determining initial response in many patients with chronic myelogenous leukemia. However, patients in complete cytogenetic remission may still have disease that is undetectable with these methods but sufficient to cause relapse. The degree to which disease can be reduced during therapy appears to relate to outcome; thus, increasingly sensitive methods for detection of minimal residual disease have been developed. Methods such as fluorescence *in situ* hybridization and nested PCR are sensitive, but not quantitative. To this end, there has been a shift from using qualitative PCR assays toward real-time quantitative techniques that allow monitoring of the kinetics of residual disease over time. The method used for the detection of bcr/abl mRNAs involves one probe and one pair of primers that can be used to amplify the two common fusion gene transcripts (e13a2 and e14a2). The exon2/exon3 junction of abl mRNA is used as reference transcript for relative quantification, and the final results are expressed as bcr/abl to abl ratios.

References

Faderl S, Hochhaus A, Hughes T. Monitoring of minimal residual disease in chronic myeloid leukemia. Hematol Oncol Clin North Am. 2004;18:657–70.

Schuler F, Dolken G. Detection and monitoring of minimal residual disease by quantitative real-time PCR. Clin Chim Acta. 2006;363:147.

Answer to question 7: A

Educational objective

To understand the potential uses of microarray chips to identify expression of particular genes in tumor tissue, classify tumors, and predict response to treatment and to understand that expression at the protein level is the most important factor in determining phenotype

Critique

Based on the information provided in this question, the researchers intend to compare expression of particular genes in patients who do and do not respond to chemotherapy. This information has many potential uses, one of which is to predict which patients should receive standard chemotherapy and could be predicted to respond. Expression of particular genes can point to up-regulation of cellular pathways but does not necessarily imply cause. Purity of the cell population is essential for these analyses, so contamination of samples with normal lymph node tissue could significantly alter results. Although DNA microarray analysis can investigate the relative level of messenger RNA expression of 25,000 or more genes, there are other factors that affect cell phenotype. Some expressed genes do not lead to proteins because downstream regulation can occur within the cell. This is why the study of proteomics is important. Changes in gene expression do not always correlate with protein abundance, and in fact the correlation is relatively weak. New techniques that can rapidly identify protein expression patterns are being developed and will likely contribute to therapy in the same way that gene microarrays are contributing now.

References

Freeman WM, Robertson DJ, Vrana KE. Fundamentals of DNA hybridization arrays for gene expression analysis. Biotechniques. 2000;29:1042.

Staudt LM. Molecular diagnosis of the hematologic cancers. N Engl J Med. 2003;348:1777.

Answer to question 8: C

Educational objective

To understand the concept of clonality as it applies to lymphoid malignancies and how Southern blotting can be used to demonstrate clonality

Critique

Southern blotting is a procedure for transferring denatured DNA from an agarose gel to a nitrocellulose filter where it can be hybridized with a complementary labeled nucleic acid probe for detection. If specific κ and λ light-chain probes are used for detection, one would expect to find both κ and λ genes in the germ line configuration in granulocytes (where these genes do not rearrange). If one examines normal lymphocytes from an individual, there will be a mixture of patterns of κ and λ rearrangement, reflecting the polyclonal nature of normal lymphocytes. On the κ and λ blots, this will be reflected as a smear with a discrete band at the germ line position reflecting those cells that have not rearranged the κ or λ gene on one (or in the case of some B cells) both λ chromosomes. When a similar blot is done with chronic lymphocytic leukemia cells, however, all cells will be clonal and thus derived from the same parent cell. Depending on the gene rearrangement in the malignant parent cell from each individual, one could observe the following:

1. κ gene rearranged, 1 κ gene germ line, and 2 λ genes germ line;
2. κ genes rearranged and 2 λ genes germ line;
3. κ genes rearranged, 1 λ gene rearranged, and 1 λ gene germ line;
4. κ genes rearranged and 2 λ genes rearranged.

Reference

Beishuizen A, Verhoeven MA, Mol EJ, et al. Detection of immunoglobulin kappa light-chain gene rearrangement patterns by Southern blot analysis. Leukemia. 1994;8:2228.

Answer to question 9: C

Educational objective

To understand that microRNAs control gene expression by inducing digestion of messenger RNA (mRNA) or suppression of translation

Critique

MicroRNAs are short 20–22-nucleotide RNA molecules that have been shown to regulate the expression of other genes in a variety of eukaryotic systems. MicroRNAs are formed from larger transcripts that fold to produce hairpin structures and serve as substrates for the cytoplasmic dicer. MicroRNAs are then incorporated into an RNA-induced silencing complex to induce translation suppression or degradation, depending of the degree of complementary with the target mRNA. Deletion or amplification of microRNAs has been predicted to promote cancer by interfering with regulation of cell proliferation, apoptosis, angiogenesis, and invasion. A recent analysis of the genomic location of human microRNA genes suggested that 50% of microRNA genes are located in cancer-associated genomic regions or in fragile sites.

References

Calin GA, Ferracin M, Cimmino A, et al. A microRNA signature associated with prognosis and progression in chronic lymphocytic leukemia. N Engl J Med. 200;353:1793.

Sevignani C, Calin GA, Siracusa LD, et al. Mammalian microRNAs: a small world for fine-tuning gene expression. Mamm Genome. 2006;17:189.

Answer to question 10: B

Educational objective

To recognize that mutations in noncoding regions of DNA can also lead to changes in phenotype including splice site mutations, regulatory region mutations, and mutations in microRNAs that control gene expression

Critique

Sequencing of cDNA to identify mutations has limitations in that only the coding sequence of the gene may be identified and sequenced. If mutations occur in introns, abnormal splicing may result. Abnormal splicing may result in retention of intron sequence, splicing out of exon sequence, and/or creation of a new stop codon. If new and early stop codons are created (as in this case), messenger RNA (mRNA) from one allele will be truncated. If the new stop codon occurs early in the coding sequence, the mRNA may be destroyed by a mechanism known as nonsense-mediated decay. In this situation, the truncated mRNA (complementary DNA) may never be detected. Similarly, mutations in regulatory regions of the gene may also affect expression of mRNA although the coding region itself is normal. Recent discovery of microRNA has led to the recognition that gene expression may also be regulated by mechanisms that have nothing to do with the sequence of a gene.

References

Maquat LE, Carmichael GG. Quality control of mRNA function. Cell. 2001;104:173.

Zamore PD, Haley B. Ribo-gnome: the big world of small RNAs. Science. 2005;309:1519.

Answer to question 11: B

Educational objective

To understand the challenges and risks associated with gene therapy for inherited diseases including insertional mutagenesis, risk that a viral vector will regain replication competence or induce an undesirable host immune response, and loss of transduced gene expression over time

Critique

The gene therapy proposed in this case does not involve the use of a retrovirus. Recent data on retroviral gene therapy has suggested that retroviruses have a preferred insertion site in the genome that is within oncogenes. This has resulted in development of leukemia in 2 boys with severe combined immune deficiency who received autologous bone marrow cells treated with retrovirus. Leukemia could develop only if marrow cells were treated with the retrovirus. Because the patient in this case is receiving his own fibroblasts, he would not require immune suppression to prevent rejection. The biggest risk in this trial, which does not use a viral vector for introduction of the new gene, is that the transduced gene will not persist. Thus, even if the therapy is initially successful, there is high likelihood that expression of factor IX will decline over time.

References

Kessler CM. New perspectives in hemophilia treatment. In: Hematology: ASH Education Program Book. Washington DC: American Society of Hematology; 2005:429.

Nathwani AC, Davidoff AM, Linch DC. A review of gene therapy for haematological disorders. Br J Haematol. 2005;128:3.

CHAPTER

02

Cellular basis of hematopoiesis and marrow failure syndromes

Answer to question 1: C

Educational objective

To understand somatic mosaicism in the diagnostic workup of Fanconi anemia

Critique

This patient presents with pancytopenia and a hypoplastic marrow. Because she has a matched sibling donor, bone marrow transplant is a potential therapeutic option. Although the testing for Fanconi anemia on peripheral blood is negative, she carries several physical features suggestive of Fanconi anemia (thumb malformation, short stature, café-au-lait spots). Peripheral blood lymphocytes and other hematopoietic progenitors can undergo spontaneous correction of the Fanconi anemia gene mutation, so testing a bone marrow sample would not be sufficient to rule out mosaicism. Because Fanconi anemia is a recessive disorder, only one copy of a functional Fanconi anemia gene is sufficient. These corrected cells grow better than their Fanconi cell counterparts and may mask the diagnosis. In this case, the diagnosis of Fanconi anemia may be made by testing skin fibroblasts. Reversion to wild type has also been observed in marrow precursor cells. Because Fanconi anemia patients are sensitive to genotoxic agents, they require reduced-intensity conditioning regimens, so it is important to rule out this diagnosis prior to initiating a hematopoietic stem cell transplant. Because testing skin fibroblasts from a punch biopsy requires 1 to 2 months, it is prudent to initiate testing early rather than to wait and follow serial blood counts until the counts fall further.

References

Gregory JJ Jr, Wagner JE, Verlander PC, et al. Somatic mosaicism in Fanconi anemia: evidence of genotypic reversion in lymphohematopoietic stem cells. Proc Natl Acad Sci USA. 2001;98:2532–7.

Shahidi NT, Dokal I, Roberts I, et al. Somatic mosaicism in Fanconi anemia: molecular basis and clinical significance. Eur J Hum Genet. 1997;5:137–48.

Waisfisz Q, Morgan NV, Savino M, et al. Spontaneous functional correction of homozygous Fanconi anaemia alleles reveals novel mechanistic basis for reverse mosaicism. Nat Genet. 1999;22:379–83.

Answer to question 2: A

Educational objective

To recognize that malignancy or myelodysplasia (MDS) may be the presenting clinical manifestation of Fanconi anemia

Critique

Fanconi anemia may present with MDS, leukemia, or solid tumors as the initial clinical manifestation without antecedent bone marrow failure. Clonal cytogenetic abnormalities associated with MDS of leukemia are often complex in patients with Fanconi anemia. A sibling with clinical stigmata suggestive of Fanconi anemia increases concern for this diagnosis. Reduced-intensity conditioning regimens are required to avoid undue toxicity in patients with Fanconi anemia. The clinical manifestations of Fanconi anemia may vary widely even between family members, so if the patient's diepoxybutane test is positive, both her sister and brother should also be tested. The absence of renal abnormalities would not rule out the diagnosis of Fanconi anemia. If her sister also has Fanconi anemia, a search for a matched unrelated donor may be indicated.

References

Giampietro PF, Adler-Brecher B, Verlander PC, et al. The need for more accurate and timely diagnosis in Fanconi anemia.

A report from the international Fanconi Anemia Registry. Pediatr. 1993;91:1116–20.
Giampietro PF, Verlander PC, Davis JG, et al. Diagnosis of Fanconi anemia in patients without congenital malformations: an International Fanconi Anemia Registry study. Am J Med Genet. 1997;68:58–61.

Answer to question 3: A

Educational objective

To understand the potential long-term complications of aplastic anemia

Critique

Treatment with antithymocyte globulin (ATG) and cyclosporin often does not return the blood counts to normal, and macrocytosis may persist. The goal is to achieve blood counts sufficient for transfusion independence and avoid a high risk of infection. Patients treated with ATG and cyclosporin for aplastic anemia remain at risk for subsequent relapse and for the development of clonal marrow disease such as myelodysplasia or acute myelogenic leukemia. Thus, a bone marrow aspirate and biopsy with cytogenetics would be an appropriate diagnostic test. Although hypothyroidism is associated with macrocytic anemia, it is unlikely to cause pancytopenia. Relapse may respond to reinstitution of cyclosporin alone or may require a second round of ATG and cyclosporin.

References

Frickhofen N, Gluckman E, Tichelli A. Late clonal diseases of treated aplastic anemia. Semin Hematol. 2000;37:91–101.
Schrezenmeier H, Marin P, Raghavachar A, et al. Relapse of aplastic anaemia after immunosuppressive treatment: a report from the European Bone Marrow Transplantation Group SAA Working Party. Br J Haematol. 1993;85:371–7.

Answer to question 4: A

Educational objective

To consider myelodysplasia (MDS) in the diagnostic workup for aplastic anemia

Critique

The differential diagnosis of pancytopenia with a hypocellular marrow includes hypoplastic MDS. Marrow cytogenetics is a useful test in the identification of clonal marrow disease. Although pancytopenia may be associated with severe B_{12} or folate deficiency, the absence of megaloblastic features makes this diagnosis less likely. Hypothyroidism may be associated with macrocytic anemia, but it is not typically associated with pancytopenia.

Reference

Marsh JC, Ball SE, Darbyshire P, et al. Guidelines for the diagnosis and management of acquired aplastic anaemia. Br J Haematol. 2003;123:782–801.

Answer to question 5: A

Educational objective

To recognize posthepatitis aplastic anemia

Critique

Posthepatitis aplastic anemia typically occurs several weeks after the resolution of the hepatitis. The hepatitis viral testing is typically negative for hepatitis A, B, and C. Aplastic anemia associated with cytomegalovirus is typically seen in patients with immunocompromise. Parvovirus is typically associated with pure red cell aplasia rather than aplastic anemia. A liver biopsy is not helpful in the initial diagnostic workup of pancytopenia in this patient.

Reference

Brown KE, Tisdale J, Barrett AJ, et al. Hepatitis-associated aplastic anemia. New Engl J Med. 1997;336:1059–64.

Answer to question 6: A

Educational objective

To understand the treatment of acquired idiopathic aplastic anemia

Critique

Untreated idiopathic severe aplastic anemia carries a dismal prognosis, and spontaneous remission is uncommon. Treatment options include bone marrow transplant and immunosuppressive therapy with antithymocyte globulin (ATG) and cyclosporin (CYA). The decision between these 2 treatment modalities depends largely on the age and general health of the patient. A matched sibling bone marrow transplant carries a relatively low up-front risk of morbidity and mortality for a young patient and constitutes curative treatment. Treatment with ATG and CYA is not generally curative, and the patient remains at risk for relapse or late clonal disease indefinitely. In contrast, significantly higher morbidity and mortality is associated with bone marrow transplants performed in older patients (>40 or 50 years of age), and the potential life span over which the older patient remains at risk for relapse or clonal disease following ATG/CYA is shorter than that of a child. Granulocyte colony-stimulating factor alone has not been shown to improve overall survival for severe aplastic anemia.

References

Bacigalupo A, Brand R, Oneto R, et al. Treatment of acquired severe aplastic anemia: bone marrow transplantation compared with immunosuppressive therapy – the European Group for Blood and Marrow Transplantation experience. Semin Hematol. 2000;37:69–80.

Brodsky RA, Jones RJ. Aplastic anaemia. Lancet. 2005;365: 1647–56

Answer to question 7: D

Educational objective

To recognize congenital amegakaryocytic thrombocytopenia (CAMT) as a cause for bone marrow failure (aplastic anemia) in children and to understand its underlying pathogenesis

Critique

CAMT is a rare autosomal recessive disorder characterized by absent or a markedly reduced number of megakaryocytes in the bone marrow. These patients typically present with severe isolated thrombocytopenia. Other blood counts are initially within the normal range. However, in a high percentage of patients, pancytopenia develops over the course of years with gradual reduction in trilineage marrow cellularity, often progressing to full aplastic anemia. Recently, the molecular pathogenesis of this disorder was identified as inactivating mutations in the receptor (c-*mpl*) for thrombopoietin (TPO), the major cytokine regulator of megakaryopoiesis and thrombopoiesis. The gradual bone marrow failure seen in these patients likely reflects the recently recognized role of TPO/c-*mpl* signaling in the maintenance/expansion of multipotent hematopoietic progenitor and stem cells. Indeed, $CD34^+$ cells from CAMT patients show significantly lower myeloid, erythroid, and megakaryocytic colony-forming activity in semisolid, collagen-based media (in the presence of stem cell factor, TPO, interleukin 3 [IL-3], IL-6, and erythropoietin) compared with healthy controls, and this worsens during the course of the bone marrow failure. Although one might also expect inactivating mutations in TPO to result in a subset of CAMT patients, to date none have been reported. Bone marrow transplantation is the only currently known curative treatment of CAMT.

Mutations or deletions involving the Wiskott–Aldrich gene (WAS) cause a thrombocytopenia with very small platelets (not seen in this patient) and typically do not result in complete bone marrow failure. Mutations in *GATA-1* typically cause X-linked macrothrombocytopenia and often are accompanied by dysplastic features of the megakaryocytes, erythroid lineage, and/or β thalassemia. They are also not known to progress to aplastic anemia. Finally, *MYH9* mutations typically cause macrothrombocytopenia, such as in the May–Hegglin anomaly, and do not progress to bone marrow failure.

References

Ballmaier M, Germeshausen M, Krukemeier S, et al. Thrombopoietin is essential for the maintenance of normal hematopoiesis in humans: development of aplastic anemia in patients with congenital amegakaryocytic thrombocytopenia. Ann NY Acad Sci. 2003;996:17–25.

Gandhi MJ, Pendergrass TW, Cummings CC, et al. Congenital amegakaryocytic thrombocytopenia in three siblings: molecular analysis of atypical clinical presentation. Exp Hematol. 2005;33:1215–21.

Kaushansky K. Thrombopoietin and the hematopoietic stem cell. Ann NY Acad Sci. 2005;1044:139–41.

Answer to question 8: B

Educational objective

To recognize hematopoietic stem cell transplantation as curative therapy for congenital amegakaryocytic thrombocytopenia (CAMT)

Critique

This patient best fits the clinical description of CAMT. This is a genetic deficiency of the thrombopoietin receptor. In addition to having severe thrombocytopenia, these patients are at high risk for developing full bone marrow failure, typically over the course of several years. This is likely due to a requirement of thrombopoietin (TPO) signaling to maintain or expand multipotent progenitors and/or hematopoietic stem cells. Allogeneic stem cell transplant has been shown to be curative for CAMT and is the treatment of choice if a suitable donor is available. Immunosuppressive therapy with corticosteroids is not effective. Intravenous immunoglobulin (IVIg) is helpful for immune thrombocytopenic purpura (ITP), but the pancytopenia and paucity of megakaryocytes in the bone marrow argue against this diagnosis. Use of IVIg in CAMT is not effective. Treatment with recombinant TPO would not be expected to help because these patients have a deficiency in the receptor and typically already have elevated TPO levels. In addition, use of a pegylated recombinant form of TPO has been linked to the development of inhibitory antibodies against endogenous TPO. Desmopressin (DDAVP) has been shown to enhance the hemostatic function of platelets in certain conditions, such as uremia, but does not have a role in the management of CAMT.

References

Al-Ahmari A, Ayas M, Al-Jefri A, et al. Allogeneic stem cell transplantation for patients with congenital amegakaryocytic thrombocytopenia (CAT). Bone Marrow Transplant. 2004;33:829–31.

Lackner A, Basu O, Bierings M, et al. Haematopoietic stem cell transplantation for amegakaryocytic thrombocytopenia. Br J Haematol. 2000;109:773–5.

Answer to question 9: A

Educational objective

To recognize Diamond-Blackfan anemia (DBA) as a cause of bone marrow failure in infancy and to be aware of diagnostic workup

Critique

The isolated severe anemia and reticulocytopenia present in this infant suggest a selective erythroid production defect. The differential diagnosis in this age group includes DBA, a bone marrow failure syndrome. The median age of diagnosis of DBA is 2–3 months. This contrasts with transient erythroblastopenia of childhood (TEC), a disorder of temporary erythroid hypoplasia, typically occurring in older children (median age 23 months). Although the anemia of DBA can be normocytic, it is more commonly macrocytic. Adenosine deaminase (ADA), a critical enzyme in the purine salvage pathway, is often elevated in patients with DBA. Although elevated ADA is not specific to DBA, it is typically not found in TEC and can be helpful in distinguishing acute DBA from TEC. Over a third of patients with DBA have been reported to have physical abnormalities including triphalangeal thumbs, micrognathia, cleft lip or palate, short stature, and genitourinary abnormalities. Mutations in the gene encoding the ribosomal protein RPS19 have been found in ~25% of cases with DBA. Additional genetic loci appear involved, including a region mapping to 8p23.2–p22.

Iron studies would be less helpful in this patient because iron deficiency is rare in this age group and would not be expected to produce a macrocytic anemia. Coombs, osmotic fragility testing, and Heinz body preparation would be more helpful in anemias associated with increased reticulocytosis, suggesting a destructive process.

References

Federman N, Sakamoto KM. The genetic basis of bone marrow failure syndromes in children. Mol Gen Metab. 2005;86:100–9.

Glader BE, Backer K. Elevated red cell adenosine deaminase activity: a marker of disordered erythropoiesis in Diamond-Blackfan anaemia and other haematologic diseases. Br J Haematol. 1988;68:165.

Lackner A, Basu O, Bierings M, et al. Haematopoietic stem cell transplantation for amegakaryocytic thrombocytopenia. Br J Haematol. 2000;109:773–5.

Answer to question 10: C

Educational objective

To understand treatment options for patients with Diamond-Blackfan anemia

Critique

Overall, about 50% of patients with DBA respond to corticosteroid treatment. Recommended initial dosing is with prednisone at 2 mg/kg/d. This is continued until an adequate hemoglobin level is reached and then slowly tapered as tolerated to reduce the long-term side effects of corticosteroid therapy. A variety of responses have been reported ranging from (i) rapid response and remission, (ii) eventual steroid independence, (iii) requirement for large daily doses and relapse with lowered doses, and (iv) steroid dependence with later failure to respond to the same or higher doses. For very young children, consideration may be given to delaying corticosteroid therapy (while supporting with red blood cell transfusions) until the child is 1–2 years of age to avoid potential adverse effects of corticosteroids during early development. Other therapies have been reported to produce responses in a small number of patients and include androgens and 6-mercaptopurine. Spontaneous remission has been reported in as many as 15–20% of patients. Bone marrow transplantation can be curative, but the risks and benefits must be weighed for each patient.

Levels of erythropoietin (Epo), folate, and vitamin B_{12} are often elevated in patients with DBA. Further supplementation with Epo, folate, or vitamin B_{12} does not play a role in treatment of DBA. Intravenous immunoglobulin has been shown to be ineffective for treatment of DBA. Antithymocyte globulin and cyclosporine are often used for patients with aplastic anemia who do not have an HLA-matched sibling bone marrow donor. Transient responses using antilymphocyte globulin or cyclosporine, in combination, with other medications have been reported, but this is not considered first-line therapy.

References

Allen DM, Diamond LK. Congenital (erythroid) hypoplastic anemia. Am J Dis Child. 1961;102:416.

Lipton JM, Atsidaftos E, Zyskind I, et al. Improving clinical care and elucidating the pathophysiology of Diamond Blackfan anemia: an update from the Diamond Blackfan Anemia Registry. Pediatr Blood Cancer. 2005.

Ohga S, Mugishima H, Ohara A, et al. Aplastic Anemia Committee, Japanese Society of Pediatric Hematology. Int J Hematol. 2004;79:22–30.

Answer to question 11: E

Educational objective

To recognize congenital dyserythropoietic anemia (CDA) in the differential diagnosis of anemia in adolescents and adults and to understand the clinical pathologic findings

Critique

The clinical vignette describes a patient with CDA type II. This is also known as HEMPAS (for *h*ereditary *e*rythroblastic *m*ultinuclearity with a *p*ositive *a*cidified *s*erum test). The characteristic findings in this disorder are a high proportion (10–40%) of bi- and multinucleated erythroblasts on bone marrow examination and red cell lysis after incubating with acidified normal donor serum (but not the patient's own serum). The internuclear chromatin bridges and large number of giant multinucleated erythroblasts seen in CDA types I and III, respectively, are not present. The anemia in patients with CDA type II is variable, and patients can present anywhere from infancy to adulthood. Red cell life span is shorter than normal, and some patients with CDA type II benefit from splenectomy.

The red blood cell morphology and normal mean corpuscular hemoglobin concentration are not consistent with a diagnosis of hereditary spherocytosis. Therefore, osmotic fragility testing would not be helpful. Direct antiglobulin test is not the most appropriate next diagnostic test because the peripheral blood cell and bone marrow morphology are not consistent with an autoimmune hemolytic anemia. Viral hepatitis is not expected to produce the hematologic abnormalities described, and therefore serologic testing is not indicated at this time. The slightly elevated mean corpuscular volume, hyperbilirubinemia, and bone marrow morphology are not consistent with iron deficiency. Therefore, determination of iron saturation is not the next best diagnostic step.

References

Fokuda MN. Congenital dyserythropoietic anemia type II (HEMPAS) and its molecular basis. Baillieres Clin Haematol. 1993;6:493.

Heimpel H. Congenital dyserythropoietic anemias: epidemiology, clinical significance, and progress in understanding their pathogenesis. Ann Hematol. 2004;83:613–21.

Answer to question 12: B

Educational objective

To recognize dyskeratosis congenita in the differential diagnosis of graft-versus-host disease (GVHD)

Critique

This patient has a family history suggestive of an inherited marrow failure syndrome. Dyskeratosis congenita (DC) is associated with a reticular skin rash, dystrophic nails, and leukoplakia, but these symptoms develop over time with increasing age. Additional features variably associated with dyskeratosis congenita include dry eyes and pulmonary fibrosis. The X-linked recessive form of DC is associated with mutations in *DKC1*, and the autosomal dominant form of DC is associated with *TERC* mutations. The absence of gene mutations does not rule out the diagnosis of DC because there are additional forms of DC for which gene mutations have not yet been identified. However, the most appropriate next step in the management of this case is to send a buccal swab for *DKC1* and *TERC* sequencing.

Sending a blood sample for genetic analysis is incorrect because this patient has undergone a bone marrow transplant, and the results would reflect the donor's genetics. The 10-year delay between his bone marrow transplant and the onset of his symptoms is not typical for GVHD, and therefore treatment with increased immunosuppression is not the next best step in the patient's management. The family history of childhood marrow failure and this constellation of clinical findings are more suspicious for an inherited marrow failure syndrome than a rheumatologic disorder. Therefore, referral to a rheumatologist is not the best choice for the next step in this patient's management.

References

Ivker RA, Woosley J, Resnick SD. Dyskeratosis congenita or chronic graft-versus-host disease? A diagnostic dilemma in a child eight years after bone marrow transplantation for aplastic anemia. Pediatr Dermatol. 1993;10:362–5.

Ling NS, Fenske NA, Julius RL, et al. Dyskeratosis congenita in a girl simulating chronic graft-versus-host disease. Arch Dermatol. 1985;121:1424–8.

CHAPTER 03

Hematopoietic growth factors

Answer to question 1: D

Educational objective

To understand the time frame and chance of response to an erythroid growth factor in patients with myelodysplasia

Critique

This patient has angina, likely exacerbated by his severe anemia. Transfusion of 2 U of packed red blood cells will promptly increase his hematocrit. Patients with myelodysplasia have an approximately 20% chance of responding to an erythroid growth factor with a 1–2 g/dL increase in the hemoglobin, but response is usually seen during the second month of therapy. The use of an erythroid growth factor plus filgrastim increases the chance of response to approximately 40%, but again the time frame is within 4–8 weeks. Prednisone would not be appropriate therapy for this patient.

Reference

Kasper C, Zahner J, Sayer HG. Recombinant human erythropoietin in combined treatment with granulocyte- or granulocyte-macrophage colony-stimulating factor in patients with myelodysplastic syndromes. J Cancer Res Clin Oncol. 2002;128:499–502.

Answer to question 2: B

Educational objective

To understand the differential diagnosis of thrombocytopenia in human immunodeficiency virus (HIV)-positive patients

Critique

This patient has a slightly reduced white blood cell count, mild anemia, and profound thrombocytopenia. Although pancytopenia may be due to HIV-induced suppression, the striking thrombocytopenia is more likely due to peripheral destruction of platelets. Idiopathic thrombocytopenic purpura (ITP) is very common in patients with HIV. An increase in megakaryocytes is likely to be found on marrow examination. Hemolytic uremic syndrome usually presents with more severe anemia in addition to renal insufficiency. No schistocytes are noted on smear. Folic acid deficiency more commonly presents with macrocytic anemia. Although medications used for HIV-positive patients have a plethora of side effects, they more commonly cause anemia than thrombocytopenia.

Initiation of highly active antiretroviral therapy is an effective way to increase the platelet count in patients with HIV-associated ITP. The platelet count usually improves within 1 to 2 months. Transfused platelets have a short survival in ITP and would not be indicated in this nonbleeding patient. Because other therapeutic interventions are often successful for HIV-associated ITP, the option of splenectomy would be reserved for later in this patient's clinical course. Fresh frozen plasma and plasma exchange would not be effective for this patient.

Reference

Scaradavou A. HIV-related thrombocytopenia. Blood Rev. 2002;16:73–6.

Answer to question 3: D

Educational objective

To understand the clinical effects of cytokines in peripheral blood stem cell transplantation

Critique

Following chemotherapy, filgrastim effectively mobilizes increased numbers of $CD34^+$ peripheral blood progenitor cells and/or stem cells, which leads to more rapid engraftment in both autologous and allogeneic transplantation. Filgrastim administered posttransplant is not necessary when peripheral blood stem cells (PBSCs) are used in the transplant procedure. Side effects attributable to filgrastim are usually mild and manageable with conventional analgesics but occur in up to 30% of patients. No definite evidence of filgrastim-associated leukemia has been noted among normal donors. No increased incidence of chronic graft-versus-host disease (GVHD) has been seen with filgrastim-mobilized allografts compared with bone marrow. Although granulocyte recovery is more rapid with mobilized PBSCs, overall mortality is not improved. The duration of treatment of chronic GVHD among patients who received PBSCs compared with bone marrow appears to be longer. Although pegylated filgrastim is not routinely used for stem cell mobilization, it has been shown in reports to have the same mobilization effect as filgrastim.

References

Bensinger WI, Martin PJ, Storer B, et al. Transplantation of bone marrow as compared with peripheral-blood cells from HLA-identical relatives in patients with hematologic cancers. N Engl J Med. 2001;344:175–81.

Flowers ME, Parker PM, Johnston LJ, et al. Comparison of chronic graft-versus-host disease after transplantation of peripheral blood stem cells versus bone marrow in allogeneic recipients: long-term follow-up of a randomized trial. Blood. 2002;100:415–9.

Ho VT, Mirza NQ, Junco Dd D, et al. The effect of hematopoietic growth factors on the risk of graft-vs-host disease after allogeneic hematopoietic stem cell transplantation: a meta-analysis. Bone Marrow Transplant. 2003;32:771–5.

Steidl U, Fenk R, Bruns I, et al. Successful transplantation of peripheral blood stem cells mobilized by chemotherapy and a single dose of pegylated G-CSF in patients with multiple myeloma. Bone Marrow Transplant. 2005;35:33–6.

Answer to question 4: E

Educational objective

To understand the role of filgrastim in the treatment of serious infections in nonneutropenic patients

Critique

Filgrastim is not indicated for the treatment of nonneutropenic fever or infection, as shown by several randomized controlled trials. In a systematic review, use of filgrastim appeared to be safe, with no increase in the incidence of total serious adverse events or organ dysfunction. However, the use of filgrastim was not associated with improved 28-day mortality. Epoetin alfa will have little effect on improving the patient's hematocrit in the short term. For rare patients who refuse blood products for religious or other reasons, beginning epoetin alfa early in the course of treatments may be useful. Her thrombocytopenia is likely related to sepsis; platelet transfusions in the absence of severe thrombocytopenia and bleeding are not indicated. Granulocyte transfusions are indicated for the rare situation where patients with neutropenia and persistent culture-positive infection fail to clear the infection despite appropriate antibiotics (adequate drug levels/appropriate sensitivities to organisms in question).

References

Cheng AC, Stephens DP, Currie BJ. Granulocyte-colony stimulating factor (G-CSF) as an adjunct to antibiotics in the treatment of pneumonia in adults. Cochrane Database Syst Rev. 2003;4:CD004400.

Hartmann P, Lammertink J, Mansmann G, et al. A randomized, placebo-controlled study of the use of filgrastim in non neutropenic patients with nosocomial pneumonia. Eur J Med Res. 2005;10:29–35.

Nelson S, Heyder AM, Stone J, et al. A randomized controlled trial of filgrastim for the treatment of hospitalized patients with multilobar pneumonia. J Infect Dis. 2000;182:970–3.

Answer to question 5: B

Educational objective

To recognize a rare, serious complication of filgrastim

Critique

The most likely diagnosis is splenic rupture, a rare complication of filgrastim described in both normal donors and patients with hematologic malignancies. Filgrastim has been shown to increase splenic size frequently in normal stem cell donors. In almost all cases, the enlargement has been asymptomatic and with no clinical consequences. The rapid decline in the donor's hematocrit without evidence for gastrointestinal bleeding or hemolysis supports a diagnosis of intraabdominal blood loss. Infectious causes for his abdominal pain would be less likely. Filgrastim occasionally produces mild to moderate bone pain. Peptic ulcer disease does not result from filgrastim therapy. Appendicitis is a possibility but unlikely in the absence of fever and prior gastrointestinal symptoms. A computed tomographic scan would confirm the diagnosis.

References

Becker PS, Wagle M, Matous S, et al. Spontaneous splenic rupture following administration of granulocyte colony-stimulating factor (G-CSF): occurrence in an allogeneic donor of peripheral blood stem cells. Biol Blood Marrow Transplant. 1997;3:45–9.

Stroncek D, Shawker T, Follmann D, et al. G-CSF-induced spleen size changes in peripheral blood progenitor cell donors. Transfusion. 2003;43:609–13.

Answer to question 6: B

Educational objective

To understand issues related to regimen selection, dose modification, and cytokine support for the treatment of patients with various malignant diseases

Critique

Filgrastim used preventatively is indicated when the risk of febrile neutropenia is 20% or greater according to National Comprehensive Cancer Network guidelines. Filgrastim shortens the absolute period of neutropenia, reduces the incidence of febrile neutropenia, and reduces hospital days without improvement in mortality and disease-free survival. Although a number of randomized controlled trials are testing the efficacy of dose escalation or dose density in a variety of solid tumors, there is no evidence to date that these approaches have led to improved survival. When 2 or more chemotherapy regimens have equal antitumor effects and survival rates for a particular malignancy/stage of disease, a regimen that does not rely on filgrastim for support (less myelotoxic) is preferred (ie, rituximab, cyclophosphamide, doxorubicin, vincristine, and prednisone [R-CHOP] over etoposide, methylprednisolone, cytarabine, and cisplatin [ESHAP] as initial therapy). Dose reduction as opposed to maintaining dose is favored initially after patients develop fever and neutropenia. Although the patient has extensive disease, his time in the intensive care unit with sepsis would suggest that this complication be avoided with future treatments. Dose reduction with his second cycle would be appropriate, and, if tolerated well, one could cautiously consider increasing his dose again if clearing lymphoma from his marrow increased his marrow reserve. Although R-CHOP has a 10–20% chance of fever and neutropenia, other risk factors increase the likelihood of this complication including age, lactate dehydrogenase levels, diagnosis of lymphoma, marrow involvement, prior radiation to bone marrow sites, diabetes, and initially low white blood cell counts.

References

Berghmans T, Paesmans M, Lafitte JJ, et al. Role of granulocyte and granulocyte-macrophage colony-stimulating factors in the treatment of small-cell lung cancer: a systematic review of the literature with methodological assessment and meta-analysis. Lung Cancer. 2002;37:115–23.

Clark OA, Lyman G, Castro AA, et al. Colony stimulating factors for chemotherapy induced febrile neutropenia. Cochrane Database Syst Rev. 2003;3:CD003039.

Savarese D, Hsieh C, Stewart FM. Clinical impact of chemotherapy dose escalation. J Clin Oncol. 1997;158:2981–95.

Answer to question 7: C

Educational objective

To understand the potential advantages of pegfilgrastim compared to filgrastim as adjuncts to myelosuppressive chemotherapy

Critique

The results from several randomized double-blind phase III clinical trials in patients with breast cancer and in patients with lymphoma treated with myelosuppressive chemotherapy showed that a single dose of pegfilgrastim provides neutrophil support comparable with that provided by an average of 11 days of filgrastim. These studies have shown also that the safety profiles of both cytokines are comparable. Pegfilgrastim given once per cycle may improve patient quality of life because it is easier for patients to receive and results in better compliance with treatment because no doses are missed. The total cost per course is similar between pegfilgrastim and filgrastim. CAE (cytoxan, adriamycin, etoposide) may not be the best regimen for this patient. Earlier consideration of alternative, less myelotoxic, but equally efficacious regimens may have been a more optimal strategy.

References

Bohlius J, Reiser M, Schwarzer G, et al. Impact of granulocyte colony-stimulating factor (CSF) and granulocyte-macrophage CSF in patients with malignant lymphoma: a systematic review. Br J Haematol. 2003;122:413–23.

Holmes FA, O'Shaughnessy JA, et al. Blinded, randomized, multicenter study to evaluate single administration pegfilgrastim once per cycle versus daily filgrastim as an adjunct to chemotherapy in patients with high risk stage II or stage III/IV breast cancer. J Clin Oncol. 2002;20:727–31.

Vose JM, Crump H, et al. Randomized, multicenter, open-label study of pegfilgrastim compared with daily filgrastim after chemotherapy for lymphoma. J Clin Oncol. 2003;21:514–9.

Answer to question 8: A

Educational objective

To recognize that lack or loss of response to erythropoietin could be the result of concomitant iron deficiency

Critique

The anemia in the patient is multifactorial and likely the result of chemotherapy and iron deficiency. Although treatment with recombinant erythropoietin (rh-Epo) is a reasonable approach for the treatment of chemotherapy-induced anemia, the patient is less likely to respond if she is iron deficient. Similarly, dose escalation of rh-Epo, although recommended for patients who do not respond after 4 weeks of therapy with rh-Epo (or after 6 weeks if treating with darbepoetin alfa), will not result in a measurable improvement in the hemoglobin for the reasons mentioned, namely, iron deficiency. By measuring iron studies and ferritin, the diagnosis could be established, at which time, searching for a gastrointestinal source of blood loss is indicated. Replenishing her iron stores is likely to result in normalization of her hemoglobin. There is no need to perform a bone marrow biopsy because her physical examination would suggest that she is responding to chemotherapy.

Reference

Rizzo JD, et al. Use of epoetin in patients with cancer: evidence-based clinical practice guidelines of the American Society of Clinical Oncology and the American Society of Hematology. J Clin Oncol. 2002;20:4083–107.

Answer to question 9: B

Educational objective

To recognize chemotherapy-induced anemia and when to initiate therapy

Critique

Anemia resulting from cancer therapy is an important clinical problem, for which therapeutic options are available. Newer and more intense chemotherapeutic combinations have made this type of anemia more prevalent. The use of recombinant human erythropoietin is recommended for patients with chemotherapy-associated anemia and a hemoglobin concentration that has declined to a level <10 g/dL. Red blood cell transfusion is also an option, depending on the severity of anemia or clinical circumstances. Dose reduction is not recommended because the patient seems to tolerate chemotherapy well with the exception of anemia that can be corrected with the use of epoetin.

There is no need to perform a bone marrow biopsy because the platelets and the white cell count are both normal. Finally, there is no clinical utility to measuring erythropoietin level. It should be noted, however, that patients who develop anemia secondary to chemotherapy will have a blunted erythropoietin response relative to their degree of anemia. This in part would explain the success of erythropoiesis-stimulating agents in correcting this type of anemia.

Reference

Rizzo JD, et al. Use of epoetin in patients with cancer: evidence-based clinical practice guidelines of the American Society of Clinical Oncology and the American Society of Hematology. J Clin Oncol. 2002;20:4083–107.

Answer to question 10: A

Educational objective

To recognize the need for prophylactic use of myeloid growth factors in elderly patients receiving chemotherapy with a curative intent

Critique

Prophylactic use of myeloid growth factors is defined as the administration of a growth factor to prevent febrile neutropenia (FN). "Primary prophylaxis" denotes their use following the first cycle of chemotherapy prior to any occurrence of FN. The term "secondary prophylaxis" refers to the use of growth factors to prevent a subsequent episode of FN in a patient who had already experienced FN in a previous cycle.

A 2006 update of recommendations for the use of myeloid growth factors is in favor of primary prophylaxis with colony-stimulating factors for patients with diffuse aggressive lymphoma who are ≥65 years old and treated with curative intent (with cyclophosphamide, doxorubicin, vincristine, and prednisone [CHOP] or more aggressive regimens) to reduce the incidence of febrile neutropenia and infections. Therefore, given the patient's age and existing cytopenias, which are likely the result of bone marrow infiltration with malignant lymphoma, administration of full-dose rituximab-CHOP (R-CHOP) in combination with either filgrastim or pegfilgrastim is recommended.

References

National Comprehensive Cancer Network. Practice Guidelines in Oncology. Vol. 1. Jenkintown, PA: NCCN; 2006.

Smith TJ, et al. Update of recommendation for the use of white blood cell growth factors: an evidence-based clinical practice guideline. J Clin Oncol. 2006;24:3187–205.

Answer to question 11: A

Educational objective

To recognize recombinant human erythropoietin as a therapeutic modality in patients with myelodysplasia and that the efficacy of this agent highly depends on baseline (or endogenous) erythropoietin level

Critique

The patient has myelodysplastic syndrome (refractory anemia) with an International Prognostic Scoring System (IPSS) risk categorization of 0. Given his low erythropoietin level for his level of anemia and low transfusion requirements (defined as <2 U every 4 weeks), his chances of responding to recombinant human erythropoietin are high, approximating 74%.

He is not likely to benefit from chelation therapy, given his current ferritin level, nor is he a candidate for immediate allogeneic transplantation, given his IPSS score.

Reference

Hellstrom-Lindberg E, Negrin R, Stein R, et al. Erythroid response to treatment with G-SCF plus erythropoietin for the anaemia of patients with myelodysplastic syndromes: proposal for a predictive model. Br J Haematol. 1997;99:344–51.

CHAPTER

04

Iron metabolism, iron overload, and the porphyrias

Answer to question 1: D

Educational objective

To identify transfusional iron overload as an indication for chelation therapy with deferasirox

Critique

Iron overload affects those individuals with chronic severe anemia who have received repeated red cell transfusions. Each unit of red cells contains 200–250 mg of iron, which is retained by the reticuloendothelial system as the red cells senesce, and no physiologic mechanism exists for the excretion of iron. Iron accumulation is therefore inevitable, and patients develop marked elevations in transferrin saturations and ferritin levels. Chelation therapy with oral deferasirox has been shown to lower hepatic iron stores and ferritin values in transfusional iron overload. Patients who are dependent on transfusions for their anemia cannot be treated with phlebotomy. The *HFE* genotype of the patient would not impact her plan of care at this time. Magnetic resonance imaging is not yet standard to quantify hepatic iron levels.

References

Greenberg PL. Myelodysplastic syndromes: iron overload consequences and current chelating therapies. J Natl Compr Canc Netw. 2006;4:91–6.

Tefferi A. Iron chelation for myelodysplastic syndrome: if and when. Mayo Clin Proc. 2006;81:197–8.

Answer to question 2: E

Educational objective

To understand indications and complications of chelation therapy for transfusional iron overload

Critique

The management of secondary causes of hemochromatosis remains difficult. Anemia often exists, and red cell transfusion may be required, making phlebotomy impractical. Deferoxamine is an effective but inconvenient and costly iron chelating agent used extensively in these conditions. Deferoxamine is administered by nightly continuous subcutaneous infusion (40 mg/kg) over an 8–12-hour period. Higher doses are required if end-organ complications already exist. Local skin complications of deferoxamine are frequent and include pain, swelling, and pruritis at the injection site. These complications can be minimized by rotation of injection sites and addition of hydrocortisone, antihistamines, or local measures. Ocular and auditory complications secondary to deferoxamine mandate annual audiologic and ophthalmologic evaluation.

Recently, deferasirox became the first oral iron chelator to receive the Food and Drug Administration's approval for treatment of transfusion-related iron overload in patients older than 2 years. In dosing, 20–30 mg/kg of deferasirox daily is at least as effective as deferoxamine in reducing liver iron concentrations and serum ferritin levels. The most frequent side effects included nausea, vomiting, diarrhea, abdominal pain, skin rash, and increases in serum creatinine. About one third of deferasirox-treated patients experienced dose-dependent increases in serum creatinine, and it is recommended that serum creatinine be assessed before initiating therapy and monitored monthly thereafter to determine if dose modification or discontinuation is necessary. Liver function should be monitored monthly, and if there is an unexplained, persistent, or progressive increase in serum transaminase levels, deferasirox should be interrupted or discontinued. As with deferoxamine, cases of ocular and auditory disturbances have been reported.

References

Hershko C. Treating iron overload: the state of the art. Semin Hematol. 2005;2:S2–4.

Neufeld EJ. Oral chelators deferasirox and deferiprone for transfusional iron overload in thalassemia major: new data, new questions. Blood. 2006;107:3436–41.

Answer to question 3: A

Educational objective

To recognize the clinical features of infectious agents to which iron-overloaded patients are susceptible

Critique

Patients with iron overload are at increased susceptibility to a number of bacterial organisms that use iron as a necessary growth factor. Additionally, iron overload in macrophages can decrease phagocytosis. Infectious agents to which iron-overloaded patients are more susceptible include *Vibrio vulnificus*, *Yersinia enterocolitica*, *Rhizopus oryzae* (the agent of mucormycosis), and *Clostridium perfringens*. Infection with *Vibrio vulnificus* produces a septicemia characterized by hypotension and the presence of bullous skin lesions. Many patients succumb to this infection, and long hospital stays and prolonged debilitation are common in survivors.

Reference

Kraffert CA, Hogan DL. Vibrio vulnificus infection and iron overload. J Am Acad Dermatol. 1992:26:140.

Answer to question 4: C

Educational objective

To understand the role of hepcidin in the anemia of inflammation

Critique

Hepcidin is a 25 amino acid polypeptide with antibacterial properties that has been shown to be critical in regulating iron balance. Hepcidin levels are up-regulated by several cytokines, including interleukin 6 (IL-6), IL-1, and tumor necrosis factor. Hepcidin levels fall in the presence of anemia and iron deficiency. Hepcidin will bind to ferroportin and lead to its internalization and degradation. Ferroportin is responsible for egress of iron out of hepatocytes and macrophages as well as absorption of iron from the gut enterocyte into the plasma. In this patient with several active infections, hepcidin levels should be markedly elevated, and gut iron absorption should decrease, as should mobilization of iron stores in hepatocytes and macrophages.

References

Fleming RE, Bacon BR. Orchestration of iron homeostasis. N Engl J Med. 2005;352:1741–4.

Haurani FL. Hepcidin and the anemia of chronic disease. Ann Clin Lab Sci. 2006;36:3–6.

Weiss G, Goodnough LT. Anemia of chronic disease. N Engl J Med. 2005;352:1011–23.

Answer to question 5: C

Educational objective

To understand optimal strategies for screening first-degree relatives of patients with hemochromatosis

Critique

Hereditary hemochromatosis, also called genetic hemochromatosis, is an inherited disorder in which mutations in the *HFE* gene, and very rarely other genes, cause increased intestinal iron absorption, apparently via an interaction with the transferrin receptor. Although the disorder in a newly diagnosed patient may be far advanced, screening of other family members (or populations) may allow diagnosis at an early stage, before there has been irreversible organ damage. A cost-effectiveness analysis compared the following strategies:

- Serum iron studies.
- Genetic testing of the proband. If the proband is homozygous for *C282Y*, genetic testing is done to determine whether the spouse is also a carrier for a mutation. If the spouse is heterozygous for *C282Y*, the children undergo genetic testing.
- Genetic testing of the proband. If the proband is homozygous, relatives undergo genetic testing.
- Direct genetic testing of relatives.

The most cost-effective strategy for screening a single child was HFE testing of the proband ($508 per life year saved). The most cost-effective strategy for screening 2 or more children was HFE testing of the proband followed by testing of the spouse (incremental cost-effectiveness ratio $3665 per life year saved). All screening strategies were cost effective compared with no screening in siblings. Strategies using HFE testing were less costly than those using serum iron studies. These strategies are reasonable provided that the proband is an HFE homozygote. In this question, the patient (ie, the proband) has 3 children. Therefore, it is most cost effective to screen the patient and his wife.

Reference

El-Serag HB, Inadomi JM, Kowdley KV. Screening for hereditary hemochromatosis in siblings and children of affected patients. A tcost-effectiveness analysis. Ann Intern Med. 2000;132:261–9.

Answer to question 6: C

Educational objective

To understand the goal of phlebotomy in patients with hereditary hemochromatosis

Critique

Phlebotomy has been shown to be effective in reducing iron stores in patients with hereditary hemochromatosis. The simplest, cheapest, and most effective way to remove iron is by therapeutic phlebotomy. Each 500 mL of whole blood removed contains 200–250 mg of iron. The marrow, in providing replacement for the lost hemoglobin, mobilizes iron from tissue stores, thereby reducing the degree of iron overload. Many hepatologists recommend weekly phlebotomy until iron stores are normalized (defined as a serum ferritin concentration below 50 ng/mL and transferrin saturation below 50%). It may be necessary to discontinue phlebotomy temporarily if anemia occurs. The induction of iron deficiency is not viewed as necessary. These recommendations were agreed upon by a panel of experts in a conference sponsored by the National Institutes of Health in May 1998.

Reference

Bacon BR, Powell LW, Adams PC, et al. Molecular medicine and hemochromatosis: at the crossroads. Gastroenterology. 1999;116:193–207.

Answer to question 7: D

Educational objective

To recognize juvenile hemochromatosis and its genetic basis

Critique

Juvenile hemochromatosis is a rare condition in which iron overload occurs at a much earlier age than in the more common hereditary hemochromatosis. Patients present with symptoms of cardiac and endocrine dysfunction at an early age. The gene for this disorder had been mapped to chromosome 1 and was initially identified as *HFE2* but then renamed "hemojuvelin." Hemojuvelin is a coreceptor for bone morphogenetic protein (BMP) and signals through BMP. Hemojuvelin mutants exhibit decreased BMP signaling, which then lowers hepcidin expression, leading to an increase in iron absorption across the gut enterocyte.

HFE is the gene mutated in the majority of classic hemochromatosis cases. Ferroportin is responsible for facilitating export of iron out of gut enterocytes or hepatocytes into the circulation. Its action is regulated by hepcidin and hephaestin. Mutations in ferroportin and hephaestin have been associated with rare cases of hemochromatosis. Hepcidin is up-regulated in the anemia of chronic disease.

References

Babitt JL, et al. Bone morphogenetic protein signaling by hemojuvelin regulates hepcidin expression. Nat Genet. 2006;38:531–9.

Franchini M. Hereditary iron overload: update on pathophysiology, diagnosis, and treatment. Am J Hematol. 2006;81:202–9.

Answer to question 8: B

Educational objective

To understand the goals of therapeutic phlebotomy in patients with hereditary hemochromatosis

Critique

Many of the complications of iron overload in hereditary hemochromatosis can be prevented or ameliorated by phlebotomy. Cardiomyopathy, hypogonadism, hyperpigmentation, and diabetes mellitus can be improved by phlebotomy. Cirrhosis, once present, is irreversible. Phlebotomy is performed by removing 500 mL of whole blood at weekly intervals until the ferritin is <50 μg/L, and then maintenance phlebotomy every 3 months is performed as necessary.

Reference

Barton JC, McDonnell SM, Adams PC, et al. Management of hemochromatosis. Ann Intern Med. 1998;129:932.

Answer to question 9: A

Educational objective

To appreciate the utility of using rapid PGB screening to recognize the hepatic porphyrias

Critique

Although the nonsurgical causes of abdominal pain are numerous, the combination of mental confusion, constipation, abdominal pain, elevated blood pressure and tachycardia are very suggestive of acute intermittent porphyria (AIP). The presence or history of a photosensitive rash is not associated with AIP, but is seen in variegate and coproporphyria both of which are also associated with abdominal pain. All 3 have a marked increase in PBG excretion during an acute attack. Additional features in this patient that strongly suggest porphyria are the new onset of hypertension, hyponatremia, and proximal muscle weakness. A history of passing red or dark urine was not given by this patient, but would complete the picture. Porphyria is often missed or the diagnosis is delayed until an extensive work up ruling out other causes has been completed. An expert panel recently suggested that screening urine for PBG should be undertaken early when porphyria is suspected. A strongly positive Watson-Schwarz, Hoesch, or related test would justify earlier and more specific therapy. A kit (PBG-trace kit, Thermo Trace/DMA, Arlington, TX) is now available that is rapid and gives a semi-quantitative result. Twenty 4 hour stool and urine collections and plasma determinations are used to sort out AIP, variegate, and coproporphyria. However, waiting for the results of these tests would delay treatment. RBC PBG deaminase determination is an important test for confirming the diagnosis of AIP, but results are usually not immediately available. Given the patient's shallow respirations, one could make a case that another important test do now is a peak respiratory flow to determine the need for intubation. Muscle weakness leading to respiratory failure occurs in patients with porphyria and close monitoring of respiratory status is recommended. Molecular diagnosis of the porphyrias is increasing in importance as an aid to genetic counseling of families.

References

Deacon AC, Peters TJ. Identification of acute porphyria: evaluation of a commercial screening test for urinary porphobilinogen. Ann Clin Biochem. 1998;35(pt 6):726–32.

Nordmann Y, Puy H. Human hereditary hepatic porphyrias. Clin Chim Acta. 2002;325:17–37.

Answer to question 10: C

Educational objective

To understand the approach to treatment of acute intermittent porphyria

Critique

An expert panel recently advocated the use of hemin infusion in patients with neurovisceral porphyria. Treatment with dextrose infusions may be sufficient for patients with mild pain and who do not have muscle weakness. Hemin is a negative feedback inhibitor of aminolevulinoc acid (ALA) synthase, thereby reducing the overproduction of porphyrin intermediates, and is the best choice for patients who have severe manifestations of porphyria. Starvation can initiate a porphyric crises, and dextrose infusions may ameliorate this. Dextrose also inhibits ALA synthase. However, hyponatremia caused by porphyria may be aggravated by 5% dextrose infusions. Infusion of 3% normal saline can improve the hyponatremia, but too rapid correction of the sodium is undesirable. Propranolol is a useful adjunctive therapy to treat hypertension and tachycardia associated with porphyria. Prior to diagnosis, many porphyria patients undergo inappropriate abdominal procedures in a futile attempt to identify a surgical cause of abdominal pain.

Reference

Anderson KE, Bloomer JR, Bonkovsky HL, et al. Recommendations for the diagnosis and treatment of the acute porphyrias. Ann Intern Med. 2005;142:439–50.

Answer to question 11: E

Educational objective

To recognize the factors that precipitate porphyria attacks

Critique

Patients with hepatic porphyrias have autosomal dominant mutations that produce a 50% (approximately) reduction in enzymatic activity. This activity is sufficient to provide needed porphyrins without a buildup of toxic intermediate compounds. Heme synthesis is up-regulated when cytochrome P450 synthesis is stimulated by many drugs or smoking. Dilantin and phenobarbital are 2 of the many drugs that may exacerbate porphyria. Stress, starvation, and alcohol also are associated with porphyria symptoms. Symptoms related to hepatic porphyrias rarely occur before the onset of puberty. Women are more often affected than men. This suggests a role for estrogen and progestins in symptoms of porphyria. Some women with hepatic porphyrias have symptoms associated with the luteal phase of the menstrual cycle. Such patients improve when given an inhibitor of gonadotropin-releasing hormone. Pregnancy, however, can be tolerated relatively well by women with hepatic porphyria. In one study of 176 deliveries, 92% of women had no symptoms related to porphyria during their pregnancies.

References

Herrick AL, McColl KE. Acute intermittent porphyria. Best Pract Res Clin Gastroenterol. 2005;19:235–49.

Kauppinen R, Mustajoki P. Prognosis of acute porphyria: occurrence of acute attacks, precipitating factors, and associated diseases. Medicine (Baltimore). 1992;71:1–13.

Answer to question 12: B

Educational objective

To understand the need to screen for hepatoma in older patients with hepatic porphyrias

Critique

Several studies document the increased incidence of hepatoma in patients with neurovisceral porphyrias. In a large Danish cohort, there was a 70-fold increased risk for hepatoma in acute intermittent porphyria and a 21-fold risk in porphyria cutanea tarda. Therefore, yearly measurements of α-fetoprotein and imaging of the liver are recommended for patients who are past 50. Some patients develop hypertension and renal insufficiency as a consequence of porphyria. It is not necessary to follow porphobilinogen or aminolevulinoc acid in patients—many do not have increased urinary excretion of porphyrins until they have significant symptoms. Although neuropathy can be an important source of discomfort and disability in porphyria, it is not necessary to do yearly nerve conduction studies.

References

Andersson C, Lithner F. Hypertension and renal disease in patients with acute intermittent porphyria. J Intern Med. 1994;236:169–75.

Linet MS, Gridley G, Nyren O, et al. Primary liver cancer, other malignancies, and mortality risks following porphyria: a cohort study in Denmark and Sweden. Am J Epidemiol. 1999;149:1010–5.

Answer to question 13: A

Educational objective

To understand how to diagnosis acute intermittent porphyria (AIP)

Critique

AIP is strongly suggested by the history, and the increased urinary excretion of aminolevulinoc acid (ALA) and porphobilinogen (PBG) without increase in coproporphyrins or protoporphyrins should be present in coproporphyria or variegate porphyria, respectively. The level of PBG deaminase in AIP is typically about 50% of normal. But 2 isoforms of PBG deaminase exist as a result of alternative splicing of messenger RNA. One these is erythroid specific; the other is expressed in many nonerythroid cells. The typical PBG deaminase mutations affect the red blood cell (RBC) enzymes, and PBG deaminase activity in the patient's RBCs is decreased. About 10% of patients/kindreds with AIP have a mutation affecting only the nonerythroid isoform. These patients have disease because of the low PBG deaminase expression in the liver, but their RBC PBG deaminase is normal. PBG deaminase may also be low due to prolonged storage of the blood sample. Reticulocytes have an increased PBG deaminase level. Porphyria patients who are recovering from bleeding or mounting a reticulocyte response for any reason will have a normal activity. RBC PBG deaminase activities have a wide range of values in normal individuals, and these may overlap with levels found in patients with AIP. Lead toxicity can be confused with porphyria. Patients may have abdominal pain and neuropathy due to plumbism. Lead, however, is associated with increase in ALA, but not PBG levels, and thus resembles ALA dehydratase deficiency. Plumbism often has an associated anemia with the finding of coarse basophilic stippling of the RBCs in the peripheral blood smear.

References

Bonkovsky HL. Neurovisceral porphyrias: what a hematologist needs to know. In: Hematology: ASH Education Program Book. Washington DC: American Society of Hematology; 2005:24–30.

Warren MJ, Cooper JB, Wood SP, et al. Lead poisoning, haem synthesis and 5-aminolaevulinic acid dehydratase. Trends Biochem Sci. 1998;23:217–21.

Answer to question 14: E

Educational objective

To recognize the presentation and risk factors for porphyria cutanea tarda (PCT)

Critique

The patient has PCT associated with uroporphyrinogen III decarboxylase (UROD) deficiency. Mutations in cytochrome and transferrin receptor 1 have also been reported in PCT. Patients are often asymptomatic until they develop hepatitis C, human immunodeficiency virus, alcoholism, or renal failure requiring dialysis. They may also have inherited *HFE* mutations associated with hemochromatosis. Patients with PCT have an increased risk for hepatoma that is independent of other risk factors such as hepatitis C. Typical sunscreens do not block the wavelengths associated with photosensitivity due to PCT—opaque creams are required. Protoporphyria and congenital erythropoietic porphyria present much earlier and have more disabling skin lesions. Coproporphyria and variegate porphyria demonstrate photosensitivity but also have abdominal pain.

References

Egger NG, Goeger DE, Payne DA, et al. Porphyria cutanea tarda: multiplicity of risk factors including HFE mutations, hepatitis C, and inherited uroporphyrinogen decarboxylase deficiency. Dig Dis Sci. 2002;47:419–26.

Fracanzani AL, Taioli E, Sampietro M, et al. Liver cancer risk is increased in patients with porphyria cutanea tarda in comparison to matched control patients with chronic liver disease. J Hepatol. 2001;35:498–503.

CHAPTER

05 Acquired underproduction anemias

Answer to question 1: B

Educational objective

To recognize zinc toxicity as a cause of copper deficiency and sideroblastic anemia

Critique

This patient was ingesting excess zinc as part of a cold remedy. Excess dietary zinc interferes with copper absorption, leading to its deficiency. Copper is necessary for proper iron absorption via 2 metalloproteins. Copper deficiency may lead to a microcytic anemia as well as to sideroblastic changes on bone marrow biopsy. Copper deficiency is important to consider in the differential diagnosis of acquired sideroblastic anemia. Myelodysplasia, although in the differential, would be less likely in an 18-year-old man unless other etiologies were first excluded. A complete blood count was normal at age 15 years, making inherited bone marrow failure syndromes unlikely. Vitamin C and selenium toxicity would not lead to anemia.

References

Fiske DN, McCoy HE III, Kitchens CS. Zinc-induced sideroblastic anemia: report of a case, review of the literature, and description of the hematologic syndrome. Am J Hematol. 1994;46:147–50.

Gregg XT, Reddy V, Prchal JT. Copper deficiency masquerading as myelodysplastic syndrome. Blood. 2002;100:1493–5.

Answer to question 2: D

Educational objective

To recognize the typical laboratory findings in the anemia of chronic inflammation/disease

Critique

The anemia of chronic inflammation/disease is a common cause of moderate anemia in patients with, but not exclusive to, chronic inflammatory conditions. The etiology is multifactorial, but recently a central role of hepcidin has been recognized. Hepcidin inhibits mobilization of iron from tissue macrophages and absorption of iron from the gastrointestinal tract. The anemia of chronic inflammation/disease is typically characterized by a mild to moderate hypoproliferative (low reticulocyte count) microcytic or normocytic anemia, with low total iron-binding capacity (TIBC), low iron saturation, and variable ferritin levels. This patient's laboratory values are classic for the anemia of chronic inflammation/disease and may respond to the administration of erythropoietic agents. In classic iron deficiency, the TIBC is often high normal to elevated, with a decreased iron level, iron saturation, and ferritin. Although myelodysplasia remains in the differential diagnosis, the presence of rheumatoid arthritis and the accompanying iron studies make the anemia of chronic inflammation/disease the more likely diagnosis. Furthermore, a bone marrow biopsy would be necessary to confirm the diagnosis of myelodysplasia. α Thalassemia is unlikely because the degree of anemia is lower than would be expected with only 1 or 2 gene deletions, and the microcytosis is not severe enough for 3 or 4 gene deletions. Although autoimmune hemolytic anemia is seen with increased frequency in rheumatoid arthritis, the normal lactose dehydrogenase and bilirubin levels do not support ongoing hemolysis.

References

Roy CN, Andrews NC. Anemia of inflammation: the hepcidin link. Curr Opin Hematol. 2005;12:107–11.

Weiss G, Goodnough LT. Anemia of chronic disease. N Engl J Med. 2005;352:1011–23.

Answer to question 3: A

Educational objective

To understand the pathophysiology leading to the anemia of chronic inflammation/disease

Critique

Significant progress has recently been made in our understanding of the pathophysiology of the anemia of chronic inflammation/disease. Although the blunted response to erythropoietin, decreased absorption of intestinal iron, decreased mobilization of iron from tissue macrophages, and increased levels of specific cytokines (ie, interleukin 1 [IL-1] and tumor necrosis factor α) have long been recognized, the true cause of decreased iron mobilization remained elusive. Recently, the antimicrobial peptide hepcidin was discovered and thought to be a key mediator of iron regulation, with an important role in the anemia of chronic inflammation/disease. In fact, hepcidin may be a key link between infection, inflammation, and iron metabolism. In certain inflammatory states, hepcidin production is up-regulated by IL-6. Hepcidin has been found to decrease mobilization of tissue iron and absorption of iron from the gut. In the face of infection, this process is thought to be an adaptive response, leading to sequestration of iron away from invading organisms. Alternatively, in iron deficient or hypoxic states, hepcidin levels are depressed, leading to an adaptive increase in iron availability.

References

Weinstein DA, Roy CN, Flemming MD, et al. Inappropriate expression of hepcidin is associated with iron refractory anemia: implications for the anemia of chronic disease. Blood. 2002;100:3776–81.

Weiss G, Goodnough LT. Anemia of chronic disease. N Engl J Med. 2005;352:1011–23.

Answer to question 4: D

Educational objective

To recognize the role of intravenous iron in dialysis patients who lose their response to red cell growth factors

Critique

This patient's anemia was originally explained by the underproduction of erythropoietin secondary to his worsening renal failure. As expected, the patient's hemoglobin level improved with darbopoetin supplementation. His worsening anemia while continuing to receive darbopoetin, however, is due to a functional iron deficiency. This phenomenon has been described in patients receiving erythropoietic agents. These patients respond best to intravenous iron, despite the fact that iron studies do not demonstrate obvious iron deficiency. Increasing the dose of darbopoetin will not be effective, and the dose suggested is higher than would be recommended. There is no evidence that switching erythropoietic agents (ie, erythropoietin) is effective when there is no response to one agent. Oral iron is less effective than intravenous iron in this setting. It is unlikely a patient who is already receiving twice daily ferrous sulfate would respond to an increased dose.

References

Eschbach JW. Iron requirements in erythropoietin therapy. Best Pract Res Clin Haematol. 2005;18:347–61.

Silverstein SB, Rodgers GM. Parenteral iron therapy options. Am J Hematol. 2004;76:74–8.

Answer to question 5: C

Educational objective

To recognize the correct management of uncomplicated iron deficiency anemia

Critique

This patient presents with uncomplicated iron deficiency anemia likely secondary to her past history of heavy menstrual periods and 5 previous pregnancies. Recent colonoscopy was negative. The most appropriate treatment for uncomplicated iron deficiency anemia is oral iron replacement. Each dose of oral iron sulfate will contain approximately 45–60 mg of elemental iron. The iron content of typical multivitamins would be insufficient to correct iron deficiency anemia. Intravenous iron formulations lead to a quicker response than oral iron but are not more effective, assuming a normal ability to absorb oral iron. Additionally, intravenous iron dextrans carry the risk of anaphylactic reactions and are much more costly. Iron sucrose, although likely safer than iron dextran, is more expensive and total dose infusion is not recommended (as presented in this problem set). Intravenous iron formulations can be considered if the patient is intolerant or does not respond to an adequate trial of oral iron.

References

Cook JD. Diagnosis and management of iron-deficiency anaemia. Best Pract Res Clin Haematol. 2005;18:319–32.

Silverstein SB, Rodgers GM. Parenteral iron therapy options. Am J Hematol. 2004;76:74–8.

Umbreit J. Iron deficiency: a concise review. Am J Hematol. 2005;78:225–31.

Answer to question 6: C

Educational objective

To recognize and evaluate celiac sprue as a cause of refractory iron deficiency

Critique

The diagnosis of celiac sprue should be considered in iron deficient patients, especially those without a reason for iron deficiency and those refractory to oral iron supplementation. In fact, celiac disease has been noted in a high proportion of patients undergoing endoscopy for evaluation of iron deficiency anemia. Endomyseal and transglutaminase antibodies have high specificity for the disease, although duodenal biopsy should be performed to ensure the diagnosis. This patient's abdominal symptoms and history of insulin-dependent diabetes mellitus (IDDM; another autoimmune disorder) is a clue to the correct diagnosis. A bone marrow biopsy is not necessary in this case that is consistent with iron deficiency. B_{12} deficiency, folate deficiency, and hypothyroidism do not lead to a microcytic anemia. Target cells were not noted on the peripheral blood smear, and globin gene synthesis studies to evaluate for α thalassemia are unnecessary in this iron-deficient patient.

References

Dewar DH, Ciclitira PJ. Clinical features and diagnosis of celiac disease. Gastroenterology. 2005;128(suppl 1):S19–24.

Hershko C, Hoffbrand AV, Keret D, et al. Role of autoimmune gastritis, Helicobacter pylori and celiac disease in refractory or unexplained iron deficiency anemia. Haematologica. 2005;90:585–95.

Lee SK, Green PHR. Celiac sprue (the great modern-day imposter). Curr Opin Rheumatol. 2006;18:101–7.

Answer to question 7: B

Educational objective

To recognize and evaluate parvovirus as a cause of pure red cell aplasia in an immunocompromised patient

Critique

This patient is chronically immunosuppressed and developed a severe hypoproliferative anemia. He had recent exposure to a sick grandchild, whose fever and rash were most likely due to a parvovirus infection. Patients on chronic immunosuppression may not be able to clear parvovirus, and pure red cell aplasia may ensue. Anemia with severe reticulocytopenia is characteristic of pure red cell aplasia (suggested by the bone marrow biopsy report). Because immunocompromised hosts may not be able mount an effective immune response, parvovirus DNA testing (instead of immunoglobulin G [IgG] and IgM studies) should be pursued. Intravenous immunoglobulin has proven to be effective therapy in this condition. There is no suggestion of hemolysis, and therefore a Coombs test is not indicated. Antierythropoietin antibodies have been described with the use of erythropoietic agents but remain exceedingly rare, especially with darbopoetin. Antibody testing could be considered only if parvovirus testing and other evaluations returned normal. An ANA would not help in the evaluation of anemia in this patient with known lupus.

References

Abkowitz JL. Acquired pure red cell aplasia: physiology and therapy. In: Young NS (Chair), Abkowitz JL, Luzzatto L. New Insights Into the Pathophysiology of Acquired Cytopenias. Hematology Am Soc Hematol Educ Program. 2000:18–38.

Frickhofen N, Chen ZJ, Young NS, et al. Parvovirus B19 as a cause of acquired chronic pure red cell aplasia. Br J Haematol. 1994;87:818–24.

Young NS, Brown KE. Parvovirus B19. N Engl J Med. 2004;350:586–97.

Answer to question 8: D

Educational objective

To choose appropriate therapy in a patient with idiopathic pure red cell aplasia

Critique

Acquired pure red cell aplasia (PRCA) is characterized by severe anemia, reticulocytopenia, and an absence of red blood cell precursors in the bone marrow. Although the etiology of pure red aplasia remains diverse, including viruses and drugs, many cases are immunologic in origin.

Initial therapy, if an underlying etiology is not found on investigation, usually includes immune suppression such as steroids, cyclosporine, cyclophosphamide, or antithymocyte globulin. Although thymoma may be found in 5–8% of cases of acquired PRCA, prophylactic thymectomy is not indicated unless a thymoma is found on evaluation. Splenectomy is not considered a first-line therapy for pure red cell aplasia unless a lymphoproliferative disorder (ie, splenic lymphoma) exists. Erythropoietin levels are usually very high in pure red cell aplasia. Exogenous administration of erythropoietin is generally not effective and does not address the underlying pathophysiology.

References

Abkowitz JL. Acquired pure tred cell aplasia: physiology and therapy. In: Young NS (Chair), Abkowitz JL, Luzzatto L. New Insights Into the Pathophysiology of Acquired Cytopenias. Hematology Am Soc Hematol Educ Program. 2000:18–38.

Fisch P, Handgretinger R, Schaefer HE. Pure red cell aplasia. Br J Haematol. 2000;111:1010–22.

Answer to question 9: D

Educational objective

To recognize the association of pernicious anemia with other autoimmune disorders (ie, hypothyroidism)

Critique

In cobalamin deficiency, repletion of cobalamin with a standard dose as in this patient will result in a reticulocytosis beginning within days of initiating therapy. Gradual correction of anemia is noted over a period of several weeks. After 4 weeks of adequate therapy, this patient did not have an appropriate reticulocyte response or correction of her anemia, suggesting a second problem. Patients with pernicious anemia are at increased risk of having other autoimmune disorders, including thyroiditis. Hypothyroidism can result in macrocytic anemia due to inadequate bone marrow production. Iron deficiency is unlikely because adequate iron stores were noted in the bone marrow. A concomitant hemolytic anemia with a high lactose dehydrogenase or positive Coombs test would be expected to result in reticulocytosis after B_{12} was administered.

References

Carmel R, Spencer C. Clinical and subclinical thyroid disorders associated with pernicious anemia. Observations on abnormal thyroid-stimulating hormone levels and on a possible association of blood group O with hyperthyroidism. Arch Intern Med. 1982;142:1465–9.

Ottesen M, Feldt-Rasmussen U, Andersen J, et al. Thyroid function and autoimmunity in pernicious anemia before and during cyanocobalamin treatment. J Endocrinol Invest. 1995;18:91–7.

Answer to question 10: A

Answer to question 11: C

Educational objective

To recognize that megaloblastic anemia may be associated with pancytopenia and that vitamin B_{12} deficiency leads to hyperhomocysteinemia and possibly increased thrombotic risk

Critique

If untreated, many patients with megaloblastic anemias will gradually develop pancytopenia. Rarely, patients with megaloblastic states may even present with thrombocytopenia as the first cell line affected in the bone marrow. The hypersegmentation noted on the smear makes cobalamin deficiency the most likely diagnosis of the options presented. Paroxysmal nocturnal hemoglobinuria may be associated with pancytopenia and thrombosis but is not associated with hypersegmentation of neutrophils. Although iron deficiency from chronic blood loss is a consideration given the low platelets and oral anticoagulation, this would not explain the peripheral blood smear findings or elevated mean corpuscular volume. Warm antibody hemolytic anemia and anemia of chronic inflammation/disease would not be associated with neutrophil hypersegmentation.

In the second part to this question, one must recognize the association of high homocysteine blood levels with cobalamin deficiency and the possible associated risk of vascular thrombosis. Given the likelihood of vitamin B_{12} deficiency in the first part of the question, hyperhomocysteinemia is the most likely diagnosis. It remains uncertain if lowering the homocysteine levels through administration of vitamin B_{12}, vitamin B_6, and folic acid will lead to a decreased thrombotic risk. Antithrombin deficiency and protein C deficiency states are rare and generally associated with a strong family history of thrombosis. Plasminogen activator inhibitor-1 deficiency would result in a bleeding diathesis.

References

Quere I, Gris JC, Dauzat M. Homocysteine and venous thrombosis. Semin Vasc Med. 2005;5:183–9.

Remecha AF, Souto J, Ramila E, et al. Enhanced risk of thrombotic disease in patients with acquired vitamin B12 and/or folate deficiency: role of hyperhomocyteinemia. Ann Hematol. 2002;81:616–21.

Answer to question 12: B

Educational objective

To recognize appropriate treatment strategies for anemia in human immunodeficiency virus (HIV)-infected patients

Critique

There is a high prevalence of anemia in HIV-infected patients, and the prevalence increases with progression of HIV disease. There are often multiple causes of anemia, particularly as patients experience complications of advancing HIV disease with concomitant opportunistic infections. Several studies have shown that control of HIV with highly active antiretroviral therapy (HAART) significantly correlates with improvement in anemia. The symptom presentation in this patient along with an increasing HIV viral load necessitates treatment of HIV disease with HAART. It would thus be reasonable, in the absence of other clear-cut causes of anemia, to delay use of erythropoietin and follow hemoglobin levels for improvement over the first 6 months of HAART. If the anemia did not improve with HAART therapy, then epoetin alfa can be considered. Numerous controlled and uncontrolled studies have shown that epoetin alfa is safe and effective in the treatment of anemia in HIV-infected patients, particularly in those with endogenous erythropoietin levels of <500 mU/ml. At least one randomized study has shown that epoetin alfa in a single weekly dose of 40,000 units is equivalent to epoetin alfa 100 U/kg three times weekly. Parenteral iron would not initially be necessary as an adjunct to erythropoietin therapy because the serum ferritin is >200 ng/mL.

References

Belperio P, Rhew D. Prevalence and outcomes of anemia in individuals with human immunodeficiency virus: a systematic review of the literature. Am J Med. 2004; 116:S27–43.

Berhane K, Karim R, Cohen MH, et al. Impact of highly active antiretroviral therapy on anemia and relationship between anemia and survival in a large cohort of HIV-infected women: Women's Interagency HIV Study. JAIDS. 2004; 37:1245–52.

Volberding P, Levine A, Dieterich D, et al. for the Anemia in HIV Working Group. Anemia in HIV infection: clinical impact and evidence-based management strategies. Clin Infect Dis. 2004;38:1454–63.

Answer to question 13: C

Educational objective

To understand appropriate evaluation strategies for anemia in an elderly patient

Critique

As many as 11% of men over the age of 65 have a hemoglobin ≤13 g/dl. There are numerous causes for anemia that are prevalent in this age group such as blood loss, iron deficiency anemia, chronic inflammatory conditions, and renal insufficiency. A clear-cut etiology, however, may not be obvious in as many as a third of elderly patients with anemia.

In this case, the presence of an elevated mean corpuscular volume (MCV) suggests that the anemia is more likely related to alcohol use, liver disease, hypothyroidism, or even early myelodysplasia. One particular concern is that alcohol abuse in the elderly is often overlooked and may need to be addressed directly with the patient. Inflammatory states as reflected by an increased erythrocyte sedimentation rate and C-reactive protein level would not explain a macrocytic anemia. Iron deficiency is unlikely given the elevated MCV. An erythropoietin level is not usually part of the initial evaluation of a macrocytic anemia.

References

Guralnik J, Eisenstaedt R, Ferrucci L, et al. Prevalence of anemia in persons 65 years and older in the United States: evidence for a high rate of unexplained anemia. Blood. 2004;104:2263–8.

Latvala J, Parkkila S, Niemela O. Excess alcohol consumption is common in patients with cytopenias: studies in blood and bone marrow cells. Alcohol Clin Exp Res. 2004;28:619–24.

Answer to question 14: B

Educational objective

To recognize folate deficiency as a cause of acute hypoproliferative crisis in a patient with a chronic hemolytic anemia.

Critique

Any insult that results in decreased erythrocyte production will lead to a rapid decrease in the hemoglobin in a patient with chronic hemolysis. Common causes include viral infections, particularly parvovirus B19, which selectively infects red cell precursors; however, other viruses such as cytomegalovirus can also suppress bone marrow production. Folate and B_{12} deficiency can result in megaloblastic changes and inadequate red cell production. Folate deficiency is most commonly seen in alcoholics due to inadequate dietary intake or in patients with chronic hemolytic anemias, as in this case. Although the mean corpuscular volume (MCV) increases in association with folate deficiency, it is important to note that the MCV may not be abnormally elevated in patients with baseline microcytosis such as this patient with S/β^+ thalassemia.

Disseminated fungal infections can result in marrow suppression but are most commonly seen in the setting of human immunodeficiency virus infection. Although other conditions such as Hodgkin disease, myelofibrosis, and myelodysplasia may cause hypoproliferative anemia, they have no particular association with hemoglobinopathies or substance abuse and are therefore less likely.

References

Das Gupta A. Abrogation of macrocytosis in pernicious anemia by beta-thalassemia does not mask the diagnosis of vitamin B12 deficiency. Am J Hematol. 2002;71:61–2.

Mazzone A, Vezzoli M, Ottini E. Masked deficit of B-12 and folic acid in thalassemia. Am J Hematol. 2001;67:274.

Answer to question 15: C

Educational objective

To recognize subclinical cobalamin deficiency in an elderly patient and understand appropriate treatment

Critique

As many as 12% of elderly patients living in the community have "subclinical" cobalamin deficiency. Elevation of homocysteine and methylmalonic acid often precedes declining cobalamin levels. In the present case, the increase in homocysteine and methylmalonic acid is secondary to subclinical cobalamin deficiency. Treatment for this patient requires adequate replacement of cobalamin in order to halt the progression of neurologic symptoms. Doses of oral vitamin B_{12} <500 μg each day have been shown to be unpredictable for adequate replacement. If oral therapy is to be attempted, 1000 μg each day should be initiated. Patients given a trial of oral cobalamin replacement must be followed carefully with monitoring of cobalamin levels as well as homocysteine levels. If oral therapy is not successful, intramuscular replacement should be given. Intramuscular B_{12} is typically given at a dose of 1000 μg each month but is often initiated with daily or weekly administration. Replacement with oral folate will not correct subclinical B_{12} deficiency, and neurologic symptoms will progress. Combination therapy with oral vitamin B_{12}, folate, and vitamin B_6 has been used in the treatment of hyperhomocysteinemia but is not necessary in this patient.

References

Andres E, Affenberger S, Vinzio S, et al. Food-cobalamin malabsorption in elderly patients: clinical manifestations and treatment. Am J Med. 2005;118:1154–9.

Eussen SJ, de Groot LC, Clarke R, et al. Oral cyanocobalamin supplementation in older people with vitamin B12 deficiency: a dose-finding trial. Arch Intern Med. 2005;165:1167–72.

Wolters M, Stroble A, Hahn A. Cobalamin: a critical vitamin in the elderly. Prev Med. 2004;39:1256–66.

CHAPTER

06

Hemolytic anemias

Answer to question 1: D

Educational objective

To understand the role of supplemental erythropoietin in treating hemolytic anemia caused by ribavirin in hepatitis C virus-infected patients

Critique

A major adverse effect of ribavirin therapy is hemolytic anemia, which may be related to low levels of erythrocyte membrane protein sulfhydryl concentrations. Although hemolytic anemia due to ribavirin has been historically treated with dose reduction, this results in diminished response rates to therapy. High-dose vitamin E has been studied as an antioxidant to reduce hemolysis but has not been proved effective. Although interferon α can cause marrow suppression, it does not cause hemolytic anemia. Supplemental erythropoietin has proven effective for ribavirin-induced hemolytic anemia and has allowed patients to remain on treatment with sustained virologic response.

References

Kowdley KV. Hematologic side effects of interferon and ribavirin therapy. J Clin Gastroenterol. 2005;39(suppl):S3–8.

Lebray P, Nalpas B, Vallet-Prichard A, et al. The impact of haematopoietic growth factors on the management and efficacy of antiviral treatment in patients with hepatitis C virus. Antivir Ther. 2005;10:769–76.

Saeian K, Bajaj JS, Franco J, et al. High-dose vitamin E supplementation does not diminish ribavirin-associated haemolysis in hepatitis C treatment with combination standard alpha-interferon and ribavirin. Aliment Pharmcol Ther. 2004;20:1189–93.

Answer to question 2: C

Educational objective

To identify patients with paroxysmal cold hemoglobinuria (PNH) who are at high risk for thrombosis and understand the role of prophylaxis for clotting

Critique

Patients with PNH are at a high risk of thrombosis, with venous thrombosis being the most common cause of death in this population. Patients with large PNH clones (eg, affecting greater than 50% of granulocytes) carry a thrombotic risk of over 40%, which is 8 times higher than the risk in patients with smaller clones. Therefore, anticoagulation is indicated in this patient. A prospective study has shown that patients with a large PNH clone, with no contraindication to anticoagulation, treated with prophylactic warfarin had a reduction in their thrombotic risk to zero with acceptable risks of bleeding. There are no data on primary prophylaxis with aspirin, low-molecular-weight heparin, or the combination of these 2 agents for patients with PNH.

Reference

Hall C, Richards S, Hillmen P. Primary prophylaxis with warfarin prevents thrombosis in paroxysmal nocturnal hemoglobinuria (PNH). Blood. 2003;102:3587–91.

Answer to question 3: D

Educational objective

To identify malaria on a blood smear and identify proper therapy

Critique

The peripheral smear is indicative of infection with plasmodium, which has led to this patient's hemolysis. Plasmodium vivax can have a delayed clinical presentation with vague complaints. Anemia and thrombocytopenia have been seen in US soldiers returning from Afghanistan with an attack rate of 52.4 cases per 1000 personnel. This may be related to suboptimal compliance with prophylactic therapy. Chloroquine is typically used to treat vivax infections, although azithromycin may also have some efficacy. Prednisone, intravenous immune globulin, and plasmapheresis do not have a role in the treatment of hemolytic anemia secondary to malaria.

References

Dunne MW, Singh N, Shukla M, et al. A double-blind randomized study of azithromycin compared to chloroquine for the treatment of plasmodium vivax malaria in India. Am J Trop Med Hyg. 2005;73:1108–11.

Kotwal RS, Wenzel RB, Sterling RA, et al. An outbreak of malaria in US Army Rangers returning from Afghanistan. JAMA. 2005;293:212–6.

Answer to question 4: C

Educational objective

To recognize valve-mediated hemolysis on a peripheral smear

Critique

The peripheral smear shown reveals evidence of red cell fragmentation, likely caused by an improperly functioning mechanical aortic valve. This is most commonly secondary to paravalvular leakage. Treatment would involve replacement of the malfunctioning valve. Although the patient has chronic lymphocytic leukemia, which may be associated with autoimmune hemolytic anemia, the smear does not show spherocytes that would be seen in autoimmune hemolysis. Additionally, hemolysis in a glucose-6-phosphate dehydrogenase deficient patient exposed to oxidant drugs like sulfa or phenazopridine may cause eccentrocytes, blister cells, or bite cells but would not show red cell fragmentation. Prednisone is used to treat autoimmune hemolytic anemia, which this patient does not have. Plasmapheresis is used to treat thrombotic thrombocytopenic purpura (TTP), which may have a similar peripheral smear, but the patient does not have the clinical characteristics of TTP.

Reference

Suedkamp M, Lercher AJ, Mueller-Riemenschneider F, et al. Hemolysis parameters of St. Jude Medical: Hemodynamic Plus and Regent valves in aortic position. Int J Cardiol. 2004;95:89–93.

Answer to question 5: D

Educational objective

To recognize babesiosis on the peripheral smear and identify therapy for this infection

Critique

The peripheral smear shows erythrocytes infected with *Babesia microti*, a protozoan infection which is endemic in parts of Nantucket Island, Cape Cod, Long Island, and northern California. Infection is transmitted by the *Ixodes* tick, which is also the vector for Lyme disease. Coinfection with both organisms is associated with more severe disease. Babesiosis has been associated with erythrocyte transfusion, as in this case. Symptoms typically include fever, malaise, and myalgias along with renal and hepatic insufficiency. The disease is much more severe in splenectomized persons, in whom it can lead to respiratory distress syndrome and death. Treatment is with either clindamycin and quinine or azithromycin and atovaquone, the latter of which is probably better tolerated.

References

Cable RG, Leiby DA. Risk and prevention of transfusion-transmitted babesiosis and other tick-borne diseases. Curr Opin Hematol. 2003;10:405–11.

Krause PJ. Babesiosis diagnosis and treatment. Vector Borne Zoonotic Dis. 2003;3:45–51.

Answer to question 6: B

Educational objective

To be able to interpret a red cell antibody panel in a patient with a delayed transfusion reaction

Critique

A red cell panel includes red cells of known antigenicity. In the case provided, 11 red cell concentrates (rows) are used. The panel also includes 20 antigens (columns). A red cell panel is typically performed in 3 stages. The first, the immediate spin crossmatch, involves mixing patient serum with the red cell pattern. Because this is performed at room temperature, it most frequently identifies a cold agglutinin. The second phase involves warming the serum to body temperature and adding low isotonic saline as an enhancing medium. This typically identifies a warm antibody. The third phase involves the addition of Coombs reagent (antihuman immunoglobulin G [IgG]), which promotes agglutination of cells coated with IgG. As we can see, this patient's cells agglutinated with erythrocytes in panels 1, 2, 5, and 11. The only common antigen in this selection of cells is C, a member of the Rh antigen system. This patient has therefore developed antibodies, likely of the IgG subtype, to the C antigen, which was found on transfused erythrocytes. An indirect Coombs test would also be positive in this patient as a result of IgG antibody formation.

Reference

Coombs RR. Historical note: past, present and future of the antiglobulin test. Vox Sang. 1998;74:67–73.

Answer to question 7: A

Educational objective

To understand the pathophysiology of paroxysmal cold hemoglobinuria (PNH) and use this information to formulate potential therapeutic strategies

Critique

PNH can be thought of as a primary aplastic anemia with cytokine-induced or cytotoxic T-cell-induced apoptotic signaling being transmitted through glycosyl phosphatidylinositol (GPI)-linked proteins. This results in a growth advantage for cells lacking these molecules and a relative expansion of cells lacking GPI-linked proteins. Because GPI-linked proteins transmit the apoptotic signal, any treatment strategy that would add GPI molecules to cells could potentially lead to aplastic anemia. This includes options B, C, and D. Eculizumab, a humanized monoclonal antibody that binds C5 complement protein, has been shown to reduce hemolysis successfully, improve symptoms, and improve quality of life in patients with PNH with relatively few side effects.

References

Chen G, Zeng W, Maciejewski JP, et al. Differential gene expression in hematopoietic progenitors from paroxysmal nocturnal hemoglobinuria patients reveals an apoptosis/immune response in 'normal' phenotype cells. Leukemia. 2005;19:862–8.

Hill A, Hillmen P, Richards SJ, et al. Sustained response and long-term safety of eculizumab in paroxysmal nocturnal hemoglobinuria. Blood. 2005;106:2559–65.

Sloand EM, Mainwaring L, Kayvanfar K, et al. Transfer of glycosylphosphatidylinositol-anchored proteins to deficient cells after erythrocyte transfusion in paroxysmal nocturnal hemoglobinuria. Blood. 2004;104:3782–8.

Answer to question 8: D

Educational objective

To recognize signs of pulmonary hypertension in patients with sickle cell disease and identify pulmonary hypertension as a major cause of mortality in these patients

Critique

Recently, pulmonary hypertension has been identified as a major cause of death and mortality in patients with sickle cell disease. Pulmonary hypertension may be a consequence of *in situ* thrombosis of the pulmonary vasculature or may result from nitric oxide scavenging by free hemoglobin, occurring as a result of chronic hemolysis. Pulmonary hypertension is diagnosed by Doppler echocardiography and is resistant to hydroxyurea therapy. On physical examination, pulmonary hypertension is suggested by signs of right heart failure including pedal edema. It is also characterized by hypoxia and shortness of breath. Elevated hemoglobin F is protective against organ damage in patients with sickle cell disease. The degree of anemia and presence of nucleated red blood cells are not directly linked to mortality in sickle cell patients.

Reference

Gladwin MT, Sachdev V, Jison ML, et al. Pulmonary hypertension as a risk factor for death in patients with sickle cell disease. N Engl J Med. 2004;350:886–95.

Answer to question 9: D

Educational objective

To recognize acquired α thalassemia in a patient with myelodysplasia

Critique

Although typically congenital, α thalassemia may be acquired secondary to myelodysplasia or myeloproliferative abnormalities. At the molecular level, this is due to mutations in the *ATRX* gene. *ATRX* is a transacting chromatin-associated factor. Mutations in *ATRX* cause dramatic down-regulation of α-globin gene expression. Hemoglobin H is an unstable hemoglobin composed of 4 β-globin subunits. It can be detected by supravital staining or hemoglobin electrophoresis. In the present case, microcytic anemia in the presence of hemoglobin H and signs of mild iron overload are diagnostic of thalassemia. The peripheral smear corroborates this diagnosis. Hemoglobin C disease is characterized by precipitated hemoglobin C clusters on peripheral smear. Cobalamin deficiency is associated with normal iron studies and macrocytosis. Patients with myelofibrosis typically have tear drop cells on smear and would not show the presence of hemoglobin H.

Reference

Costa DB, Fisher CA, Miller KB, et al. A novel mutation in the last exon of ATRX in a patient with alpha-thalassemia myelodysplastic syndrome. Eur J Hematol. 2006;76:432–5.

Answer to question 10: B

Educational objective

To recognize paroxysmal cold hemoglobinuria (PCH) in a child and understand the immunology of this condition

Critique

PCH is perhaps the most common cause of immune hemolysis in children and frequently follows an infectious illness. It is characterized by signs and symptoms of hemolysis including hemoglobinuria. The pathophysiology of the illness is related to the presence of a Donath–Landsteiner (DL) antibody, which is an immunoglobin G (IgG) that recognizes the P antigen on erythrocytes. The P antigen is a glycosphingolipid globoside that is similar to glycolipids found in bacteria. The DL antibody binds to erythrocytes at cooler temperatures but causes complement fixation at warmer temperatures. Diagnosis of PCH involves incubating erythrocytes with serum and a source of complement at 4°C for 30 minutes, then warming them to 37°C for 30 minutes. Hemolysis indicates a positive test. In PCH, the direct antiglobulin test (DAT) is often negative at room temperature because the IgG binds only at lower temperatures. Warm antibody mediated hemolytic anemia is characterized by IgG that binds to Rh antigens at body temperature. In this condition, the DAT is positive for IgG. Cold agglutinin disease is characterized by IgM which binds to I/i antigens at temperatures lower than body temperature and causes complement fixation and hemolysis. The DAT is positive for C3 in this condition. ABO mismatch occurs following blood transfusion and is associated with life-threatening hemolysis and shock.

Reference

Sokol RJ, Booker DJ, Stamps R. Erythropoiesis: paroxysmal cold hemoglobinuria: a clinical-pathological study of patients with a positive Donath-Landsteiner test. Hematology. 1999;4: 137–64.

Answer to question 11: C

Educational objective

To recognize the clinical manifestations of methemoglobinemia from nicotinamide-adenine-dinucleotide (NADH)–diaphorase deficiency

Critique

The patient is cyanotic with normal oxygen saturation. Possible etiologies for this patient's cyanosis include sulfhemoglobinemia, hemoglobin M, low-oxygen-affinity hemoglobins, and NADH-diaphorase deficiency. Patients with low-oxygen-affinity hemoglobins typically are anemic due to decreased erythropoietin levels. In the case of high-affinity hemoglobin, patients are often polycythemic due to erythropoietin excess. Sulfhemoglobinemia usually occurs secondarily to ingestion of drugs such as sulfonamides and is not a chronic condition. Hemoglobin M and NADH-diaphorase deficiency both lead to methemoglobinemia. In the case of hemoglobin M, a mutation in the hemoglobin molecule causes iron to resist reduction to the divalent state, which in turn impedes oxygen binding. NADH diaphorase normally reduces cytochrome b5, which in turn reduces methemoglobin to hemoglobin. Deficiency of the enzyme is another cause of methemoglobinemia. NADH-diaphorase deficiency is autosomal recessive and is therefore uncommon in parents of affected individuals. Hemoglobins M are autosomal dominant. This patient's family history makes NADH-diaphorase deficiency the most likely diagnosis.

Reference

Prchal JT, Gregg XT. Red cell enzymes. Hematology Am Soc Hematol Educ Program. 2005:19–23.

CHAPTER 07

Myeloid disorders

Answer to question 1: D

Educational objective

To recognize the clinical features that distinguish reactive neutrophilia from myeloproliferative disease

Critique

Definitive criteria distinguishing reactive leukocytosis from a primary myeloid disorder are lacking. Though there is some evidence that extreme leukocytosis (>45,000 cells/μL) may suggest an underlying malignancy, moderate neutrophilia, as in this case, is more often associated with infection. Left-shifted leukocyte differentials and monocytosis are frequently seen with reactive leukocytosis. The leukocyte alkaline phosphatase score is high in reactive neutrophilia and usually low in myeloproliferative disease. Though occasionally seen in inflammatory conditions such as parasitic infections, basophilia is most commonly associated with myeloproliferative disease or myelodysplasia. Consequently, basophilia generally warrants consideration for bone marrow evaluation.

References

Arnalich F, Lahoz C, Larrocha C, et al. Incidence and clinical significance of peripheral and bone marrow basophilia. J Med. 1987;18:293–303.

Reding MT, Hibbs JR, Morrison VA, et al. Diagnosis and outcome of 100 consecutive patients with extreme granulocytic leukocytosis. Am J Med. 1998;104:12–6.

Answer to question 2: B

Educational objective

To recognize the natural history of drug-induced agranulocytosis

Critique

The clinical presentation is highly suspicious for drug-induced neutropenia. Though highly variable, drug-induced neutropenia typically resolves within 10 days, but usually not before 4 days, after discontinuing the offending drug. A number of nonrandomized clinical trials have suggested that granulocyte colony-stimulating factor (G-CSF) treatment may shorten the duration of neutropenia. However, chronic G-CSF therapy is virtually never required. There is no evidence that drug-induced neutropenia predisposes to leukemia or aplastic anemia. Moreover, the normal red blood cell and platelet counts argue against aplastic anemia.

References

Andres E, Kurtz JE, Martin-Hunyadi C, et al. Nonchemotherapy drug-induced agranulocytosis in elderly patients: the effects of granulocyte colony-stimulating factor. Am J Med. 2002;112:460–4.

Beauchesne MF, Shalansky SJ. Nonchemotherapy drug-induced agranulocytosis: a review of 118 patients treated with colony-stimulating factor. Pharmacotherapy. 1999;19:299–305.

Answer to question 3: C

Educational objective

To appreciate that serum tryptase may not always be elevated in patients with systemic mastocytosis (SM) and measurement of 24-hour histamine excretion in the urine may be helpful

Critique

This patient has pathologic findings highly suggestive of SM, but the serum tryptase is normal. A polymorphism that results in low tryptase levels is fairly common (45% of Caucasians have a deleted α-tryptase gene in one report), so some patients with SM may have normal total tryptase even on repeated measurements. In this instance, a 24-hour urine measurement for histamine may be more sensitive. CD2 and/or CD25 coexpression with CD117 on bone marrow or peripheral blood mast cells is indicative of SM, but not just CD2 or CD25 on monocytes. *C-kit* mutations may be found in the neoplastic clone in SM but should not involve granulocytes. Red cell hexokinase is an enzyme in the glycolytic pathway and has no relevance to the diagnosis of SM, and there are no known mutations relevant to SM at 19q23.

Reference

Schwartz LB, Irani AM. Serum tryptase and the laboratory diagnosis of systemic mastocytosis. Hematol Oncol Clin North Am. 2000;14:641–57.

Answer to question 4: C

Educational objective

To appreciate that aggressive therapy for Langerhans cell histiocytosis (LCH) may be warranted, despite limited disease, if the involved site is at central nervous system risk

Critique

This young woman has an LCH that involves a craniofacial bone and the pituitary with probable diabetes insipidus (DI). Although local therapies such as radiation and curettage may be sufficient for localized LCH at other locations, the involvement of craniofacial bones and DI are associated with a relatively poor prognosis, and single-agent therapy is not recommended. The Histiocytic Society recommends more aggressive systemic treatment in these patients. The agents that have been used in higher risk patients include combination of vinblastine and prednisone for 6 to 12 months, or a combination of vinblastine, prednisone, and 6-mercaptopurine with or without methotrexate. Etoposide has been included in other regimens. Response rates vary from 67% to 90%, depending on risk category and organ dysfunction, with recurrence rates of 12–42% after 1 year of therapy. Interferon-α has been used, but is considered nonstandard therapy. Cladarabine and a combination of vincristine and cytosine arabinoside have been used for salvage therapy. There is no known role for concurrent cisplatin and radiation therapy for LCH.

Reference

Grois N, Potschger U, Prosch H, et al. Risk factors for diabetes insipidus in langerhans cell histiocytosis. Pediatr Blood Cancer. 2005.

Answer to question 5: A

Educational objective

To appreciate that cases of systemic mastocytosis (SM) are associated with the *D816V* mutation in *c-kit*

Critique

A somatic mutation of *c-kit* has been found in the neoplastic cells of some patients with SM. These mutations are different from those found in gastrointestinal stromal tumors. The most common one in SM is the *D816V* mutation. This mutation is in an activating loop of the kinase domain, and transfection studies have revealed ligand-independent constitutive receptor activation. Patients in whom this mutation is detected tend to have more severe disease and more commonly have osteosclerotic bone lesions, immunoglobulin dysregulation, and peripheral blood abnormalities with evidence for either a myelodysplastic or myeloproliferative disorder. Other mutations have been described that confer similar functional changes. The *bcr-abl* mutation, while also activating of a tyrosine kinase, is found in chronic myelogenous leukemia. The *AML-ETO* rearrangements are found in acute leukemia. The *MLL* gene on 11q23 does partner with several genes in both acute myeloid and lymphoid leukemias but has not been reported in SM. The *C282Y* mutation is found in hereditary hemochromatosis.

Reference

Worobec AS, Semere T, Nagata H, et al. Clinical correlates of the presence of the Asp816Val c-kit mutation in the peripheral blood mononuclear cells of patients with mastocytosis. Cancer. 1998;83:2120–9.

Answer to question 6: B

Educational objective

To know that imatinib mesylate (Gleevec) appears to work only in those patients with systemic mastocytosis (SM) without the *C816V c-kit* mutation

Critique

This man has classic manifestations, pathologic findings, and laboratory evidence of SM. An activation mutation of the *c-kit* receptor gene has been found in the neoplastic cells from many of these patients, and the *D816V* mutation in about 25%. These patients tend to have a more severe disease, often with underlying myelodysplasia or myeloproliferative syndrome. Although it was hoped that imatinib (Gleevec)—which inhibits the adenosine triphosphate binding site of mutated *bcr-abl*, platelet-derived growth factor, and some mutations of *c-kit* in gastrointestinal stromal tumors—would have a beneficial effect in SM patients who had activation mutations of *c-kit*, it does not appear to have activity in SM harboring the *D816V* mutation. The other therapies mentioned would all help in the symptomatic treatment of this patient through inhibiting mast cell degranulation or inhibiting the effects of the secreted products.

Reference

Pardanani A, Elliott M, Reeder T, et al. Imatinib for systemic mast-cell disease. Lancet. 2003;362:535–6.

Answer to question 7: B

Educational objective

To be able to describe the diagnostic criteria for hemophagocytic lymphohistiocytosis (HLH)

Critique

HLH is a multisystem disease that can mimic manifestations of many other disease entities. Because the differential diagnosis is broad and manifestations are nonspecific, diagnosis is often delayed. However, prompt diagnosis and therapy are associated with improved outcomes. Therefore, it is important for the clinician to consider the diagnosis when a patient presents with suggestive symptoms. Fever, anemia, splenomegaly, and a low fibrinogen are typical findings. Although adenopathy may be present, it is not included in the formal diagnostic criteria. Demonstration of low or absent natural-killer cell activity or mutations of the genes that code for perforin provides strong laboratory evidence for HLH but is not generally available in routine clinical labs. Some experts divide HLH into familial and secondary forms, but the distinction can be clinically difficult, and initial treatment is not different. Although systemic lupus erythematosus can be associated with many of these findings, elevated triglycerides (TGs) and low fibrinogen are not typically found. There is no mention of joint swelling or tenderness for juvenile rheumatoid arthritis, and exacerbations are usually marked by hyperfibrinogenemia and thrombocytosis. Diffuse adenopathy, organomegaly, and pancytopenia can be seen with multicentric Castleman disease, but again the TGs and fibrinogen would be atypical, and this patient does not have a known underlying immunodeficiency. Infectious mononucleosis can have very similar manifestations, but there is no mention of a sore throat or a monospot test. The TGs and fibrinogen are once again not typical. However, HLH may complicate infectious mononucleosis.

Reference

Janka GE, Schneider EM. Modern management of children with haemophagocytic lymphohistiocytosis. Br J Haematol. 2004;124:4–14.

Answer to question 8: D

Educational objective

To appreciate that stem cell transplantation is associated with the best outcomes for patients with hemophagocytic lymphohistiocytosis (HLH)

Critique

This boy has a hereditary (familial) form of HLH associated with homozygosity for mutations in the *PRF1* gene. This is associated with a grave prognosis. Prior to the use of aggressive multiagent therapy, mortality was over 90%. Combinations of dexamethasone, etoposide, and cyclosporin have improved this to over 50% at 3 years. Although most of the suggested therapies would be associated with a reasonable likelihood of response, the best overall cure rates are associated with allogeneic stem cell transplantation. Overall survivals of between 58% and 68% have been reported, with a median of 4 to 6 years of follow-up. Although cladarabine combined with CAMPATH-1H might have disease activity, there are no reports of this combination in HLH.

Reference

Arico M, Janka G, Fischer A, et al. Hemophagocytic lymphohistiocytosis. Report of 122 children from the International Registry. FHL Study Group of the Histiocyte Society. Leukemia. 1996;10:197–203.

Answer to question 9: A

Educational objective

To understand that S-100 and CD1a staining are characteristic of Langerhans cells in Langerhans cell histiocytosis (LCH)

Critique

Involvement of a single bone with LCH is not unusual. The diagnosis requires histologic confirmation of Langerhans cells, and this is aided by immunohistochemical stains. Classically, electron microscopy was utilized to demonstrate Birbeck bodies, but due to expense and the need for special processing, this is now rarely done. CD1a, S-100, and langerin are commonly expressed by Langerhans cells. Plasma cells in myeloma would not express either antigen; Ewing sarcoma may express S-100 but not CD1a. The cells in Rosai–Dorfman can express S-100 but should not be CD1a positive.

Reference

Howarth DM, Gilchrist GS, Mullan BP, et al. Langerhans cell histiocytosis: diagnosis, natural history, management, and outcome. Cancer. 1999;85:2278–90.

Answer to question 10: C

Educational objective

To appreciate that eosinophilic granuloma of bone presenting as a solitary lesion is typically self-limited and regression is not unusual

Critique

Important prognostic information in the management of Langerhans cell histiocytosis includes the number and extent of organ involvement and whether organ involvement is associated with organ dysfunction. Although there is some controversy regarding the appropriate treatment of monostotic involvement of the appendicular skeleton, it is generally agreed that such disease has a low likelihood of progression. In fact, regression is well documented. Risk factors for progression include multiorgan involvement or organ dysfunction, multiple bone lesions, and at-risk organ involvement including craniofacial bones, lung, liver, or bone marrow.

Reference

Howarth DM, Gilchrist GS, Mullan BP, et al. Langerhans cell histiocytosis: diagnosis, natural history, management, and outcome. Cancer. 1999;85:2278–90.

Answer to question 11: D

Educational objective

To recognize the clinical features of cyclic neutropenia and the importance of genetic testing for *ELA2* in establishing the diagnosis

Critique

Cyclic neutropenia presents in early childhood with recurrent episodes of infection, typically stomatitis and oral ulcers. Neutrophil counts cycle from normal to <500 cells/ μL. Cyclic neutropenia is usually inherited in an autosomal dominant fashion. The father's history of stomatitis as a child is suggestive of cyclic neutropenia; clinical symptoms in cyclic neutropenia often improve with age. Virtually all patients with cyclic neutropenia have mutations of *ELA2*. Genetic testing for *ELA2* mutations should be done to establish the diagnosis. Antineutrophil antibodies are used to help establish the diagnosis of primary autoimmune neutropenia. Antinuclear antibody testing is not indicated in the absence of symptoms of systemic lupus erythematosus or other autoimmunity syndrome. Though most patients will respond to granulocyte colony-stimulating factor (G-CSF) treatment, so will most other neutropenic syndromes; thus, a trial of G-CSF is not likely to be diagnostic.

References

Horwitz M, Benson KF, Person RE, et al. Neutrophil elastase mutations define a 21-day biological clock in cyclic hematopoiesis. Nat Genet. 1999;23:433–6.

Omar S, Salhadar A, Wooliever DE, et al. Genetics, phenotype, and natural history of autosomal dominant cyclic hematopoiesis. Am J Med Gen. 1996;66:413–22.

Answer to question 12: C

Educational objective

To be able to interpret neutrophil function testing in the diagnosis of chronic granulomatous disease (CGD)

Critique

Serious recurrent infections in a patient with normal levels of circulating neutrophils merit an evaluation for a neutrophil function disorder. The impaired nitroblue tetrazolium (NBT) reduction and oxidation of dihydrorhodamine by neutrophils are diagnostic for CGD. CGD presents in early childhood with recurrent, usually bacterial, infections. Cyclic neutropenia presents with episodic neutropenia; neutrophil function is essentially normal. In Chediak–Higashi syndrome, the neutrophils have characteristic giant inclusion bodies, and neutropenia is common. In myeloperoxidase deficiency, most patients are asymptomatic, and neutrophil NBT reduction is normal. Patients with severe combined immunodeficiency typically present with viral infections, and neutrophil function is normal.

References

Dinauer MC. Chronic granulomatous disease and other disorders of phagocyte function. In: Hematology: ASH Education Program Book. Washington DC: American Society of Hematology; 2005:89–95.

Winklestein JA, Marino MC, Johnston RB Jr, et al. Chronic granulomatous disease: report on a national registry of 368 patients. Medicine. 2000;79:155–69.

Answer to question 13: E

Educational objective

To understand the natural history of primary autoimmune neutropenia

Critique

Primary autoimmune neutropenia usually presents in the first year of life with severe neutropenia (absolute neutrophil count <500/αL), but bacterial infections are usually minor. Antibodies against the neutrophil antigens HNA-1a or HNA-2b are observed in the majority of patients. The clinical course is usually benign, with spontaneous recovery of neutrophil counts in most patients within 2 years. Other than possibly prophylactic antibiotics, no specific therapy is required. Genetic testing for *ELA2* mutations is appropriate where cyclic neutropenia is suspected. The absence of cycling of neutrophils in the blood or accumulation of granulocytic precursors in the bone marrow argues against these diagnoses.

References

Bruin MC, von dem Borne AE, Tamminga RY, et al. Neutrophil antibody specificity in different types of childhood autoimmune neutropenia. Blood. 1999;94:1797–802.

Bux J, Behrens G, Jaeger G, et al. Diagnosis and clinical course of autoimmune neutropenia in infancy: analysis of 240 cases. Blood. 1998;91:181.

Answer to question 14: C

Educational objective

To recognize the clinical features of Shwachman–Diamond syndrome (SDS) and the importance of genetic testing for *SBDS* mutations in establishing the diagnosis

Critique

This patient presents with classic features of SDS including exocrine pancreatic insufficiency (chronic diarrhea), hematopoietic abnormalities (most commonly neutropenia), and short stature. Fatty infiltration of the pancreas is characteristic of SDS. Other causes of congenital neutropenia are less likely because neither severe congenital neutropenia nor WHIM (warts, hypogammaglobulinemia, infections, and myelokathexis) syndrome is associated with exocrine pancreatic insufficiency. More than 90% of cases of SDS are associated with mutations of the *SBDS* gene; thus, genetic testing for *SBDS* mutations is indicated in patients with suspected SDS. Mutations of *ELA2* and *CXCR4* are seen in cyclic neutropenia/severe congenital neutropenia and WHIM syndrome, respectively.

References

Boocock GR, Morrison JA, Popovic M, et al. Mutations in SBDS are associated with Shwachman-Diamond syndrome. Nat Genet. 2003;33:97–10.

Ginzberg H, Shin J, Ellis L, et al. Shwachman syndrome: phenotypic manifestations of sibling sets and isolated cases in a large patient cohort are similar. J Pediatr. 1999;135:81–8.

Answer to question 15: C

Educational objective

To understand that cutaneous mastocytosis is children is generally a self-limited disease that requires only symptomatic treatment

Critique

This boy has urticaria pigmentosa (UP) and has no evidence for systemic mastocytosis (eg, mast cells in the bone marrow or other organ involvement, elevated serum tryptase). UP is typically a self-limited disease that responds to symptomatic treatment with drugs that inhibit mast cell degranulation. The other therapies described might be appropriate for systemic mastocytosis (SM). Imatinib has been shown to have activity in only a minority of patients with SM, generally those without the activating *c-kit* mutation. Regardless, this patient does not require systemic therapy.

Reference

Valent P, Sperr WR, Schwartz LB, et al. Diagnosis and classification of mast cell proliferative disorders: delineation from immunologic diseases and non-mast cell hematopoietic neoplasms. J Allergy Clin Immunol. 2004;114:3–11. Quiz 12.

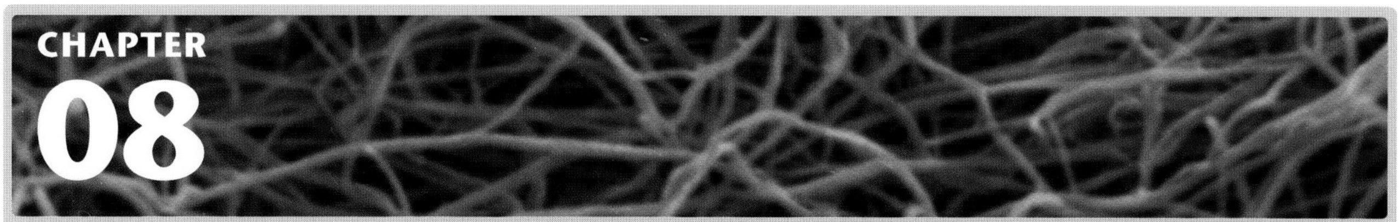

CHAPTER 08 Myeloproliferative disorders

Answer to question 1: D

Educational objective

To recognize mast cell disease associated with a clonal hematologic disorder

Critique

This patient has evidence for both a chronic myeloid disorder (myelodysplastic syndrome with some myeloproliferative features such as megakaryocyte clustering) and mast cell proliferation, including liver involvement with cells exhibiting a typical mast cell phenotype. Mastocytosis can be limited to the skin (cutaneous mastocytosis) or may involve viscera and bone marrow (systemic mastocytosis). Systemic mast cell proliferation can be indolent or aggressive and may also be associated with a coexisting clonal hematologic disorder such as myelodysplastic syndrome or a myeloproliferative disease. *FIP1L1-PDGFRA* gene fusion (due to an interstitial deletion of chromosome 4 and assayed with a fluorescence *in situ* hybridization probe for *CHIC2*) is associated with hypereosinophilia. Although systemic mastocytosis can occasionally be associated with eosinophilic proliferation and the presence of this mutation, in this case, eosinophilia is absent, making involvement of the FIP1L1-PDGFRA tyrosine kinase unlikely. JAK2 V617F is most commonly associated with polycythemia vera and less frequently with essential thrombocythemia and myelofibrosis. Although JAK2 V617F can also occur rarely in other hematologic disorders including mast cell diseases, JAK2 mutations are very uncommonly detectable in myelodysplastic syndrome (<5% of cases), and other mutations are more likely to be present in association with systemic mastocytosis. FLT3 "activation loop" mutations at D835 are associated with acute myeloid leukemia (AML) and found in about 7% of *de novo* AML cases; likewise, FLT3 internal tandem duplications are found in approximately 20% of AML patients. However, FLT3 mutations are rarely detected in chronic myeloid disorders. C-Kit mutations are the most common molecular lesions associated with mastocytosis—both D816V and D816H mutations occur—and these mutations are associated with imatinib resistance. The PDGFRB-EVI6 fusion kinase results from a t(5;12)(q33;p13) translocation and is observed in a rare cases of chronic myelomonocytic leukemia. In contrast to C-Kit D816, chronic myeloid disorders with PDGFRB-EVI6 usually respond to imatinib.

References

Pardanani A. Systemic mastocytosis: bone marrow pathology, classification, and current therapies. Acta Haematol. 2005;114: 41–51.

Pullarkat VA, Bueso-Ramos C, Lai R, et al. Systemic mastocytosis with associated clonal hematological non-mast-cell lineage disease: analysis of clinicopathologic features and activating c-kit mutations. Am J Hematol. 2003;73:12–7.

Answer to question 2: B

Educational objective

To identify appropriate initial management of patients with essential thrombocythemia

Critique

This patient probably has essential (primary) thrombocythemia (ET). The normal C-reactive protein makes an occult inflammatory disorder contributing to reactive thrombocytosis less likely, and chronic myeloid leukemia has been appropriately ruled out by a *BCR-ABL* molecular assay. She is over 60 years of age and now has a thrombotic history, so she is at quite a high risk for a recurrent thromboembolic event. In addition to minimizing other prothrombotic risk factors (eg, smoking) and treating acute clots with the usual anticoagulation, it is important to initiate cytoreductive therapy to decrease the likelihood of future thrombotic events. Hydroxyurea and anagrelide, in combination with low-dose aspirin, were compared head to head with 809 patients in the UK Medical Research Council's Primary Thrombocythaemia 1 study. All endpoints except venous thrombosis favored hydroxyurea, which is also less expensive than anagrelide. Therefore, hydroxyurea is currently considered the first-line drug for ET. This patient has no laboratory evidence of acquired von Willebrand disease, there is no bleeding, and her platelet count is only moderately elevated, so plateletpheresis is unnecessary. Low-dose aspirin (75–250 mg per day) is appropriate, but higher doses of aspirin have been associated with increased bleeding risk, especially in elderly patients. Additionally, it may be better to wait until patients have been treated appropriately for the venous thrombosis and are off warfarin before initiating aspirin therapy. Interferon-α is most appropriate in younger patients who wish to become pregnant or are concerned about the uncertain long-term leukemogenicity of hydroxyurea. Older patients usually find it difficult to tolerate the doses of interferon necessary to achieve adequate platelet suppression.

References

Barbui T, Finazzi G. When and how to treat essential thrombocythemia. N Engl J Med. 2005;353:85–6.

Cortelazzo S, Finazzi G, Ruggeri M, et al. Hydroxyurea for patients with essential thrombocythemia and a high risk of thrombosis. N Engl J Med. 1995;332:1132–6.

Harrison CN, Campbell PJ, Buck G, et al; United Kingdom Medical Research Council Primary Thrombocythemia 1 Study. Hydroxyurea compared with anagrelide in high-risk essential thrombocythemia. N Engl J Med. 2005;353:33–45.

Landolfi R, Marchioli R, Kutti J, et al; European Collaboration on Low-Dose Aspirin in Polycythemia Vera Investigators. Efficacy and safety of low-dose aspirin in polycythemia vera. N Engl J Med. 2004;350:114–24.

Answer to question 3: A

Educational objective

To recognize the role of radiotherapy in the treatment of extramedullary hematopoiesis in myelofibrosis with myeloid metaplasia

Critique

The development of pulmonary hypertension in a patient with a myeloproliferative disorder is associated with a life expectancy of less than 18 months. This complication is most common in chronic idiopathic myelofibrosis (IMF) and can be due to extramedullary hematopoiesis, chronic thromboembolic disease, or both. Rarely, it is present at the time of initial diagnosis of the myeloid disorder. In this case, a nuclear medicine bone marrow scan suggests extensive extramedullary hematopoiesis in the lungs. Responses to hydroxyurea in extramedullary hematopoiesis may be observed but are inconsistent and usually take at least several weeks. In this setting, whole-lung radiotherapy can result in striking, rapid clinical improvement, sometimes normalizing pulmonary pressures. Radiotherapy can also be considered in IMF when extramedullary hematopoiesis threatens the spinal column or other vital tissues, or when patients have indications for splenectomy but are poor surgical candidates. In this patient, there is no evidence of embolic disease, although sometimes only angiography or lung biopsy can define this clearly. Thrombolytic therapy, therefore, is not indicated. Induction chemotherapy with one of the regimens typically used for patients with acute myeloid leukemia is generally ineffective in IMF because any remissions achieved are not durable and marrow aplasia is often prolonged. Epoprostenol is often used for idiopathic (primary) pulmonary hypertension, but its role in secondary pulmonary hypertension, such as that complicating myeloproliferative disorders, is unclear.

References

Dingli D, Utz JP, Krowka MJ, et al. Unexplained pulmonary hypertension in chronic myeloproliferative disorders. Chest. 2001;120:801–8.

Mesa RA, Tefferi A. Surgical and radiotherapeutic approaches for myelofibrosis with myeloid metaplasia. Semin Oncol. 2005;32:403–13.

Rumi E, Passamonti F, Boveri E, et al. Dyspnea secondary to pulmonary hematopoiesis as presenting symptom of myelofibrosis with myeloid metaplasia. Am J Hematol. 2006;81:124–7.

Steensma DP, Hook CC, Stafford SL, et al. Low-dose, single-fraction, whole-lung radiotherapy for pulmonary hypertension associated with myelofibrosis with myeloid metaplasia. Br J Haematol. 2002;118:813–6.

Answer to question 4: D

Educational objective

To understand the role of JAK2 V617F molecular testing in the evaluation of erythrocytosis

Critique

The first task in evaluating erythrocytosis is to determine whether the red cell mass is truly elevated. In the absence of extreme volume depletion, a hemoglobin of 19.2 g/dL is too high to be consistent with relative polycythemia; therefore, formal demonstration of an elevated red cell mass by nuclear medicine testing is unnecessary in this case. The next task in evaluating erythrocytosis is to exclude secondary causes, such as hypoxia or physiologically inappropriate exposure to endogenous/exogenous erythropoietin. The low-normal serum erythropoietin levels in this patient make chronic hypoxia or an erythropoietin-producing tumor unlikely. Although the patient's history of competitive cycling raises the possibility of blood doping with an erythropoietic product, the elevated white count and platelet count are more consistent with a primary hematologic disorder. Ideally, the diagnosis of polycythemia vera (PV) would be confirmed with marrow examination, but JAK2 mutation testing can be performed on peripheral blood if necessary. JAK2 V617F testing may be suitable as a first-intention diagnostic test in the evaluation of erythrocytosis, and some investigators believe this test can spare the majority of patients from further investigations if the results are abnormal. Elevated granulocyte *PRV-1* expression is more common in PV than in secondary erythrocytosis, but this finding provides supportive rather than definitive evidence for a clonal myeloid disorder.

References

James C, Delhommeau F, Marzac C, et al. Detection of JAK2 V617F as a first intention diagnostic test for erythrocytosis. Leukemia. 2006;20:350–3.

Tefferi A, Pardanani A. Mutation screening for JAK2(V617F): when to order the test and how to interpret the results. Leuk Res. 2006;30:739–44.

Answer to question 5: C

Educational objective

To understand the role of molecular testing in the evaluation of thrombocytosis and initiate appropriate initial therapy for a myeloproliferative disorder in a patient desiring pregnancy

Critique

It has long been recognized that chronic myelogenous leukemia (CML) can present with isolated thrombocytosis, but the advent of molecular testing for *BCR-ABL* fusion and the availability of new drugs has made decision making in this setting more challenging. Whether cases of marked isolated thrombocytosis expressing low levels of the *BCR-ABL* fusion gene in the absence of the Philadelphia chromosome are best considered as CML or a variant form of essential thrombocytosis (ET) has long been controversial. (In this patient, the thrombocytosis is probably exacerbated by iron deficiency.) At least one study reported an incidence of 48% of the *BCR-ABL* transcript in 25 Philadelphia-chromosome–negative ET patients, and there were neither clinical nor laboratory differences compared with *BCR-ABL*–negative ET patients. However, other reports have cast doubt on the frequency and clinical relevance of this finding. Responses of these patients when treated with imatinib have often been incomplete. The level of expression of *BCR-ABL* messenger RNA is often much lower in patients presenting with thrombocytosis than in those presenting with a more typical CML picture. BCR-ABL fusion and JAK2 mutations appear to be mutually exclusive. The results of an additional RT-PCR assay would not change initial management. The patient is symptomatic and requires therapy. Because of the patient's desire to become pregnant, interferon-α would be a consideration, and interferon should result in myelosuppression regardless of the underlying diagnosis. Imatinib could also be considered, but hydroxyurea is potentially teratogenic and should not be used in a young woman who is trying to conceive.

References

Blickstein D, Aviram A, Luboshitz J, et al. BCR-ABL transcripts in bone marrow aspirates of Philadelphia-negative essential thrombocytopenia patients: clinical presentation. Blood. 1997;90:2768–71.

Heller P, Kornblihtt LI, Cuello MT, et al. BCR-ABL transcripts may be detected in essential thrombocythemia but lack clinical significance. Blood. 2001;98:1990.

Hsu HC, Tan LY, Au LC, et al. Detection of bcr-abl gene expression at a low level in blood cells of some patients with essential thrombocythemia. J Lab Clin Med. 2004;143:125–9.

Rice L, Popat U. Every case of essential thrombocythemia should be tested for the Philadelphia chromosome. Am J Hematol. 2005;78:71–3.

Answer to question 6: B

Educational objective

To recognize the role of radiophosphorus in treating frail elderly patients with polycythemia vera (PV)

Critique

This patient has high-risk PV that is poorly controlled (the goal hematocrit for men with PV is <45%, and ideally his platelet count would also be lower than it is), and he is at risk for a thrombotic event. Although radiophosphorus was shown to be leukemogenic in long-term randomized studies by the Polycythemia Vera Study Group, it may still play an important cytoreductive role in elderly patients with PV, especially those who have difficulty taking other treatments. Increasing the dose of hydroxyurea would normally be expected to cause further myelosuppression, but this drug has not controlled the patient's blood counts well in the past, and nonhealing ankle ulcers or other skin toxicity that may be associated with hydroxyurea are cause for concern. Anagrelide is likely to be tolerated poorly by this man because it frequently causes fluid retention, and he has a history of heart failure; anagrelide also does little to control other lineages besides the platelet count. The role of anagrelide in PV therapy is unclear. Splenectomy would be very high risk given his general medical condition and might actually worsen the blood counts. Elderly patients tolerate interferon-α poorly.

Reference

Berlin NI. Treatment of the myeloproliferative disorders with 32P. Eur J Haematol. 2000;65:1–7.

Answer to question 7: C

Educational objective

To identify subtypes of hypereosinophilia that are likely to respond to treatment with imatinib mesylate

Critique

This patient has symptoms typical of a hypereosinophilic syndrome (HES) with end-organ involvement due to tissue infiltration by eosinophils, and the presence of a clonal gene rearrangement suggests that his illness is best classified as chronic eosinophilic leukemia (CEL). The most prominently affected organ here is the heart, with Löffler fibroplastic endocarditis and probably an intramural thrombus. There may be involvement of the lung and gut by eosinophilic infiltrates as well. The clinical presentation of HES/CEL is quite variable, and minimal diagnostic criteria and subtype classification are controversial. Even though this patient does not yet meet the formal World Health Organization definition for HES (eosinophil elevation documented for >6 months), he requires urgent treatment. The *FIP1L1-PDGFRA* fusion, due to an interstitial deletion on chromosome 4, predicts responsiveness to imatinib. Doses of imatinib used in this setting are generally lower than those required for treatment of chronic myeloid leukemia, and some patients with CEL will experience a complete hematologic response at a dose of 100 mg daily. Many physicians start corticosteroids at the same time as imatinib in this group of patients. Interferon-α, hydroxyurea, vincristine, 2-CDA, and other therapies could be considered if he were refractory to imatinib and steroids.

References

Gotlib J, Cools J, Malone JM III, et al. The FIP1L1-PDGFRalpha fusion tyrosine kinase in hypereosinophilic syndrome and chronic eosinophilic leukemia: implications for diagnosis, classification, and management. Blood. 2004;103:2879–91.

Vandenberghe P, Wlodarska I, Michaux L, et al. Clinical and molecular features of FIP1L1-PDFGRA (+) chronic eosinophilic leukemias. Leukemia. 2004;18:734–42.

Answer to question 8: E

Educational objective

To distinguish clonal myelofibrosis with myeloid metaplasia from reactive marrow fibrosis and to treat reactive marrow fibrosis

Critique

Marrow fibrosis can be reactive or it can be a consequence of a clonal hematologic disorder. In this patient with a long-standing history of difficult-to-control lupus, high-titer antinuclear antibody, normal marrow karyotype, and negative tests for molecular abnormalities, the possibility of reactive myelofibrosis due to her autoimmune disease is high. The first step would be to adjust her immunosuppressive regimen, including increasing her dose of glucocorticoids, because marrow fibrosis in connective tissue disease is often steroid responsive. Intravenous γ-globulin has also been used in this setting. Hydroxyurea, interferon-α, thalidomide, and marrow transplantation would all be options more suitable for a clonal hematologic disorder such as chronic idiopathic myelofibrosis.

References

Durupt S, David G, Durieu II, et al. Myelofibrosis in systemic lupus erythematosus: a new case. Eur J Intern Med. 2000;11:98–100.

Kiss E, Gal I, Simkovics E, et al. Myelofibrosis in systemic lupus erythematosus. Leuk Lymphoma. 2000;39:661–5.

Paquette RL, Meshkinpour A, Rosen PJ. Autoimmune myelofibrosis. A steroid-responsive cause of bone marrow fibrosis associated with systemic lupus erythematosus. Medicine (Baltimore). 1994;73:145–52.

Answer to question 9: D

Educational objective

To distinguish essential thrombocytosis from other conditions associated with an elevated platelet count

Critique

The pertinent clinical findings in this patient include weight loss, gastrointestinal symptoms, refractory iron deficiency anemia, numerous Howell–Jolly bodies, and thrombocytosis. Howell–Jolly bodies and mild to moderate thrombocytosis suggest hyposplenism. In a patient who has never undergone splenectomy, celiac disease is the leading cause of functional hyposplenism, and celiac disease can also be associated with iron malabsorption. A gluten-free diet should lead to marked clinical improvement, though the hyposplenism may not resolve. The thrombocytosis here is probably a result of both the iron deficiency and the hyposplenism. Anagrelide and hydroxyurea would be considerations if the patient had essential thrombocythemia. Aspirin is not usually necessary for thrombosis prevention in reactive/secondary thrombocytosis. Autologous transplantation could be considered if the patient had systemic amyloidosis, another potential cause of cryptic functional hyposplenism, but the likelihood of sprue is higher, especially with normal serum and urine monoclonal protein studies.

References

Di Sabatino A, Rosado MM, Cazzola P, et al. Splenic hypofunction and the spectrum of autoimmune and malignant complications in celiac disease. Clin Gastroenterol Hepatol. 2006;4:179–86.

Tefferi A, Hanson CA, Inwards DJ. How to interpret and pursue an abnormal complete blood cell count in adults [review]. Mayo Clin Proc. 2005;80:923–36.

Answer to question 10: D

Educational objective

To understand the methods for following a chronic myeloid leukemia (CML) patient initiated on imatinib therapy

Critique

Careful follow-up of patients after they have been started on imatinib is important to identify nonresponding patients or disease relapse. Qualitative polymerase chain reaction (PCR) for the *BCR-ABL* fusion can be used for initial CML diagnosis but cannot be used to follow patients. Standard G-banding cytogenetics is not sensitive enough to follow CML patients in the modern therapeutic era, and cytogenetics would reliably identify only >1 in 100 Philadelphia-chromosome–positive cells, depending on the number of cells analyzed. Fluorescence *in situ* hybridization can be used to follow CML patients, but real-time quantitative reverse transcription PCR is the most sensitive method and has been recommended as the method to follow a patient's clinical response to imatinib.

Reference

Hughes TP, Deininger MW, Hochhaus A, et al. Monitoring CML patients responding to treatment with tyrosine kinase inhibitors—review and recommendations for 'harmonizing' current methodology for detecting BCR-ABL transcripts and kinase domain mutations and for expressing results. Blood. 2006;108:28–37.

Answer to question 11: D

Educational objective

To identify chronic myeloid leukemia (CML) myeloid blast crisis and to initiate therapy correctly

Critique

The patient is diagnosed with acute myeloid leukemia and appropriately begins standard induction chemotherapy. The cytogenetic findings demonstrate that this patient actually has CML in blast phase. Trisomy 8 is observed in myelodysplastic syndromes and other chronic myeloid disorders but is also found in patients with blast phase CML. The goal of blast phase CML therapy is to achieve a second chronic phase and then to proceed to allogeneic stem cell transplant if a suitable donor can be identified; there is no clear benefit from autologous transplantation. Imatinib alone at doses of 600 to 1000 mg/d can achieve a transient hematologic remission in 52% of patients in CML blast phase. Imatinib is the most active agent so far identified for CML patients in blast crisis.

References

Ilaria RL Jr. Pathobiology of lymphoid and myeloid blast crisis and management issues. In: Hematology: ASH Education Program Book. Washington DC: American Society of Hematology; 2005:188–94.

Kantarjian HM, Cortes J, O'Brien S, et al. Imatinib mesylate (STI571) therapy for Philadelphia chromosome-positive chronic myelogenous leukemia in blast phase. Blood. 2002;99:3547–53.

Sawyers CL, Hochhaus A, Feldman E, et al. Imatinib induces hematologic and cytogenetic responses in patients with chronic myelogenous leukemia in myeloid blast crisis: results of a phase II study. Blood. 2002;99:3530–9.

Shimoni A, Kroger N, Zander AR, et al. Imatinib mesylate (STI571) in preparation for allogeneic hematopoietic stem cell transplantation and donor lymphocyte infusions in patients with Philadelphia-positive acute leukemias. Leukemia. 2003;17:290–7.

Answer to question 12: A

Educational objective

To understand that Philadelphia-chromosome–negative chronic myeloid leukemia (CML) must be diagnosed via BCR-ABL–specific molecular probes (FISH or RT-PCR)

Critique

A minority of patients with CML (approximately 5–10%) lack the Philadelphia chromosome; that is, they have no detectable t(9:22) karyotypic abnormality by conventional cytogenetic assays. One third of patients with clinical and laboratory abnormalities typical of CML but who have a normal karyotype actually have the *BCR-ABL* rearrangement detectable at the molecular level. Two assays can appropriately diagnose these cases: polymerase chain reaction to identify the fusion gene or transcripts of the fusion gene, and fluorescence *in situ* hybridization analysis of interphase nuclei. The clinical presentation here with splenomegaly, immature myeloid forms, and basophils on the peripheral smear as well as long-standing leukocytosis makes CML or another myeloproliferative disorder very likely. Imatinib is effective for Ph-negative, BCR-ABL–positive CML because the drug acts to block the tyrosine kinase function of the $p210^{BCR\text{-}ABL}$ oncoprotein; thus, it is important to distinguish whether this molecular lesion is present. This patient is afebrile, has had an elevated white blood count for at least 6 months, and has elevated numbers of basophils on her peripheral smear, making an infection unlikely. The leukocyte alkaline phosphatase (LAP) score could provide helpful supportive evidence, but LAP scores lack sensitivity and specificity for the diagnosis of CML. The lack of the JAK2 V617F mutation and low hemoglobin make the diagnosis of polycythemia vera less likely; therefore, endogenous erythroid colony assays would have a low yield.

Reference

Goldman JM, Melo JV. Chronic myeloid leukemia–advances in biology and new approaches to treatment. N Engl J Med. 2003;349:1451–64.

Answer to question 13: B

Educational objective

To understand the need to adjust the dose of imatinib in a patient with chronic myeloid leukemia (CML) who does not achieve cytogenetic or molecular remission

Critique

Careful follow-up in patients with CML by performing quantitative reverse transcriptase polymerase chain reaction (RT-PCR) every 3 months can identify the development of imatinib resistance at an early stage. An increasing *BCR-ABL* transcript level by quantitative PCR assay identifies patients with the probable development of imatinib resistance, which is generally due to point mutations in the target molecule. Increasing the dose of imatinib in such a patient might induce a response if the particular mutation results in modest resistance or in overexpression of the BCR-ABL protein. However, the responses are usually not durable, so evaluating the patient for allogeneic transplant is reasonable. Holding or stopping the imatinib would not improve the chances of reachieving a remission and might lead to acceleration of the disease. Hydroxyurea is a palliative cytoreductive medication in CML and is not indicated in this situation in which the patient remains in a hematologic remission with only molecular evidence of relapse. The use of newer agents such as dasatinib or referral for a clinical trial would be reasonable, but increasing the dose of imatinib should always be attempted first. This recommendation could change as studies with the newer agents become available.

Reference

Kantarjian HM, Talpaz M, O'Brien S, et al. Dose escalation of imatinib mesylate can overcome resistance to standard-dose therapy in patients with chronic myelogenous leukemia. Blood. 2003;101:473–5.

Answer to question 14: A

Educational objective

To recognize and manage common side effects of imatinib

Critique

Mild side effects such as gastrointestinal discomfort and peripheral edema are common with imatinib therapy and are generally well tolerated with symptomatic treatment. Bone marrow suppression can be dose limiting and can involve all myeloid lineages, and cytopenias are generally more severe with advanced disease. In a study from MD Anderson, 68% of patients on imatinib therapy developed anemia, and most of these patients responded to erythropoietin therapy. Anemia occurs more frequently at higher doses of the drug. There is no clear role for dose reduction of imatinib in chronic myeloid leukemia therapy.

References

Cortes J, O'Brien S, Quintas A, et al. Erythropoietin is effective in improving the anemia induced by imatinib mesylate therapy in patients with chronic myeloid leukemia in chronic phase. Cancer. 2004;100:2396–402.

Deininger MW, O'Brien SG, Ford JM, et al. Practical management of patients with chronic myeloid leukemia receiving imatinib. J Clin Oncol. 2003;21:1637–47.

Answer to question 15: E

Educational objective

To understand the molecular causes of resistance to imatinib and the alternative treatment options available

Critique

This patient never achieved a major molecular remission (defined as >3-log decrease in transcript), and now he has evidence of cytogenetic relapse as well. The availability of a laboratory that can sequence the mutation that is responsible for the imatinib failure can provide important additional information. The T315I mutation results in a BCR-ABL protein that is highly resistant to imatinib as well as newer agents such as dasatinib and AMN107. Hydroxyurea is a palliative cytoreductive medication and is not indicated for molecular or cytogenetic relapse. An autologous stem cell collection would contain hematopoietic progenitors that harbor the T315I mutation. The best treatment option for this patient is allogeneic transplant.

Reference

Druker BJ (Chair), Deininger M, Shah N, et al. Chronic myeloid leukemia. In: Hematology: ASH Education Program Book. Washington DC: American Society of Hematology; 2005:174–94.

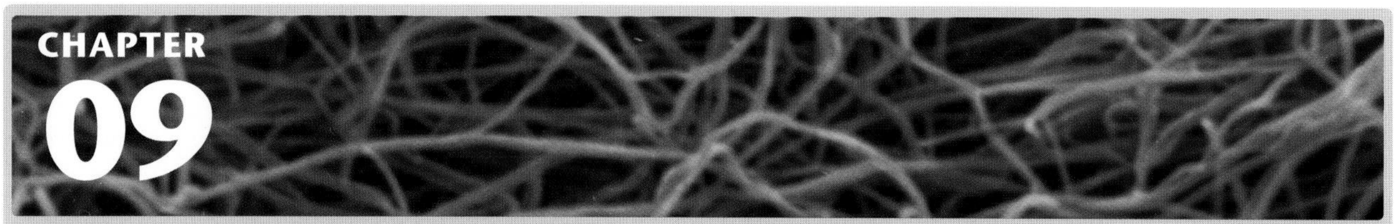

CHAPTER 09

Myelodysplastic syndrome and overlap syndromes

Answer to question 1: D

Educational objective

To understand the risk of iron overload and the potential benefits of iron chelation therapy in myelodysplastic syndrome (MDS)

Critique

Although clinically important systemic iron overload is uncommon in MDS patients at the time of diagnosis, most patients will accumulate potentially harmful levels of tissue iron after they have received 20–30 U of packed red blood cells, which contain approximately 250 mg of elemental iron per unit. The risk of developing iron overload in MDS may be greater in patients with sideroblastic anemia or one of the germ line HFE polymorphisms (eg, C282Y) that are associated with hereditary hemochromatosis. A multivariate analysis published in 2005 demonstrated for the first time that transfusional hemosiderosis designated by a ferritin level $>$1000 μg/L is associated with an increased risk of death in patients with MDS. The hazard ratio for death continues to increase as the ferritin level rises further beyond that level. Patients with higher risk forms of MDS generally do not live long enough for systemic iron accumulation to be a major factor, so the decrease in life expectancy associated with iron overload in MDS is greatest in patients with International Prognostic Scoring System (IPSS) low- and intermediate-1-risk disease, who have relatively longer life expectancies.

This patient has IPSS intermediate-1-risk MDS, which is associated with a median survival of longer than 5 years for patients under the age of 60; therefore, consideration of iron chelation therapy is quite reasonable. In the past, the only effective method of iron chelation therapy available in the United States was an 8–12-hour parenteral infusion of deferoxamine administered 5–7 nights per week. A new tridentate oral iron chelator, deferasirox, is now FDA-approved for treatment of patients older than age 2 with transfusional hemosiderosis and is currently undergoing formal clinical trials in transfusion-dependent MDS patients with IPSS low- and intermediate-1-risk disease. Because this patient has declined other therapies and enjoys travel, it seems unlikely that she would be willing to pursue a cumbersome parenteral infusion regimen, especially with deferasirox now available. So-called short deferoxamine chasers given in the clinic or hospital during or after an episode of transfusion are ineffective and a waste of resources.

References

Greenberg P. Myelodysplastic syndromes: iron overload consequences and current chelating therapies [review]. J Natl Compr Canc Netw. 2006;4:91–6.

Malcovati L, et al. Prognostic factors and life expectancy in myelodysplastic syndromes classified according to WHO criteria: a basis for clinical decision making. J Clin Oncol. 2005;23:7594–603.

Answer to question 2: C

Educational objective

To recognize an acquired disorder of red cell function in myelodysplastic syndrome (MDS) and the associated gene mutation

Critique

Frequently, patients with MDS not only have diminished numbers of fully mature blood cells, but also suffer from functional defects of those cells (eg, poor platelet aggregation or impaired neutrophil chemotaxis). One of the more phenotypically obvious acquired red cell disorders in MDS is α thalassemia, which is usually associated with microcytic and hypochromic erythrocyte indices and with somatic point mutations in ATRX, a chromatin remodeling factor encoded by the X chromosome. When a patient whose origins are in a region of the world (eg, northern and western Europe) where there is a low prevalence of the common inherited forms of thalassemia presents with microcytic/hypochromic red cell indices in the absence of iron deficiency, a mutation of ATRX or of another *trans*-acting factor (eg, GATA1) that regulates globin expression should be considered. Patients with MDS who exhibit microcytic indices and circulating hemoglobin H-containing cells (which are most easily demonstrated by supravital staining) almost always have point mutations in ATRX. This finding is not known to alter the natural history of the disease, but the acquired thalassemia can exacerbate anemia, and some investigators believe the presence of an ATRX-mutant clone may alter response to hypomethylating therapy (azacitidine or decitabine) because ATRX alters DNA methylation globally.

Overall, mutations in *RUNX1/AML1* are the most common point mutations described in MDS to date, but *RUNX1/AML1* mutations have no distinct hematologic phenotype and are most commonly associated with previous radiation exposure and with higher risk disease (especially with excess blasts). *JAK2* mutations are common in myeloproliferative disorders, especially polycythemia vera, but are present in <5% of patients with MDS. *TP53* and *NRAS* point mutations do occur in MDS but are present in <10% of cases and are also more common in advanced or secondary MDS than in early *de novo* MDS cases, such as the patient in this question.

References

Gibbons RJ, et al. Identification of acquired somatic mutations in the gene encoding chromatin-remodeling factor ATRX in the alpha-thalassemia myelodysplasia syndrome (ATMDS). Nat Genet. 2003;34:446–9.

Steensma DP, et al. Acquired alpha-thalassemia in association with myelodysplastic syndrome and other hematologic malignancies. Blood. 2005;105:443–52.

Steensma DP, List AF. Genetic testing in the myelodysplastic syndromes: molecular insights into hematologic diversity. Mayo Clin Proc. 2005;80:681–98.

Answer to question 3: E

Educational objective

To understand the role of recombinant human erythropoietin therapy in the supportive care patients with myelodysplastic syndrome (MDS)

Critique

Approximately 15–25% of unselected patients with MDS will enjoy an improvement in hemoglobin when treated with recombinant human erythropoietin, and some of these individuals will become transfusion independent. Typically, such responses last for up to 1–2 years. Combining epoetin with granulocyte colony-stimulating factor (G-CSF) or granulocyte–macrophage CSF (GM-CSF) can increase the hemoglobin response rate from 15–25% to 35–45%, but combination therapy with myeloid growth factors is often impractical in the United States because of logistical and reimbursement concerns with chronic administration of G-CSF or GM-CSF.

In view of the cost of erythropoietic growth factors and the increasing availability of alternative therapies for MDS, there is growing interest in avoiding this therapy in patients who are quite unlikely to respond. The Nordic MDS Group has generated a useful predictive model for epoetin use in MDS: patients who are transfusion dependent (defined as requiring 2 U of packed red blood cells or more per month) and those who have a serum erythropoietin level of >100 U/L (and especially >500 U/L) are less likely to respond to therapy than those without such adverse features. Patients who have both adverse features (eg, the woman described here) have the lowest response rate to epoetin, <10% overall, and for this reason Medicare does not reimburse erythropoietic growth factor therapy for patients with very high serum epoetin levels (the specific cutoff level varies by state). Additionally, patients with unilineage erythroid dysplasia (eg, refractory anemia) have a higher likelihood of response to erythropoietic growth factors than patients with refractory cytopenia with multilineage dysplasia.

Most published MDS treatment guidelines suggest that if a patient has not responded to adequate doses of an erythropoietic growth factor (ie, at least 60,000 U/week of epoetin alfa, or equivalent doses of another agent) by 8–12 weeks, the agent should be discontinued. Rare patients will respond later than 8–12 weeks, but it is currently not felt to be cost effective to treat patients for longer than this time interval in the absence of a salutary response. Recent clinical trials with darbepoetin using doses higher than suggested in the package insert (eg, 300 μg every week) have reported a hemoglobin response rate with this agent that exceeds 50%. It is not clear if this is due to a simple dose effect, differences between darbepoetin and epoetin, or selection of patients with a higher likelihood of responding to erythropoietin supplementation in modern trials compared to the original epoetin MDS trials initiated in the early 1990s. There is interest in combining erythropoietin with parenteral iron in cancer-associated anemia to overcome "functional" iron deficiency, but iron overload is a more prominent issue in MDS patients, and the risk–benefit ratio of intravenous iron would be higher in this group.

References

Hellstrom-Lindberg E, et al. A validated decision model for treating the anaemia of myelodysplastic syndromes with erythropoietin + granulocyte colony-stimulating factor: significant effects on quality of life. Br J Haematol. 2003;120:1037–46.

Mannone L, et al. High-dose darbepoetin alpha in the treatment of anaemia of lower risk myelodysplastic syndrome: results of a phase II study. Br J Haematol. 2006;133:513–9.

Answer to question 4: A

Educational objective

To recognize the role of lenalidomide in the therapy of patients with myelodysplastic syndrome (MDS) and an abnormality of chromosome 5q31

Critique

Lenalidomide improves anemia in some patients with MDS and a normal marrow karyotype, but this immunomodulatory agent seems to be particularly effective in MDS patients who have an interstitial deletion of chromosome 5q that includes band 31 (eg, q13q35), regardless of karyotypic complexity. The patient presented here has a disorder consistent with typical 5q-syndrome, as defined by the World Health Organization; therefore, she has a high likelihood of responding to lenalidomide therapy. A recent clinical trial of 148 patients with MDS and chromosome 5 deletions that included band q31 revealed that lenalidomide was associated with transfusion independence in 67% of transfusion-dependent patients, and the median hemoglobin improvement was 5.4 g/dL. Complete cytogenetic remissions were also seen. After 2 years of follow-up, the median response duration had not yet been reached. The most common adverse effects of lenalidomide therapy are neutropenia and thrombocytopenia, which require growth factor support and dose reduction in many patients. This patient has adequate baseline white blood and platelet counts (indeed, the platelet count is elevated, as is often the case in 5q-syndrome) and therefore would be a good candidate for lenalidomide therapy.

Antithymocyte globulin improves blood counts in a subset of patients with MDS but has a much lower response rate than lenalidomide, and it is difficult to predict in advance which patients will respond to antithymocyte globulin. This patient has a high endogenous erythropoietin level (typical of patients with 5q-syndrome) and would be unlikely to respond to epoetin alfa or darbepoetin alfa. Stem cell transplantation is most beneficial in MDS patients with higher risk disease, and patients with 5q-syndrome have a life expectancy >8 years with supportive care alone and therefore are not usually appropriate transplant candidates. A hypomethylating agent such as azacitidine or decitabine might be effective, but hematologic response rates in patients with a 5q deletion are much higher with lenalidomide.

References

List A, et al. Efficacy of lenalidomide in myelodysplastic syndromes. N Engl J Med. 2005;352:549–57.

List AF, et al. Lenalidomide in the myelodysplastic syndrome with chromosome 5q deletion. N Engl J Med. 2006;355:1456–65.

Answer to question 5: A

Educational objective

To recognize the clinical features of 5q-syndrome

Critique

This patient has myelodysplastic syndrome (MDS) and, more specifically, 5q-syndrome. 5q-syndrome was first described 30 years ago by Van den Berghe et al., and the World Health Organization classification of myeloid neoplasms has now recognized 5q-syndrome as a distinct type of MDS. Interstitial deletions of the long arm of chromosome 5 that include bands p31–p33 are the only cytogenetic abnormalities in 5q-syndrome.

There is a distinct female preponderance, and the median age at diagnosis is 68 years. Hematologic abnormalities associated with 5q-syndrome are macrocytic anemia, erythroid hypoplasia, and monolobulated megakaryocytes. Macrocytic anemia is frequently the only remarkable hematologic alteration. Leukopenia, when present, is mild, and platelet counts are usually normal or increased. Prognosis is favorable, and transformation to acute myeloid leukemia (AML) is less common than in other subtypes of MDS. The indolent course and chronicity of the 5q-syndrome often result in transfusion dependence in these patients, along with the associated transfusion management issues (eg, iron overload, volume management).

References

Boultwood J, et al. Blood. 1994;84:3253.

Harris NL, et al. J Clin Oncol. 1999;17:3835.

Mathew T, et al. Blood. 1993;81:1040.

Van den Berghe H, et al. Nature. 1974;251:437.

Answer to question 6: C

Educational objective

To know when to consider allogeneic transplantation as a treatment option for patients with myelodysplastic syndrome (MDS)

Critique

The International Prognostic Scoring System (IPSS) was developed to reliably estimate survival and risk of transformation to acute myeloid leukemia (AML). The IPSS assigns a score value based on the percentage of blasts in bone marrow, the initial chromosomal abnormalities, and the number of cytopenias. This patient's IPSS is calculated at 0, which would mean that he has low-risk disease.

To date, the only curative treatment for MDS is high-dose chemotherapy with allogeneic bone marrow transplantation. The optimal timing of this procedure has been evaluated in study by Cutler et al. (2004). In that study, it was shown that for low- and intermediate-1 (int-1)-risk IPSS groups, transplantation at the time of leukemic progression was associated with a higher life expectancy than was the strategy of transplantation at the time of diagnosis. For both of these risk groups, however, transplantation at a fixed interval after diagnosis (but prior to the development of AML) was the strategy that maximized overall discounted life years. For the more advanced IPSS risk groups (int-2 and high), the strategy that maximized discounted life expectancy was transplantation at the time of diagnosis. Given these data and given that the patient has low-risk disease, strategies to reduce his transfusion requirements are recommended, and allogeneic transplantation should be considered at the time of disease progression.

References

Cutler CS, et al. Blood. 2004;104:579.
Deeg HJ, et al. Blood. 2000;95:1188.
Greenberg P, et al. Blood. 1997;89:2079.

Answer to question 7: E

Educational objective

To recognize clinical and biologic features of juvenile myelomonocytic leukemia (JMML)

Critique

This patient has a classic constellation of findings that support a diagnosis of JMML. Boys are affected much more often than girls—this male predilection is present in children who develop JMML in the context of a genetic predisposition such as *NF1* (as in this case) or Noonan syndrome. Children with Fanconi anemia are at increased risk of developing myelodysplastic syndrome (MDS) and acute myeloid leukemia, but not JMML. Cell culture and cytogenetic studies can provide important additional diagnostic information. A hallmark of JMML is selective pattern of hypersensitive growth in response to the growth factor granulocyte–macrophage colony-stimulating factor. Monosomy 7 is a frequent cytogenetic finding that would also support this diagnosis. Whereas bone marrow hypercellularity, morphologic dysplasia, and peripheral cytopenias are classic features of MDS, children with JMML present with a mixed pattern of dysplasia in association with prominent myeloproliferation. Adults with chronic myelomonocytic leukemia (CMML) and atypical chronic myelogenous leukemia (CML) show similar findings. As a result, the new category of myelodysplastic/myeloproliferative disorder was developed by the World Health Organization and includes CMML, JMML, and atypical CML. The prognosis is poor in JMML, with very few patients cured without transplantation.

Reference

Lauchle JO, Braun BS, Loh ML, et al. Inherited predispositions and hyperactive Ras in myeloid leukemogenesis. Pediatr Blood Cancer. 2006;46:579–85.

Answer to question 8: C

Educational objective

To recognize the characteristic features of alkylator-induced myelodysplastic syndrome (MDS)

Critique

This unfortunate young lady has developed MDS as a result of therapeutic exposure to mutagenic chemotherapeutic agents and radiation. Cases of therapy-induced myeloid malignancies arising in adults and children share similar clinical and biologic features. In this patient, the time of disease onset and MDS presentation are most consistent with alkylator-induced MDS, which is most often associated with monosomy 7. By contrast, patients who develop therapy-related myeloid malignancies after exposure to etoposide typically present with acute leukemia after shorter latency. In most of these cases, cytogenetic analysis reveals 11q23 translocations, which fuse the *MLL* gene to multiple partner genes. There is no evidence that intensive chemotherapy improves the dismal outcome in patients with therapy-associated MDS. The most appropriate management for this child is to proceed directly to allogeneic stem cell transplantation after a suitable donor is identified.

Reference

Smith SM, Le Beau MM, Huo D, et al. Clinical-cytogenetic associations in 306 patients with therapy-related myelodysplasia and myeloid leukemia: the University of Chicago series. Blood. 2003;102:43–52.

Answer to question 9: B

Educational objective

To understand how studies of patients with inherited predispositions can provide molecular insights regarding the pathophysiology of myeloid malignancies

Critique

Children with NF1 and Noonan syndrome are predisposed to juvenile myelomonocytic leukemia (JMML) and chronic myelomonocytic leukemia (CMML). The *NF1* tumor suppressor gene encodes a protein called "neurofibromin," which accelerates hydrolysis of active GTP-bound Ras to Ras-GDP. The normal copy of the *NF1* gene is deleted in many JMML samples. Noonan syndrome is caused by point mutations in the *PTPN11* gene, which encode SHP-2 proteins with increased phosphatase activity. Somatic *PTPN11* mutations are detected in ~35% of JMML specimens from patients without Noonan syndrome. Studies in cell lines and in animal models have shown that SHP-2 is a positive effector of Ras signaling. These 2 familial cancer syndromes implicating hyperactive Ras in leukemogenesis are also consistent with the finding of RAS mutations in ~25% of JMMLs and in ~40% of CMMLs. It is of further interest that strains of mice engineered to express a mutant *Ras* allele or that have inactivated *Nf1* within the hematopoietic compartment develop myeloid disorders that model JMML and CMML. Whereas the Jak/STAT pathway is frequently activated by growth factor receptors, there is limited genetic data implicating this canonical pathway in overlap disorders. Somatic *JAK2* mutations are common in polycythemia vera, and germ line mutations have been reported in some patients. Somatic *c-kit* mutations are found in some cases of acute myeloid leukemia but have not been detected in overlap syndromes. The PI3 kinase/Akt pathway is a downstream target of Ras in many cell types, but isolated mutations of components of this pathway are not found in JMML or CMML.

Reference

Lauchle JO, Braun BS, Loh ML, et al. Inherited predispositions and hyperactive Ras in myeloid leukemogenesis. Pediatr Blood Cancer. 2006;46:579–85.

CHAPTER

10

Acute myeloid leukemia

Answer to question 1: C

Educational objective

To recognize the standard approach in treating core binding factor leukemia

Critique

The patient is a young man with inv(16), who has responded to one induction therapy course. His chances for prolonged event-free survival are favorable. His disease is very sensitive to cytarabine, and his consolidation should contain high-dose cytarabine-based courses. There is no evidence that therapy beyond a total of 4 courses is of clinical benefit. Stem cell transplant in the first complete remission is not indicated, even if a related donor is available, because the risks of transplants outweigh the benefits in this favorable acute myelogenous leukemia subtype.

References

Gibson BES, Wheatley K, Hann IM, et al. Treatment strategy and long-term results in paediatric patients treated in consecutive UK AML trials. Leukemia. 2006;19:2130–8.

Marcucci G, Mrozek K, Ruppert AS, et al. Prognostic factors and outcome of core binding factor acute myeloid leukemia patients with t(8;21) differ from those of patients with inv(16): a Cancer and Leukemia Group B study. J Clin Oncol. 2005;23:5705–17.

Schlenk RF, Benner A, Krauter J, et al. Individual patient data-based meta-analysis of patients aged 16 to 60 years with core binding factor acute myeloid leukemia: a survey of the German Acute Myeloid Leukemia Intergroup. J Clin Oncol. 2004;22:3741–50.

Answer to question 2: D

Educational objective

To manage acute myelogenous leukemia (AML) relapse

Critique

The patient has AML relapse 6 months after completing 4 courses of AML therapy. He is not a candidate for a phase I agent because he has a reasonable chance for long-term survival with chemotherapy followed by stem cell transplantation (SCT). Standard induction with 3 doses of an anthracycline combined with 7 days of cytarabine infusion can be used; however, most commonly salvage will consist of a high-dose cytarabine regimen in combination with fludarabine, anthracycline, or both (eg, FLAG, Ida-FLAG, etc.). Chance of maintaining remission is <10% using chemotherapy alone. Even when the donor is readily available, SCT should not be performed before attempting to reduce the leukemia burden.

References

Breems DA, Van Putten WLJ, Huijgens PC, et al. Prognostic index for adult patients with acute myeloid leukemia in first relapse. J Clin Oncol. 2005;23:1969–78.

Craddock C, Tauro S, Moss P, et al. Biology and management of relapsed acute myeloid leukaemia. Br J Haematol. 2005;129:18–34.

Answer to question 3: D

Educational objective

To recognize that acute myelogenous leukemia (AML) following myelodysplastic syndrome (MDS) is a clinical diagnosis and that dysplastic changes can be seen in t(8;21) AML and do not affect the diagnosis or the prognosis

Critique

The distinction between de novo AML and AML after MDS is a clinical one. This patient has no antecedent history of hematologic disorders to suggest MDS. The dysplastic features observed in the marrow have been associated with t(8;21) AML and have no influence on prognosis. The bruising is secondary to low platelets, not to disseminated intravascular coagulation, which is a common presentation in acute promyelocytic leukemia (APL). Moreover, APL is associated wit t(15;17), not t(8;21). This patient has a core binding factor leukemia, which has favorable outcome and is sensitive to cytarabine.

References

Haferlach T, Bennett JM, Loffler H, et al. Acute myeloid leukemia with translocation (8;21). Cytomorphology, dysplasia and prognostic factors in 41 cases. AML Cooperative Group and ECOG. Leuk Lymphoma. 1996;23:227–34.

Marcucci G, Mrozek K, Ruppert AS, et al. Prognostic factors and outcome of core binding factor acute myeloid leukemia patients with t(8;21) differ from those of patients with inv(16): a Cancer and Leukemia Group B study. J Clin Oncol. 2005;23:5705–17.

Answer to question 4: D

Educational objective

To recognize risk and characteristics of secondary acute myelogenous leukemia/myelodysplastic syndrome (AML/MDS) following treatment with alkylating agents

Critique

Patients with Hodgkin disease who are treated with alkylating agents, irradiation, or the combination are at increased risk of developing AML and MDS. The latency period is typically 5 to 10 years and is often preceded by myelodysplasia. Deletions or monosomies of chromosomes 5 and 7 are common. Translocations involving 11q23 are associated with AML induced by topoisomerase II inhibitors, have a shorter latency period, and usually are not preceded by dysplasia. t(12;22) is a favorable translocation present in 25% of pediatric acute lymphoblastic leukemia and is extremely rare in adolescents and young adults. Bone marrow involvement with Hodgkin disease is not likely in the absence of systemic evidence of recurrence. In addition, relapsed Hodgkin disease is unlikely after being in a complete remission for 10 years.

References

Block AMW, Carroll AJ, Hagemeijer A, et al. Rare recurring balanced chromosome abnormalities in therapy-related myelodysplastic syndromes and acute leukemia: report from an international workshop. Genes Chromosomes Cancer. 2002;33:401–12.

Josting A, Wiedenmann S, Franklin J, et al. Secondary myeloid leukemia and myelodysplastic syndromes in patients treated for Hodgkin's disease: a report from the German Hodgkin's Lymphoma Study Group. J Clin Oncol. 2003;21:3440–6.

Smith SM, LeBeau M, Huo D, et al. Clinical-cytogenetic associations in 306 patients with therapy-related myelodysplasia and myeloid leukemia: the University of Chicago series. Blood. 2003;102:43–52.

Answer to question 5: E

Educational objective

To recognize and manage leukostasis (to recognize the hyperleukocytosis syndrome in acute leukemia)

Critique

The patient has an elevated white blood cell count, resulting in leukostasis with bilateral thickening of the peribronchovasculature interstitium and interlobar septa and causing respiratory difficulty, hypoxia-induced drowsiness, and bilateral diffuse infiltrates. Transfusions would increase blood viscosity and the risk of respiratory failure and intracranial hemorrhage and should be held because the anemia is not critical. Leukapheresis is lifesaving and should be initiated as soon as possible; however, it is of only transient benefit. Diagnosis should be promptly established and treatment initiated.

References

Creutzig U, Zimmermann M, Reinhardt D, et al. Early deaths and treatment-related mortality in children undergoing therapy for acute myeloid leukemia: analysis of the multicenter clinical trials AML-BFM 93 and AML-BFM 98. J Clin Oncol. 2004;22:4384–93.

Lowe EJ, Pui CH, Hancock ML, et al. Early complications in children with acute lymphoblastic leukemia presenting with hyperleukocytosis. Pediatr Blood Cancer. 2005;45:10–5.

Novotny JR, Müller-Beiβenhirtz H, Herget-Rosenthal S, et al. Grading of symptoms in hyperleukocytic leukaemia: a clinical model for the role of different blasts types and promyelocytes in the development of leukostasis syndrome. Eur J Haematol. 2005;74:501–10.

Answer to question 6: C

Educational objective

To diagnose and treat the all-*trans* retinoic acid (ATRA) syndrome

Critique

This patient has developed ATRA syndrome manifesting with hyperleukocytosis, respiratory symptoms, fluid retention, and fever. Immediate initiation of high-dose dexamethasone is essential in controlling the potentially fatal ATRA syndrome. In addition to initiation of dexamethasone, ATRA could be held until the patient stabilizes, and an anthracycline could be added. The hyperleukocytosis is an early reaction to the differentiating agent ATRA and not an indication of progressive disease, and cytarabine has a minor role in the treatment of acute promyelocytic leukemia.

Reference

Estey E, Thall PF, Pierce S, et al. Treatment of newly diagnosed acute promyelocytic leukemia without cytarabine. J Clin Oncol. 1997;15:483–90.

Answer to question 7: C

Educational objective

To consider treatment options for elderly patients with acute myelogenous leukemia (AML)

Critique

Older patients with AML have unfavorable disease and poor tolerance to chemotherapy. Decisions about treatment options should take into account the poor prognosis as well as the patient's performance status and desire to pursue therapy. This older patient has good performance status and a desire to pursue therapy; otherwise, palliative care would have been a reasonable option. Despite his general good health, the patient should receive adjusted doses of cytarabine because of poor renal clearance and increased risk of neurotoxicity with high-dose cytarabine in the elderly. Use of investigational therapy is also reasonable because some agents (decitabine, clofarabine, gemtuzumab, etc.) are well tolerated and effective in this poor prognosis subgroup of patients. Although all-*trans* retinoic acid is active in acute promyelocytic leukemia, it is not effective in other AML subtypes lacking the *PML-RAR*α rearrangement.

References

Appelbaum FR, Gundacker H, Head DR, et al. Age and acute myeloid leukemia. Blood. 2006;107:3481–5.

Burnett AK, Mohite U. Treatment of older patients with acute myeloid leukemia—new agents. Semin Hematol. 2006;43:96–106.

Estey EH. General approach to, and perspective on clinical research in, older patients with newly diagnosed acute myeloid leukemia. Semin Hematol. 2006;43:89–95.

Answer to question 8: C

Educational objective

To treat pregnant women with acute myelogenous leukemia

Critique

The patient is in her second trimester, and it is safe to treat her leukemia. Delaying chemotherapy or reducing the doses will result in poor outcome. The patient is too far into her pregnancy to recommend a therapeutic abortion, which in the first trimester is recommended to reduce the risks of complications. Holding chemotherapy is only acceptable for a short period if the patient is stable and the delivery due.

Reference

Chelghoum Y, Vey N, Raffoux E, et al. Acute leukemia during pregnancy: a report on 37 patients and a review of the literature. Cancer. 2005;104:110–7.

Answer to question 9: D

Educational objective

To recognize the morphologic and immunophenotypic characteristics of the different acute myelogenous leukemia (AML) subtypes

Critique

The weak myeloperoxidase (MPO) and positive terminal deoxynucleotidyl transferase and CD19 are not by themselves diagnostic of acute lymphoblastic leukemia and can be seen in AML, especially in the poorly differentiated M0. Despite the MPO negativity, detection of Auer rods changes the classification to AML with minimal differentiation (M1). The megakaryocytic markers CD41 and CD61 are negative.

References

Arber DA. Realistic pathologic classification of acute myeloid leukemias. Am J Clin Pathol. 2001;115:552–60.

Harris NL, Jaffe ES, Diebold J, et al. World Health Organization classification of neoplastic diseases of the hematopoietic and lymphoid tissues: report of the clinical advisory committee meeting—Airlie House, Virginia, November 1997. J Clin Oncol. 1999;17:3835–49.

Answer to question 10: C

Educational objective

To recognize preventable causes of early death in acute myelogenous leukemia (AML) patients

Critique

Leukostasis is a clinicopathologic syndrome characterized by abnormal aggregation and clumping of circulating leukemic blasts in tissue microvasculature. The brain and lungs are the most commonly affected organs, resulting in respiratory and neurologic manifestations. Leukostasis is usually associated with a very high number of circulating blasts ($>100{,}000/\mu L$) but has been described with blast counts $<50{,}000/\mu L$. Interactions between leukemic blasts and the surface of endothelial cells, and a difference in the expression of adhesion molecules on the blast cell surfaces, may explain the higher incidence of leukostasis in AML (especially in the monocytic subtypes) versus acute lymphoblastic leukemia (ALL), although ALL is more frequently associated with hyperleukocytosis than AML. Hyperleukocytosis is a medical emergency that needs prompt cytoreductive modalities including chemotherapy and/or leukophoresis in order to prevent respiratory failure or intracranial hemorrhage. Central nervous system (CNS) involvement is not common in AML, and more common causes of altered mental status would be leukostasis, hypoxia, CNS bleed, or similar complications. Although tumor lysis can occur in AML, it is not as frequent as in B- and T-cell hematologic malignancies. Superior vena cava syndrome, a group of symptoms resulting from partial occlusion of the superior vena cava, is reported with several solid tumors, lymphomas, and T-lineage hematologic malignancies.

References

Creutzig U, Zimmermann M, Reinhardt D, et al. Early deaths and treatment-related mortality in children undergoing therapy for acute myeloid leukemia: analysis of the multicenter clinical trials AML-BFM 93 and AML-BFM 98. J Clin Oncol. 2004;22:4384–93.

Fenaux P, Chastang C, Chevret S, et al. A randomized comparison of all *trans*-retinoic acid (ATRA) followed by chemotherapy and ATRA plus chemotherapy and the role of maintenance therapy in newly diagnosed acute promyelocytic leukemia. The European APL Group. Blood. 1999;94:1192–200.

Novotny JR, Müller-Beißenhirtz H, Herget-Rosenthal S, et al. Grading of symptoms in hyperleukocytic leukaemia: a clinical model for the role of different blast types and promyelocytes in the development of leukostasis syndrome. Eur J Haematol. 2005;74:501–10.

Answer to question 11: D

Educational objective

To treat acute promyelocytic leukemia

Critique

Unlike other acute myelogenous leukemia (AML) French-American-British classification subtypes, acute promyelocytic leukemia (APL) is very sensitive to differentiating agents like all-*trans* retinoic acid (ATRA) and arsenic compounds. Maintenance therapy with ATRA and low-dose chemotherapy improves APL outcome, whereas low-dose maintenance therapy has no role in the treatment of other AML subtypes. APL is sensitive to anthracyclines. Cytarabine, which is a main component of standard AML therapy, has a minor role in APL.

References

Estey E, Thall PF, Pierce S, et al. Treatment of newly diagnosed acute promyelocytic leukemia without cytarabine. J Clin Oncol. 1997;15:483–90.

Fenaux P, Chastang C, Chevret S, et al. A randomized comparison of all *trans*-retinoic acid (ATRA) followed by chemotherapy and ATRA plus chemotherapy and the role of maintenance therapy in newly diagnosed acute promyelocytic leukemia. The European APL Group. Blood. 1999;94:1192–200.

Answer to question 12: C

Educational objective

To recognize and manage transient myeloproliferative disorders (TMDs) of the newborn

Critique

Infants with Down syndrome are prone to develop TMDs, which are undistinguishable from acute leukemia by clinical and morphologic criteria. The blasts look like acute myelogenous leukemia (AML) French-American-British classification M7, and the cytogenetics occasionally show a clonal trisomy 8 in addition to the constitutional trisomy 21. TMD usually resolves spontaneously or after minimal treatment. In this patient, observation is sufficient. Exchange transfusion is indicated to reduce or prevent hyperviscosity if the white blood cell count (WBC) increases over 100,000/μL or if there are signs of hyperviscosity or anemia. Exchange transfusion is usually sufficient, but occasionally low-dose cytarabine is also needed to control the high white count. The WBC usually normalizes over the first few weeks of life. Approximately 25% of these cases will develop AML within the first year of life, at which time they should receive AML therapy. M7 is usually associated with t(1;22) in children and with 3q abnormalities in adults.

References

Athale UH, Razzouk B, Raimondi SC, et al. Biology and outcome of childhood acute megakaryoblastic leukemia: a single institution experience. Blood. 2001;97:3727–32.

Duchayne E, Fenneteau O, Pages MP, et al. Acute megakaryoblastic leukaemia: a national clinical and biological study of 53 adult and childhood cases by the Groupe Français d'Hematologie Cellulaire (GFHC). Leuk Lymphoma. 2003;44:49–58.

Paredes-Aguilera R, Romero-Guzman L, Lopez-Santiago N, et al. Biology, clinical, and hematologic features of acute megakaryoblastic leukemia in children. Am J Hematol. 2003;73:71–80.

Webb D. Optimizing therapy for myelid disorders of Down syndrome. Br J Haematol. 2005;131:3–5.

Answer to question 13: B

Educational objective

To recognize risks and characteristics of acute myelogenous leukemia (AML) following prior treatment with topoisomerase II inhibitors

Critique

Exposure to topoisomerase II inhibitors is associated with treatment-related AML, frequently showing monocytic differentiation and a balanced 11q23 translocation with chromosomes 6, 9, or 19. The latency period is relatively short, usually between 1 to 3 years. AML induced by alkylating has a longer latency period and is associated with changes in chromosomes 5 and 7, rather than 11. Cranial irradiation is associated with secondary malignancies, usually following longer latency periods, and most commonly brain tumors, not AML, with chromosome 11 translocation.

References

Block AMW, Carroll AJ, Hagemeijer A, et al. Rare recurring balanced chromosome abnormalities in therapy-related myelodysplastic syndromes and acute leukemia: report from an international workshop. Genes Chromosomes Cancer. 2002;33:401–12.

Josting A, Wiedenmann S, Franklin J, et al. Secondary myeloid leukemia and myelodysplastic syndromes in patients treated for Hodgkin's disease: a report from the German Hodgkin's Lymphoma Study Group. J Clin Oncol. 2003;21:3440–6.

Schoch C, Schnittger S, Klaus M, et al. AML with 11q23/*MLL* abnormalities as defined by the WHO classification: incidence, partner chromosomes, FAB subtype, age distribution, and prognostic impact in an unselected series of 1897 cytogenetically analyzed AML cases. Blood. 2003;102:2395–402.

Smith SM, LeBeau M, Huo D, et al. Clinical-cytogenetic associations in 306 patients with therapy-related myelodysplasia and myeloid leukemia: the University of Chicago series. Blood. 2003;102:43–52.

Answer to question 14: B

Educational objective

To recognize the clinical and pathologic characteristics of t(9;11) acute myelogenous leukemia (AML)

Critique

The patient has AML French-American-British (FAB) classification M5 with t(9;11), which is frequently associated with hyperleukocytosis and tissue infiltration, particularly the gingiva. The phenytoin can cause gingival hypertrophy but does not account for the other symptoms and findings. Gingival hypertrophy can occur with other leukemia subtypes, including t(8;21) and inv(16), although less frequently. The myeloperoxidase negativity further points to AML FAB M5 t(9:11); the monoblasts will show intense nonspecific esterase activity.

References

Harris NL, Jaffe ES, Diebold J, et al. World Health Organization classification of neoplastic diseases of the hematopoietic and lymphoid tissues: report of the clinical advisory committee meeting—Airlie House, Virginia, November 1997. J Clin Oncol. 1999;17:3835–49.

Tallman MS, Kim HT, Paietta E, et al. J. Acute monocytic leukemia (French-American-British classification M5) does not have a worse prognosis than other subtypes of acute myeloid leukemia: a report from the Eastern Cooperative Oncology Group. Clin Oncol. 2004;22:1276–86.

Answer to question 15: D

Educational objective

To diagnose megakaryocytic leukemia

Critique

AML FAB M7 is rare and can be difficult to diagnose because of associated marrow fibrosis, limiting material available for establishing the diagnosis. Other leukemias, including acute lymphoblastic leukemia (ALL), can be associated with a difficult marrow aspirate secondary to a packed marrow. The blue round cells can also be confused with solid tumors like Ewing and neuroblastoma, especially in association with a negative myeloperoxidase and absence of ALL markers. The extensive fibrosis and cytoplasmic blebbing are characteristic, although not diagnostic, of M7. Definite diagnosis used to be made by positive platelet peroxidase on electron microscopy but has been replaced by the faster detection of the megakaryocytic markers CD41 and CD61 by flow cytometry. t(1;22) is associated with M7 in children, whereas abnormalities of chromosomes 3, 5, and 7 are more common in adults with M7.

References

Athale UH, Razzouk B, Raimondi SC, et al. Biology and outcome of childhood acute megakaryoblastic leukemia: a single institution experience. Blood. 2001;97:3727–32.

Duchayne E, Fenneteau O, Pages MP, et al. Acute megakaryoblastic leukaemia: a national clinical and biological study of 53 adult and childhood cases by the Groupe Français d'Hematologie Cellulaire (GFHC). Leuk Lymphoma. 2003;44:49–58.

Paredes-Aguilera R, Romero-Guzman L, Lopez-Santiago N, et al. Biology, clinical, and hematologic features of acute megakaryoblastic leukemia in children. Am J Hematol. 2003;73:71–80.

Tallman MS, Andersen JW, Schiffer CA, et al. ALL-*trans* retinoic acid in acute promyelocytic leukemia: long-term outcomes and prognostic factor analysis from the North American Intergroup protocol. Blood. 2002;100:4298–302.

CHAPTER 11

Acute lymphoblastic leukemia and lymphoblastic lymphoma

Answer to question 1: C

Educational objective

To recognize that Philadelphia chromosome-positive acute lymphoblastic leukemia (ALL) is not cured with standard chemotherapy and that allogeneic stem cell transplant (SCT) is the only known curative approach

Critique

This question highlights the prognostic significance of specific immunophenotypic and molecular cytogenetic subsets in ALL and the notion that treatment plans should be modified according to these characteristics. Patients A and C fall into the most favorable prognostic subsets of ALL and have excellent survival when treated according to current pediatric regimens. Young adults with precursor T-cell ALL also have expected disease-free survival (DFS) of from 60% to 83% in pediatric and adult series; allogeneic SCT in first complete remission is not recommended for these patients. However, patients with Philadelphia chromosome-positive ALL (patient C) fare poorly with traditional chemotherapeutic approaches for ALL, with expected survival of <10%. These patients have been shown to have improved outcomes if allogeneic SCT can be performed in first remission. The addition of imatinib to frontline therapies may further improve response rates and enhance DFS following allogeneic SCT. At this time, allogeneic SCT still remains the treatment of choice for eligible patients.

References

Dombret H, Gabert J, Boiron JM, et al. Outcome of treatment in adults with Philadelphia chromosome-positive acute lymphoblastic leukemia—results of the prospective multicenter LALA-94 trial. Blood. 2002;100:2357–66.

Faderl S, Jeha S, Kantarjian HM. The biology and therapy of adult acute lymphoblastic leukemia. Cancer. 2003;98:1337–54.

Ottmann OG, Wassmann B. Treatment of Philadelphia chromosome-positive acute lymphoblastic leukemia. In: Hematology: ASH Education Program Book. Washington, DC: American Society of Hematology; 2005:118–22.

Thomas DA, Faderl S, Cortes J, et al. Treatment of Philadelphia chromosome-positive acute lymphocytic leukemia with hyper-CVAD and imatinib mesylate. Blood. 2004;103:4396–407.

Answer to question 2: A

Educational objective

To recognize presenting characteristics and biologic features of mature B-cell acute lymphoblastic leukemia (ALL) and identify the most effective therapeutic approach for these patients

Critique

The patient is a young woman with a mature B-cell (Burkitt) ALL. The lymphoblasts have a characteristic morphologic appearance and have strong expression of CD20 and surface immunoglobulin (in contrast to precursor-B ALL). Mature B-cell ALL is characterized by the presence of chromosome translocations that result in overexpression of the *c-MYC* protooncogene on chromosome 8q24. These include the t(8;14), t(2;8), and t(8;22). Due to the tumor bulk and rapid cycling time of these leukemias, careful prophylaxis and monitoring for tumor lysis is mandatory. Most regimens employ a prephase of treatment to minimize risk of tumor lysis that usually includes a glucocorticoid with or without low doses of an alkylating agent. These patients have been shown to benefit from an intensive short-course (typically 16–20 weeks) of cyclic chemotherapy with fractionated doses of alkylating agents, high-dose methotrexate, and intensive central nervous system (CNS) prophylaxis due to the high risk of CNS involvement. With this approach, the majority of these patients are now enjoying prolonged disease-free survival. There has been no proven efficacy for the use of prolonged maintenance therapy for this subset of ALL. Finally, the use of the targeted tyrosine kinase inhibitor imatinib is not appropriate in this case. Imatinib targets the abl tyrosine kinase overexpressed in leukemias with the t(9;22) or the Philadelphia chromosome translocation. The patient described here has a translocation involving the *c-MYC* protooncogene. Imatinib does not target the deregulated *c-MYC*; therefore, there is no role for its use in mature B-cell ALL.

References

Patte C, Auperin A, Michon J, et al. The Societe Francaise d'Oncologie Pediatrique LMB89 protocol: highly effective multiagent chemotherapy tailored to the tumor burden and initial response in 561 unselected children with B-cell lymphomas and L3 leukemia. Blood. 2001;97:3370–9.

Rizzieri DA, Johnson H, Niedzwiecki D, et al. Intensive chemotherapy with and without cranial radiation for Burkitt leukemia and lymphoma: final results of Cancer and Leukemia Group B Study 9251. Cancer. 2004;100:1343–448.

Answer to question 3: D

Educational objective

To recognize cumulative toxicities of the agents that are used to treat acute lymphoblastic leukemia (ALL)

Critique

This question relates to toxicities of the common agents that are employed in treatment of ALL. Although all of the choices can result in some neurologic toxicity, vincristine-induced peripheral neuropathy, which is cumulative, is the most likely explanation for this patient's symptoms. Other manifestations of vincristine-induced neuropathy include dysesthesia, numbness, foot drop, constipation, and gastroparesis.

References

Faderl S, Jeha S, Kantarjian HM. The biology and therapy of adult acute lymphoblastic leukemia. Cancer. 2003;98:1337–54.

Pui C-H, Evans WE. Drug therapy: treatment of acute lymphoblastic leukemia. N Engl J Med. 2006;354:166–78.

Answer to question 4: B

Educational objective

To manage methotrexate toxicity

Critique

This question describes the methods used to manage methotrexate toxicity. This patient has failed to clear methotrexate adequately. Hydration and alkalinization facilitate methotrexate clearance by the kidneys, whereas sulfa drugs and a variety of other medications inhibit methotrexate secretion into the kidney tubules and should be avoided during methotrexate administration or when methotrexate clearance is impaired. Increasing leucovorin (folinic acid) dose may minimize system toxicities of prolonged methotrexate exposure, including mucositis and severe myelosuppression, and should be administered until the drug levels are $<5 \times 10^6$ mol/L. If methotrexate levels fail to clear quickly with these more conservative methods and the patient remains in acute renal failure after correction of dehydration and treatment of urinary tract infection, then both hemodialysis (only with a high-flux membrane) and the use of carboxypeptidase, a bacterial enzyme that rapidly hydrolyzes methotrexate to inactive metabolites that can be obtained through the National Cancer Institute on a compassionate use basis, should be considered.

References

Wall SM, Hohansen MJ, et al. Effective clearance of methotrexate using high-flux hemodialysis membranes. Am J Kidney Dis. 1996;28:846–54.

Widemann BC, Adamson PC. Understanding and managing methotrexate nephrotoxicity. Oncologist. 2006;11:694–703.

Widemann BC, Balis FM, et al. Caroxypeptidase-G2, thymidine and leucovorin rescue in cancer patients with methotrexate-induced renal dysfunction. J Clin Oncol. 1997;15:2125–34.

Answer to question 5: C

Educational objective

To understand that prognosis for acute lymphoblastic leukemia (ALL) is linked to cytogenetics and that promising new treatment strategies are focusing on new agents targeted to specific immunophenotypic or cytogenetic subsets

Critique

Approximately 50% of cases of precursor B-cell ALL in adults older than age 60 years are Philadelphia chromosome positive (Ph^+), resulting in the *BCR-ABL* fusion gene. These patients have fared poorly with traditional treatment, with a median survival of <12 months. Recently, the addition of imatinib to frontline therapy of patients with Ph^+ ALL has been demonstrated to be feasible, appears to increase remission rates, and already appears to prolong disease-free survival even in patients who do not undergo allogeneic transplant, which is rarely an option for older patients with ALL. Thus, the correct answer to this question is C.

Flt3-activating mutations occur frequently in AML but are not common in adults with ALL. Nelarabine is an agent that has received approval for relapsed precursor T-cell ALL, a subset that occurs uncommonly in older patients with ALL. Myeloablative transplants may be appropriate for only a very selected subset of older patients with ALL due to comorbid conditions present in older adults and the significant toxicity associated with myeloablative transplants and their sequelae.

References

Ottmann OG, Wassmann B. Treatment of Philadelphia chromosome-positive acute lymphoblastic leukemia. In: Hematology: ASH Education Program Book. Washington, DC: American Society of Hematology; 2005:118–22.

Thomas DA, Faderl S, Cortes J, et al. Treatment of Philadelphia chromosome-positive acute lymphocytic leukemia with hyper-CVAD and imatinib mesylate. Blood. 2004;103: 4396–407.

Answer to question 6: D

Educational objective

To identify important biologic and clinical prognostic features in pediatric and adult acute lymphoblastic leukemia (ALL)

Critique

This question incorporates knowledge of clinical and molecular cytogenetic prognostic features. Children ages 2–10 years have the most favorable outcomes of any subset of patients with ALL. In part, this is due to the presence of favorable molecular cytogenetic features in a large percentage of these children, including presence of the *TEL-AML1* fusion gene or a hyperdiploid karyotype. In contrast, infants with ALL often have abnormalities involving the *MLL* gene on chromosome band 11q23 and worse outcomes than older children with ALL. Detection of high levels of minimal residual disease following achievement of remission using either quantitative flow cytometry or polymerase chain reaction is associated with decreased disease-free survival in both pediatric and adult ALL. The Philadelphia chromosome occurs in only about 5% of children with ALL but increases in frequency with age. The outcome of patients with a t(8;14) has improved dramatically with intensive cyclic chemotherapy and is now reported to be 60–85% in both pediatric and adult series.

References

Bruggemann M, Raff T, Flohr T, et al. Clinical significance of minimal residual disease quantification in adult patients with standard-risk acute lymphoblastic leukemia. Blood. 2006;107:1116–23.

Coustan-Smith E, Ribeiro RC, Stow P, et al. A simplified flow cytometric assay identifies children with acute lymphoblastic leukemia who have a superior clinical outcome. Blood. 2006;108:97–102.

Jaffe ES, Harris NL, Stein H, et al., eds. World Health Organization Classification of Tumours of Hameotpoietic and Lymphoid Tissues. Lyon, France: IARC; 2001.

Mortuza FY, et al. Minimal residual disease tests provide an independent predictor of clinical outcome in adult acute lymphoblastic leukemia. J Clin Oncol. 2002;20:1094–104.

Pullen J, Shuster JJ, Link M, et al. Significance of commonly used prognostic factors differs for children with T cell acute lymphocytic leukemia (ALL), as compared to those with B-precursor ALL. A Pediatric Oncologoy Group (POG) study. Leukemia. 1999;13:1696–707.

Wetzler M. Cytogenetics in adult acute lymphocytic leukemia. Hematol Oncol Clin North Am. 2000;14:1237–49.

Answer to question 7: A

Educational objective

To recognize the presenting features of infant acute lymphoblastic leukemia (ALL) and the associated poor prognosis and treatment challenges in this age group

Critique

ALL diagnosed in infancy is associated with high treatment failure that is greatest in infants younger than 3 months and those with a poor early response to prednisone. A poor prognosis is associated with t(4;11) with the *MLL-AF4* fusion gene, which occurs in approximately 50% of cases in infants. Poor outcome in infants with ALL is also associated with an elevated white blood cell count (WBC), central nervous system leukemia, lack of CD10 (CALLA antigen) expression, and poor response to initial treatment. Hyperdiploidy (>50 chromosomes per cell or DNA index >1.16) generally occurs in cases with favorable prognostic factors (aged 1–9 years and a low WBC count) and is itself associated with favorable prognosis. In this case, the cells would not be hyperdiploid.

References

Pui CH, Chessells JM, Camitta B, et al. Clinical heterogeneity in childhood acute lymphoblastic leukemia with 11q23 rearrangements. Leukemia. 2003;17:700–6.

Reaman GH, Sposto R, Sensel MG, et al. Treatment outcome and prognostic factors for infants with acute lymphoblastic leukemia treated on two consecutive trials of the Children's Cancer Group. J Clin Oncol. 1999;17:445–55.

Answer to question 8: C

Educational objective

To know the indications for stem cell transplant in the treatment of childhood acute lymphoblastic leukemia (ALL)

Critique

Hematopoietic stem cell transplantation from a matched sibling donor is the treatment of choice for patients with Philadelphia chromosome-positive ALL. This is probably the one situation in newly diagnosed ALL where transplantation is the treatment of choice if a matched sibling donor is available. The t(12;21) represents the *TEL-AML* translocation and has an excellent outcome. The t(1;19) occurs in 5–6% of childhood ALL and may occur as either a balanced translocation or as an unbalanced translocation and is primarily associated with pre-B ALL. Its presence was initially associated with inferior outcome in the context of antimetabolite-based therapy. Studies have shown that the poorer prognosis associated with the t(1;19) can be largely overcome by more intensive therapy.

Patients with T-cell ALL when treated with appropriately intensive therapy have an outcome similar to that for children with B-precursor ALL. HLA-matched sibling donor transplant has not been proven to be of benefit in patients defined as high risk solely by white blood cell count, gender, and age.

References

Balduzzi A, Valsecchi MG, Uderzo E, et al. Chemotherapy versus allogeneic transplantation for very-high-risk childhood acute lymphoblastic leukaemia in first remission: comparison by genetic randomization in an international prospective study. Lancet. 2005;366:635–42.

Wheeler KA, Richards SM, Bailey CC, et al. Bone marrow transplantation versus chemotherapy in the treatment of very high-risk childhood acute lymphoblastic leukemia in first remission: results from Medical Research Council UKALL X and XI. Blood. 2000;96:2412–9.

Answer to question 9: C

Educational objective

To understand that osteonecrosis (avascular necrosis) is a potential complication of acute lymphoblastic leukemia (ALL) treatment, particularly in the adolescent age range

Critique

With current treatment approaches utilizing postinduction intensification therapy in ALL, steroid-induced osteonecrosis has emerged as a significant complication in the adolescent age group. Typical presentation is in an adolescent patient (females > males) with pain in a weight-bearing joint. Depending on the stage when the problem is first identified, the patient may have negative plain x-rays. Magnetic resonance imaging (MRI) is a more sensitive modality, and if osteonecrosis is present, then other bones need to be examined for involvement by MRI and/or bone scan. Steroids are held once diagnosis is made and analgesia is given. In extreme cases, patients may need surgery, so a high index of suspicion is important.

Reference

Mattano LA Jr, Sather HN, Trigg ME, et al. Osteonecrosis as a complication of treating acute lymphoblastic leukemia in children: a report from the Children's Cancer Group. J Clin Oncol. 2000;18:3262–72.

Answer to question 10: B

Educational objective

To know the prognostic factors associated with outcome after acute lymphoblastic leukemia (ALL) relapse

Critique

The most important factors for prognosis for a child with ALL following relapse are the length of time and the site of relapse. Marrow relapse in B-lineage ALL that occurs during treatment or within 6 months of stopping treatment, or a combined relapse within 18 months of diagnosis, has a very poor outcome (event-free survival of 10–20%). Patients with T-cell ALL who experience a bone marrow relapse with or without a concurrent extramedullary relapse at any point during treatment or off treatment have a very poor outcome. Patients with B-cell ALL who experience an isolated marrow relapse while on treatment or within 6 months of therapy discontinuation, or a combined relapse within 18 months of diagnosis, have a very poor outcome. The following groups have an intermediate prognosis: patients with an extramedullary relapse while on treatment or within 6 months of therapy discontinuation, patients with B-cell ALL and a marrow relapse with or without extramedullary relapse >6 months off therapy, and patients with B-lineage ALL and a combined relapse between 18 and 36 months from diagnosis.

References

Chessells JM, Veys P, Kempski H, et al. Long-term follow-up of relapsed childhood acute lymphoblastic leukaemia. Br J Haematol. 2003;123:396–405.

Roy A, Cargill A, Love S, et al. Outcome after first relapse in childhood acute lymphoblastic leukaemia—lessons from the United Kingdom R2 trial. Br J Haematol. 2005;130:67–75.

Answer to question 11: C

Educational objective

To know the presenting characteristics of T-cell acute lymphoblastic leukemia (ALL) in children and adolescents and the approach to diagnosis

Critique

Biopsy of the mass is not necessary in this case because a bone marrow aspirate is the first step in making this diagnosis. If the bone marrow aspirate is normal, then the pleural effusion could be tapped, and immunophenotyping and cytogenetics could be performed on the fluid to make the diagnosis. The presence of a mediastinal mass along with respiratory symptoms is considered a medical emergency, so the diagnosis should be made as quickly as possible. The most likely diagnosis is T-cell ALL or lymphoblastic lymphoma. In patients with a mediastinal mass, the rate of resolution of the tumor does not appear to have prognostic significance. Patients with T-cell disease and high tumor burden are at high risk for tumor lysis.

References

Attarbaschi A, Mann G, Dworzak M, et al. Mediastinal mass in childhood T-cell acute lymphoblastic leukemia: significance and therapy response. Med Pediatr Oncol. 2002;39:558–65.

Margolin JF, Steuber CP, Poplack DG. Acute Lymphoblastic Leukemia in Pizzo and Poplack Principles and Practice of Pediatric Oncology. Philadelphia: Lippincott Williams & Wilkins; 2006.

CHAPTER 12

Lymphoproliferative disorders

Answer to question 1: B

Educational objective

To recognize the immunophenotypic features of mantle cell lymphoma (MCL)

Critique

MCL cells are monoclonal B cells with relatively intense surface immunoglobulin M (IgM) and IgD. They are typically CD5$^+$; they are usually CD10$^-$, FMC$^+$, and CD20$^+$; and virtually all express cyclin D1. CD23 is usually negative. Follicular lymphomas are usually sIg+, bcl2$^+$, CD10$^+$, CD5$^-$, CD19$^+$, and CD20$^+$. Diffuse large B cell lymphomas express various pan-B markers such as CD19, CD20, CD22, and CD79a but may lack one or more of these. Marginal zone lymphomas have CD20$^+$, CD5$^-$, CD10$^-$, and CD23$^-$.

Reference

Jaffe ES, Harris NL, Stein H, et al., eds. WHO Classification, Tumors of Hematopoietic and Lymphoid Tissues. Lyon: IARC Press; 2001.

Answer to question 2: B

Educational objective

To recognize the role of central nervous system (CNS) prophylaxis in patients with testicular lymphoma

Critique

Testicular large cell lymphoma is associated with a particularly high risk of extranodal relapse even with localized disease at diagnosis. CNS relapse has been reported in 15% of patients. Anthracycline-based chemotherapy, CNS prophylaxis, and contralateral testicular irradiation seem to improve outcome. Although there is no randomized clinical trial that has established its benefit, prophylactic intrathecal chemotherapy is recommended in patients with testicular lymphoma. Other scenarios given are not particularly associated with an increased risk of CNS relapse.

Reference

Zucca E, Conconi A, Mughal TI, et al. Patterns of outcome and prognostic factors in primary large cell lymphoma of the testis in a survey by the International Extranodal Study Group. J Clin Oncol. 2003;21:20–7.

Answer to question 3: C

Educational objective

To understand the importance of confirming histologic diagnosis prior to initiating therapy

Critique

Many of the mediastinal tumors that present like the one in this clinical case have curative potential; therefore, histologic diagnosis should be established prior to starting therapy. Biopsy can be obtained by excision of an enlarged lymph node by mediastinoscopy, mediastinotomy, or thoracotomy. Fine needle aspirate biopsy usually does not provide adequate tissue to establish the diagnosis.

Reference

Lichtenstein AK, Levine A, et al. Primary mediastinal lymphoma in adults. Am J Med. 1980;68:509–14.

Answer to question 4: B

Educational objective

To recognize the role of systemic therapy using high-dose methotrexate in the initial therapy for younger patients with primary central nervous system lymphoma (PCNSL)

Critique

Radiotherapy alone yields only 5–10% survival after 5 years in PCNSL. Addition of chemotherapy has improved the outcome of PCNSL. High-dose methotrexate-containing regimens appear to be associated with significant survival benefit when given prior to radiation therapy. There is no evidence for the utility of monoclonal antibody rituximab in this disease. CHOP (cyclophosphamide, doxorubicin, vincristine, and prednisone) with or without rituximab is ineffective in the treatment of PCNSL because most of these agents do not cross the blood–brain barrier.

Reference

Blay JY, Conroy T, Chevreau C. High dose methotrexate for treatment of primary cerebral lymphomas: analysis of survival and late neurologic toxicity. J Clin Oncol. 1998;16:864–76.

Answer to question 5: A

Educational objective

To recognize the role of methotrexate in the genesis of Epstein–Barr virus (EBV)–positive lymphoproliferative disorders

Critique

EBV-positive lymphoproliferative disorders have been shown to be associated with prolonged use of methotrexate. There is recent evidence that methotrexate may induce EBV replication, at the same time causing immunosuppression. Withdrawing immunosuppression would be the most appropriate next step in this patient who has no B symptoms and has a low-grade histology. If there is no response or progression of disease after discontinuation of methotrexate, rituximab alone or in combination with chemotherapy would be appropriate.

References

Heslop HE. Biology and treatment of Epstein-Barr virus–associated non-Hodgkin lymphomas. In: Hematology: ASH Education Program Book. Washington DC: American Society of Hematology; 2005:260.

Menke DM, Griesser H, Moder KG, et al. Lymphomas in patients with connective tissue disease. Comparison of p53 protein expression and latent EBV infection in patients immunosuppressed and not immunosuppressed with methotrexate. Am J Clin Pathol. 2000;113:212–8.

Answer to question 6: A

Educational objective

To recognize the role of autologous stem cell transplantation in relapsed large B cell lymphoma

Critique

Outcome of autologous stem cell transplantation in relapsed large cell lymphoma has been shown to be superior to conventional salvage chemotherapy. In a randomized study of patients with intermediate- and high-grade non-Hodgkin lymphoma in relapse, 5-year overall survival was 53% and 32% for transplant and chemotherapy arms, respectively ($P = 0.038$). Similarly, the disease-free survival at 5 years was 46% with transplant compared to 12% with chemotherapy ($P = 0.001$). There is no evidence that allogeneic stem cell transplantation in this situation offers any additional benefit. Because the patient relapsed in a short period after CHOP (cyclophosphamide, doxorubicin, vincristine, and prednisone) + rituximab, repeating the chemotherapy is not advisable. There is very limited data on the efficacy and safety of use of radioimmunotherapy in relapsed large cell lymphoma.

Reference

Phillip et al. N Engl J Med. 1995;333:1540–5.

Answer to question 7: E

Educational objective

To identify the role of splenectomy in patients with splenic marginal zone lymphoma

Critique

Splenic marginal zone lymphoma is a unique entity and usually presents with splenomegaly and low blood counts. As with other low-grade lymphoma, asymptomatic patients with normal blood counts may be observed. For patients in whom treatment is indicated, as in this patient who is pancytopenic, splenectomy is the treatment of choice. Many patients do not need additional therapy. If splenectomy cannot be done because of patient preference or comorbid conditions that make the risk of the procedure unacceptable, chemotherapy with CVP (cyclophosphamide, vincristine, and prednisone), CHOP (cyclophosphamide, doxorubicin, vincristine, and prednisone), or rituximab are appropriate options.

Reference

Chacon JI, Mollejo M, Munoz E. Splenic marginal zone lymphoma: clinical characteristics and prognostic factors in a series of 60 patients. Blood. 2002;100:1648–54.

Answer to question 8: A

Educational objective

To recognize the clinical behavior and treatment options for grade IIIB follicular lymphoma (FL)

Critique

Although FL is classified as an indolent lymphoma, grade III FL (follicular large cell lymphoma) has clinical behavior similar to diffuse large B cell lymphoma. For this reason, these patients are usually treated as for diffuse large B cell lymphomas. Because this patient had no previous therapy, CHOP (cyclophosphamide, doxorubicin, vincristine, and prednisone) + rituximab is an appropriate therapy. There is no clear evidence of benefit from autologous stem cell transplant as frontline therapy or consolidation in first complete remission.

Reference

Rodriguez J, McLaughlin P, Hagemeister FB. Follicular large cell lymphoma: an aggressive lymphoma that often presents with favorable prognosis. Blood. 1999;93:2202–7.

Answer to question 9: A

Educational objective

To discuss the treatment options of an elderly patient with low-grade lymphoma who has severely compromised cardiac function and significant involvement of marrow by lymphoma

Critique

When treatment options are selected for patients with low-grade lymphomas, both the need for therapy and the patient's ability to tolerate therapy should be taken into consideration. This patient needs therapy because she is symptomatic with significant tumor mass. Because of severely compromised cardiac function, anthracycline therapy is not a good choice. Radioimmunotherapy is not a good choice particularly because its safety in patients with >25% involvement of bone marrow is not established. The patient had response that lasted for 2 years with chlorambucil and prednisone; therefore, repeating that therapy would be appropriate.

Reference

Rai KR, Peterson BL, Appelbaum FR, et al. Fludarabine compared with chlorambucil as primary therapy for chronic lymphocytic leukemia. N Engl J Med. 2000;343:1750–7.

Answer to question 10: B

Educational objective

To discuss the advantages and disadvantages of various sources of stem cells for transplantation

Critique

Autologous stem cell transplantation is the treatment of choice in relapsed Hodgkin lymphoma if the quality and the quantity of the harvested stem cells are adequate. Presence of deletion 7 chromosome abnormality in the marrow indicates likely damage to stem cells from prior therapy. In this situation, autologous stem cell transplantation is not a good choice even if the cytogenetics reverts to normal after therapy. Syngeneic transplantation is likely to be associated with less morbidity but lacks graft-versus-lymphoma effect that can be provided by transplantation using other stem cell sources. An HLA-matched sibling would be preferable as a stem cell source when available, over matched unrelated and umbilical cord stem cell transplantation.

References

VanLeeuwen FE, Klokman WJ, Hagenbeck, et al. A. Second cancer risk following Hodgkin disease. A 20-year follow-up study. J Clin Oncol. 1994;12:312–25.

Rocha V, Wagner JE, Sobocinski KA, et al. Graft-versus-host disease in children who have received a cord-blood or bone marrow transplant from an HLA-identical sibling. Eurocord and International Bone Marrow Transplant Registry Working Committee on Alternate Donor and Stem Cell Sources. N Engl J Med. 2000;342:1846–54.

Answer to question 11: B

Educational objective

To identify the appropriate therapeutic option for localized gastric mucosa-associated lymphoid tissue (MALT) lymphoma

Critique

Low-grade MALT lymphomas that are *Helicobacter pylori* positive are best treated initially with a course of antibiotics. Exceptions to this include evidence of transformation to large cell histology as well as the presence of t(11;18), which predict poor response to antibiotic therapy, although *H. pylori* can be isolated from the lesion. These patients are best treated with radiotherapy (for localized disease) or systemic chemotherapy (for advanced disease). Rituxan is effective in MALT lymphoma, but its use has not been systematically studied in this disease. Surgery has been used in the past; currently, its use is limited to gastric outlet obstruction, bleeding, or perforation.

Reference

Levy M, Copie-Bergman C, Gameiro C, et al. Prognostic value of translocations t(11;18) in tumoral response of low-grade gastric lymphoma of mucosa-associated lymphoid tissue type to oral chemotherapy. J Clin Oncol. 2005;23:5061–6.

Answer to question 12: A

Educational objective

To identify the appropriate diagnostic features and treatment options for a patient with newly diagnosed hairy cell leukemia

Critique

Cladribine has been studied extensively in hairy cell leukemia and leads to excellent outcome with more than 80% of patients in long-term remission after a single course of therapy. Rituximab has activity in this disease, but its use in frontline therapy has not been systematically studied. Fludarabine and CHOP (cyclophosphamide, doxorubicin, vincristine, and prednisone) therapies are active but are not the choice for initial therapy. Splenectomy is rarely used as a first-line therapy.

Reference

Mey U, Strehl J, Gorschluter M, et al. Advances in the treatment of hairy cell leukemia. Lancet Oncol. 2003;4:86–94.

Answer to question 13: C

Educational objective

To recognize the unique clinical behavior and treatment options for lymphocyte-predominant Hodgkin disease (LPHD)

Critique

LPHD represents a subtype of Hodgkin lymphoma (HL) with unique biologic characteristics as well as therapeutic implications. Unlike the classic HL, LPHD usually behaves like indolent non-Hodgkin lymphoma with a long natural history and a tendency to relapse frequently despite the most aggressive therapy. Hence, this disease is best approached like a low-grade non-Hodgkin lymphoma. Almost all nodular lymphocyte-predominant Hodgkin lymphomas express CD20 and are responsive to rituximab. Observation is not an appropriate option in this patient because he is symptomatic.

Reference

Ekstrans BC, Lucas JB, Horwitz SM, et al. Rituximab in lymphocyte predominant Hodgkin disease: results of a phase 2 trial. Blood. 2003;101:4285–9.

Answer to question 14: C

Educational objective

To recognize alternate treatment options for hairy cell leukemia (HCL) that relapses shortly after standard therapy

Critique

HCL responds well to 2-deoxycoformycin. The majority of patients achieve durable remission. When the disease progresses within a few months after a course of 2-deoxycoformycin, a repeat course of the same drug is unlikely to benefit. Rituximab, an anti-CD20 monoclonal antibody, as a single agent has significant activity in HCL in part because of the high levels of CD20 antigen on the surface of these tumor cells. Rituximab has been shown to be effective in patients relapsing after cladribine. Complete responses up to 53% and overall response rates of 64–80% have been reported. Rituximab has a favorable adverse event profile and would be an appropriate choice in this elderly patient. Conventional chemotherapy regimens like chlorambucil and CVP (cyclophosphamide, vincristine, and prednisone) have lower activity in HCL.

References

Hagberg H, Lundholm L. Rituximab, a chimeric anti-CD20 monoclonal antibody, in the treatment of hairy cell leukemia. Br J Hematol. 2001;115:609–11.

Thomas DA, O'Brien S, Bueso-Ramos C. Rituximab in relapsed refractory hairy cell leukemia. Blood. 2003;102:3906–11.

CHAPTER 13

Plasma cell dyscrasias

Answer to question 1: B

Educational objective

To understand staging, indications, and choices for treatment for multiple myeloma in younger patients

Critique

The stage grouping of this patient is best described as stage IIA by the Durie–Salmon and stage IA by the International Staging Systems based upon the presence of bone lesions, her β_2-microglobulin, and her serum albumin level. The patient has symptomatic bone disease and is anemic, so treatment is indicated. Initial treatment options for this patient should be based upon the fact that she is an autologous stem cell transplant candidate. Alkylator-based regimens should be avoided. VAD (vincristine, doxorubicin, dexamethasone [Dex]) and HD Dex have been shown to be less efficacious than thalidomide + Dex in comparative III studies. The combination of bortezomib + Dex, although promising in phase II studies, is still undergoing evaluation in phase III trials.

References

Cavo M, Zamagni E, Tosi P, et al. Superiority of thalidomide and dexamethasone over vincristine-doxorubicin dexamethasone (VAD) as primary therapy in preparation for autologous transplantation for multiple myeloma. Blood. 2005;106:35–9.

Durie BGM, Salmon SE. A clinical staging system for multiple myeloma. Cancer. 1975;36:842–54.

Greipp PR, San Miguel J, Durie BG, et al. International staging system for multiple myeloma. J Clin Oncol. 2005;23:6281.

Palumbo A, Bringhen S, Caravita T, et al. Oral melphalan and prednisone chemotherapy plus thalidomide compared with melphalan and prednisone alone in elderly patients with multiple myeloma. Lancet. 2006;367:825–31.

Rajkumar SV, Blood E, Vesole D, et al. Phase III clinical trial of thalidomide plus dexamethasone compared with dexamethasone alone in newly diagnosed multiple myeloma. J Clin Oncol. 2006;24:431–6.

Answer to question 2: B

Educational objective

To understand the potential implications of chromosomal abnormalities in multiple myeloma (MM)

Critique

Cyclin D1 dysregulation induced by (11;14)(q13;q32) is the most frequent event, identified in about 50% of MM patients, and is considered to be associated with a lower response rate to conventional treatments. Translocations (8;14)(q24;q32) and t(4;14)(p16;q32) occur in about 5%, 1%, and 25% of MM patients, respectively.

References

Bergsagel PL, Kuehl WM, Zhan F, et al. Cyclin D dysregulation: an early and unifying pathogenic event in multiple myeloma. Blood. 2005;106:296–303.

Kuehl WM, Bergsagel PL. Multiple myeloma: evolving genetic events and host interactions. Nat Rev Cancer. 2002;2:175–87.

Answer to question 3: E

Educational objective

To understand the best treatment options for older patients with multiple myeloma

Critique

For an older patient with symptomatic multiple myeloma, MPT (melphalan, prednisone, thalidomide) is considered an important new option and has been shown to be superior to MP alone for response rates, event-free survival, and overall survival in phase III randomized trials. VAD (vincristine, doxorubicin, dexamethasone) would be contraindicated given the cardiac history. High-dose dexamethasone would be similarly problematic given his older age and noninsulin dependent diabetes mellitus. Bortezomib and dexamethasone combination therapy is very active but remains under study in this setting.

References

Jagannath S, Durie G, et al. Bortezomib therapy alone or in combination with dexamethasone for previously untreated symptomatic multiple myeloma. Br J Haematol 2005;129:776–83.

Palumbo A, Bringhen S, Caravita T, et al. Oral melphalan and prednisone chemotherapy plus thalidomide compared with melphalan and prednisone alone in elderly patients with multiple myeloma. Lancet. 2006;367:825–31.

Answer to question 4: B

Educational objective

To appreciate the role of autologous stem cell transplant (auto-SCT) in the treatment of younger patients with multiple myeloma

Critique

After successful initial therapy in younger patients, single auto-SCT is a standard of care, resulting in a median event-free survival of 2–3 years and a median overall survival of 5 years. Tandem auto-SCT shows benefit in a subset of patients with a median improvement in event-free and overall survivals of about 1 year but remains controversial, especially given the emerging role of novel therapies and concerns regarding the impact on quality of life when compared to single transplant.

References

Attal M, Harousseau JL, Facon T, et al. Single versus double autologous stem-cell transplantation for multiple myeloma. N Engl J Med. 2003;349:2495–502.

Attal M, Harousseau JL, Stoppa AM, et al. A prospective, randomized trial of autologous bone marrow transplantation and chemotherapy in multiple myeloma. N Engl J Med. 1996;335:91–7.

Answer to question 5: D

Educational objective

To understand the emerging role of maintenance therapy post autologous SCT (post auto-SCT)

Critique

Thalidomide maintenance has shown event-free and overall survival advantages in a large randomized trial post auto-SCT. The subsets benefiting most appear to be those with partial response to auto-SCT and those with no chromosome 13 deletion. Low-dose α interferon is associated with significant side effects and limited evidence of benefit. Prednisone or dexamethasone maintenance has yet to be shown to be effective as maintenance post auto-SCT and has the potential of increased risk of infection.

References

Attal M, Harousseau JL, Leyvraz S, et al. Maintenance therapy with thalidomide improves survival in multiple myeloma patients. Blood. In press.

Berenson JR, Crowley JJ, Grogan TM, et al. Maintenance therapy with alternate-day prednisone improves survival in multiple myeloma patients. Blood. 2002;99:3163–8.

Answer to question 6: A

Educational objective

To appreciate the importance of the bone marrow microenvironment in multiple myeloma (MM) biology

Critique

Only interleukin 6 (IL-6) can trigger Ras/Raf/mitogen-activated protein kinase (MEK)/ERK cascade, Janus kinase (JAK) 2/signal transducers, and activators of the transcription (STAT) 3 signaling cascade, as well as phosphatidylinositol 3-kinase (PI3-K)/Akt signaling. It has been shown that IL-6-induced MM cell proliferation is mediated by activation of the MEK/ERK signaling cascade (1, 2). Survival of MM cells triggered by IL-6 is conferred via JAK2/STAT3 signaling through regulation of downstream antiapoptotic Bcl-XL and Mcl-1 protein expression. The PI3-K/Akt signaling cascade is a major regulator of cytokine-mediated glucose metabolism. Akt regulates cell growth through its effect on the molecular targets of rapamycin and p70 S6 kinase pathway, and modulates cell cycle and proliferation via its direct activity on the CDK inhibitors $p21^{WAF1/Cip1}$ and $p27^{Kip1}$, as well as indirectly by affecting the levels of p53 and cyclin D1. Akt is also a major mediator of cell survival by directly inhibiting proapoptotic proteins Bad and the forkhead family of transcription factors. In MM cells, IL-6 overcomes drug (dexamethasone)-induced apoptosis via activation of Akt. IGF-1, VEGF, and SDF-1α can activate MEK/ERK and PI3-K/Akt signaling pathways.

References

Hideshima T, Anderson KC. Molecular mechanisms of novel therapeutic approaches for multiple myeloma. Nat Rev Cancer. 2002;2:927–37.

Hideshima T, Podar K, Chauhan D, et al. Cytokines and signal transduction. Best Pract Res Clin Haematol. 2005;18:509–24.

Answer to question 7: C

Educational objective

To understand the activity of novel agents in multiple myeloma (MM) and its bone marrow microenvironment

Critique

The initial rationale for the use of bortezomib in tumor cells was its inhibitory effect on nuclear factor κB (NF-κB) activity in MM cells. NF-κB is a transcriptional factor that mediates expression of many proteins including cytokines, chemokines, and cell adhesion molecules, as well as those involved in antiapoptosis and cellular growth control. NF-κB is typically a heterodimer composed of p50 and p65 subunits in MM cells, and its activity is regulated by association with IκB family proteins. After stimulation, IκB is phosphorylated and subsequently polyubiquitinated, followed by proteasomal degradation, which allows p50/p65 NF-κB nuclear translocation and binding to consensus motifs in the promoter region of target genes. Inhibition of NF-κB activity is therefore a major target for antitumor activity induced by bortezomib.

References

Hideshima T, Anderson KC. Molecular mechanisms of novel therapeutic approaches for multiple myeloma. Nat Rev Cancer. 2002;2:927–37.

Hideshima T, Chauhan D, Richardson P, et al. NF-κB as a therapeutic target in multiple myeloma. J Biol Chem. 2002;277: 16639–47.

Voges D, Zwickl P, Baumeister W. The 26S proteasome: a molecular machine designed for controlled proteolysis. Annu Rev Biochem. 1999;68:1015–68.

Answer to question 8: C

Educational objective

To understand the best options for the treatment of relapsed multiple myeloma

Critique

Bortezomib has been shown to be an effective therapy in first relapse for patients with multiple myeloma, as well as in relapsed and refractory disease. Although thalidomide and dexamethasone could be recommended, bortezomib therapy has been shown in phase III studies to be superior to high-dose dexamethasone and may be preferable as the next line of therapy in this patient given her prior exposure to thalidomide, emerging bone disease, and renal dysfunction. Lenalidomide and dexamethasone have also been shown in phase III studies to be markedly superior to high-dose dexamethasone, but eligibility in these studies was limited to patients with creatinine ≤ 2. 5mg/dL. Lenalidomide is renally cleared, suggesting caution is needed in this setting until more data about its use in renal dysfunction is available.

References

Dimopoulous M, Weber D, Chen C, et al. Evaluating oral lenalidomide (Revlimid) and dexamethasone versus placebo and dexamethasone in patients with relapsed or refractory multiple myeloma. Haematologica. 2005;90:160.

Jagannath S, Barlogie B, Berenson J, et al. A phase 2 study of two doses of bortezomib in relapsed or refractory myeloma. Br J Haematol. 2004;127:165–72.

Richardson P, Barlogie B, Berenson J, et al. A phase 2 study of bortezomib in relapsed, refractory myeloma. N Engl J Med. 2003;348:2609–17.

Richardson P, Sonneveld P, Schuster MW, et al. Bortezomib or high-dose dexamethasone for relapsed multiple myeloma. N Engl J Med. 2005;352:2487–98.

Answer to question 9: B

Educational objective

To understand the importance of thromboprophylaxis when treating multiple myeloma patients with thalidomide- and lenalidomide-based therapies

Critique

Thromboembolic complications occur with thalidomide- and lenalidomide-based treatment in multiple myeloma patients with an incidence of between 5% and 20%, depending on the choice of concomitant therapy. When combined with dexamethasone, rates are between 10% and 15%, and higher with cytotoxic chemotherapy, including alkylators (eg, melphalan) and anthracyclines such as Adriamycin. Thromboprophylactic strategies include full-dose aspirin (325 mg/d), therapeutic dosing of coumadin (with a target international normalized ratio of 2–3), and prophylactic dosing of low-molecular-weight heparin (eg, enoxaparin at 40 mg/d).

References

Ghobrial I, Rajkumar S. Management of thalidomide toxicity. J Support Oncol. 2003;1:194–205.

Rajkumar S, Blood E. Lenalidomide and venous thrombosis in multiple myeloma. N Engl J Med. 2006;354:2079.

Richardson P, Anderson K. Thalidomide and dexamethasone: a new standard of care for initial therapy in multiple myeloma. J Clin Oncol. 2006;24:334–6.

Answer to question 10: B

Educational objective

To determine optimal therapeutic choices in relapsed myeloma

Critique

The combination of lenalidomide and dexamethasone is a good option for this patient. Response rates approaching 60% with this combination have been reported in advanced disease, with a median time to progression of 11 months described. Significant peripheral neuropathy is rarely seen with this combination, although thromboprophylaxis is warranted because deep venous thrombosis is an important complication. Given the patient's residual neuropathy, thalidomide- and bortezomib-based therapy would be less attractive because of the risk of increased neurotoxicity. VAD (vincristine, doxorubicin, dexamethasone) or melphalan and prednisone would likely be less effective and so would not be recommended.

References

Meletios A, Dimpopoulos A, Spencer A, et al. Study of lenalidomide plus dexamethasone versus dexamethasone alone in relapsed or refractory multiple myeloma (MM): results of a phase 3 study (MM010). Paper presented at: 47th Annual Meeting of the American Society of Hematology; December 10–13, 2005; Atlanta, GA. Abstract 6.

Weber C, Chen C, Niesvizky M, et al. Lenalidomide plus high-dose dexamethasone provides improved overall survival compared to high-dose dexamethasone alone for relapsed or refractory multiple myeloma (MM): results of a North American phase III study (MM-009). Paper presented at: 42nd Annual Meeting of the American Society of Clinical Oncology; June 2–6, 2006; Atlanta, GA. Abstract 7521.

CHAPTER 14

Stem cell transplantation

Answer to question 1: D

Educational objective

To understand the role of stem cell transplantation in chronic myelogenous leukemia (CML) therapy and the risks and benefits of particular donors when selecting a stem cell source

Critique

Option A is wrong. A patient who has failed to obtain a cytogenetic response after 12 months of treatment with imatinib is unlikely to respond to an increase in the dose. Option B, the initiation of a novel tyrosine kinase/SRC inhibitor, is reasonable, but because there is no long-term follow-up with such treatment, allogeneic transplantation should be considered even if the patient responds.

Syngeneic transplantation, ie, transplantation using an identical twin donor, is associated with considerably less graft-versus-host disease (GVHD) than transplantation from an HLA-identical sibling. Syngeneic transplantation is associated with an increased risk of disease recurrence in CML because of lack of graft-versus-leukemia effects. Whether syngeneic or allogeneic transplantation from an HLA-identical sibling is preferred in an individual patient remains a matter of debate.

GVHD can still occasionally occur in syngeneic transplantation, particularly when either the donor or recipient is a female who has been pregnant. Host (recipient) tolerance to fetal cells from prior pregnancies may be altered with myeloablative therapy, potentially explaining an association between chronic GVHD and recipient parity. In the case of a pregnant donor, allosensitization of maternal T cells to fetal antigens during pregnancy could prime cells to similar antigens in a transplant recipient. Another intriguing hypothesis originates in the finding that fetal cells persist in parous women decades after childbirth and could potentially be transferred to the recipient.

Autologous GVHD is a similar phenomenon that might occur in up to 10% of autologous transplant recipients.

References

Adams KM, Holmberg LA, Leisenring W, et al. Risk factors for syngeneic graft-versus-host disease after adult hematopoietic cell transplantation. Blood. 2004;104:1894–7.

Baccarani M, Saglio G, Goldman J, et al.; European LeukemiaNet. Evolving concepts in the management of chronic myeloid leukemia: recommendations from an expert panel on behalf of the European LeukemiaNet [review]. Blood. 2006;108:1809–20.

Answer to question 2: A

Educational objective

To identify the presentation of chronic graft-versus-host disease (cGVHD) and its risk factors

Critique

This patient has diagnostic signs of cGVHD including lichenoid changes of the mouth. According to classic criteria, cGVHD is characterized as extensive or limited and also as high risk or low risk. Limited cGVHD involves limited areas of the skin and/or is associated with mild elevations of liver function tests. Such cGVHD does not necessarily require treatment. Any more extensive involvement is called extensive cGVHD. This patient has extensive cGVHD because of the involvement of mouth and eyes.

The best predictor for survival in cGVHD is the platelet count. For reasons that remain largely unknown, patients with low platelet counts ($<100 \times 10^9$/L) are at much higher risk for death. Eosinophilia, although a typical sign of cGVHD, is not a predictor of outcome. Prolonged immune suppression with steroids is necessary as well as prophylaxis for *Pneumocystis carinii* pneumonia, mold, and encapsulated gram positives. The patient should be recommended to start Pen VK for pneumococcal prophylaxis. Based on a recent study, posaconazole, a new antifungal with broad activity against molds, might be preferable to fluconazole.

The classification of cGVHD as outlined here is far from satisfactory. A National Institutes of Health consensus group has recently proposed an entirely new set of diagnostic and prognostic categories.

References

Filipovich AH, Weisdorf D, Pavletic S, et al. National Institutes of Health consensus development project on criteria for clinical trials in chronic graft-versus-host disease: I. Diagnosis and Staging Working Group report. Biol Blood Marrow Transplant. 2005;11:945–56.

Shulman HM, Kleiner D, Lee SJ, et al. Histopathologic diagnosis of chronic graft-versus-host disease: National Institutes of Health consensus development project on criteria for clinical trials in chronic graft-versus-host disease: II. Pathology Working Group report. Biol Blood Marrow Transplant. 2006;12:31–47.

Answer to question 3: A

Educational objective

To understand the role of stem cell transplantation in low-grade lymphomas

Critique

Follicular lymphoma is a heterogeneous disease with widely variable prognosis. Duration of response to initial treatment remains the best predictor of response to subsequent treatment and of long-term survival. This patient received appropriate initial treatment but had only a very short remission. Watchful waiting is not a good strategy for this patient, who likely will become rapidly symptomatic. Rituximab monotherapy is likely to result in ever shorter remissions. Autologous transplantation after induction of response should be considered. A randomized study, the CUP study, showed a survival benefit for autologous transplantation in patients with chemotherapy-sensitive recurrences of follicular lymphoma. Most centers would consider incorporating rituximab as part of the induction chemotherapy, but its value in this situation remains somewhat uncertain. Neither the fact that the patient is >60 years of age nor the fact that he has bone marrow involvement represents contraindication for autologous transplantation. Allogeneic transplantation is another reasonable approach, with a very low recurrence rate, but has considerable treatment-related mortality.

References

Schouten HC, Qian W, Kvaloy S, et al. High-dose therapy improves progression-free survival and survival in relapsed follicular non-Hodgkin's lymphoma: results from the randomized European CUP trial. J Clin Oncol. 2003;21:3918–27.

van Besien K, Loberiza FR Jr, Bajorunaite R, et al. Comparison of autologous and allogeneic hematopoietic stem cell transplantation for follicular lymphoma. Blood. 2003;102:3521–9.

Answer to question 4: D

Educational objective

To understand the role of stem cell transplantation in the treatment of myeloma

Critique

Autologous transplantation can be performed safely in patients well into their 70s and is the treatment of choice for many patients in first remission or for patients with recurrent disease who have not previously undergone transplantation. Melphalan-containing conditioning has been shown to be safer than and superior to total body irradiation-containing regimens. Allogeneic transplantation is excessively risky in a 69-year-old patient.

Reference

Barille-Nion S, Barlogie B, Bataille R, et al. Advances in biology and therapy of multiple myeloma. In: Hematology: ASH Education Program Book. Washington, DC: American Society of Hematology; 2003:248–78.

Answer to question 5: E

Educational objective

To understand the serious complication of post-transplantation cytomegalovirus (CMV) infection as well as its treatment

Critique

This patient has CMV viremia. CMV viremia occurs in 40% to 60% of patients after allogeneic transplantation, usually in the first 100 days after transplantation or sometimes later in patients with graft-versus-host disease. It is usually a consequence of reactivation of CMV virus in patients who were previously exposed (CMV-seropositive patients). CMV-seronegative patients can contract it from exposure to blood products that contain CMV virus (a risk much reduced by leukodepleting blood products) or from the transplanted stem cells if their donor is CMV seropositive.

CMV viremia in the first 100 days after transplant is a powerful predictor of CMV pneumonia, a difficult-to-treat complication with a high fatality rate. The progression to

CMV pneumonia can be prevented almost completely by preemptive treatment with intravenous (IV) ganciclovir. IV foscarnet and per os valganciclovir are reasonable alternatives. Most centers screen weekly for CMV viremia in the first months after transplantation.

Acyclovir and its prodrug valacyclovir have minimal activity against CMV and have no role in preemptive treatment. Because of their favorable side-effect profile, they are often used for CMV prophylaxis (ie, treatment with the intent of preventing CMV viremia). CMV hyperimmune globulin is used as an adjunct treatment for CMV disease (ie, CMV pneumonia, CMV colitis, CMV retinitis, etc.) but has no role in preemptive treatment of CMV viremia.

Reference

Boeckh M, Fries B, Nichols WG. Recent advances in the prevention of CMV infection and disease after hematopoietic stem cell transplantation. Pediatr Transplant. 2004;8(suppl 5):19–27.

Answer to question 6: C

Educational objective

To review the evaluation of a patient with gastrointestinal (GI) symptoms after an allogeneic stem cell transplantation

Critique

Upper GI symptoms are common after allogeneic stem cell transplant. Most of the upper GI symptoms secondary to the high-dose chemotherapy and/or radiation should have resolved by day 28 after bone marrow transplantation. However, it could be nausea from the multiple medications that the patients take such as antibiotics or immunosuppressive therapy. Although engraftment is achieved, the patient is still at risk of opportunistic infection such as esophageal candidiasis, varicella-zoster virus, or herpes simplex virus gastritis. Cytomegalovirus gastritis is less common early after transplant. With engraftment achieved, patient is at risk of development of acute graft-versus-host disease despite absence of other organ manifestation. Upper endoscopy with multiple biopsies will help to determine the etiology of the symptoms.

References

Weisdorf DJ. Acute upper intestinal graft versus host disease: clinical significance and response to immunosuppressive therapy: Blood. 1990;76:624–9.

Weisdorf DJ, Salati LM, Ramsay NK. Graft-versus-host disease of the intestine: a protein losing enteropathy characterized by fecal alpha 1-antitrypsin. Gastroenterology. 1983;85:1076–81.

Answer to question 7: C

Educational objective

To review the surveillance for cytomegalovirus (CMV) viruses in the posttransplant period

Critique

Posttransplant CMV infections are associated with high mortality. Preemptive treatment or prophylaxis has significantly improved the transplant outcome. Universal prophylaxis with ganciclovir is effective, but this is limited by cytopenia, in particular, neutropenia, and side effects. Day 35 bronchoalveolar lavage was once used to guide preemptive treatment, but it is too cumbersome and is no longer performed. CMV polymerase chain reaction (PCR) or antigenemia monitoring followed by preemptive therapy is simple and effective. For patients who are CMV negative, the use of CMV-negative blood products reduces the risk of CMV infections, but they are difficult to find. Leukocyte-reduced blood product is an acceptable alternative with a small nonsignificant increase in the rate of infection (0% versus 2.4% in a randomized study). In this case, both the donor and the recipient are CMV^{+ve}, so there is no benefit to using CMV-negative blood products. When CMV blood culture becomes positive, this represents infection, and treatment is less effective when compared with more sensitive techniques such as antigen detection or PCR studies used together with preemptive treatment.

References

Bowden RA, Slichter SJ, Sayers M, et al. A comparison of filtered leukocyte-reduced and CMV seronegative blood products for the prevention of transfusion-associated CMV infection after marrow transplant. Blood. 1995;86:3598–603.

Zaia JA. Prevention of CMV disease in hematopoietic stem cell transplantation. Clin Infect Dis. 2002;35:999–2004.

Answer to question 8: C

Educational objective

To understand severe drug interactions in agents commonly used during stem cell transplantation (SCT)

Critique

Azoles inhibit the metabolism of cyclosporine, FK506, and sirolimus. These are all commonly used immunosuppressive drugs after allogeneic SCT. When azoles are used in patients receiving these drugs, dose adjustments are necessary and drug-level monitoring is recommended. However, the interaction between voriconazole and sirolimus is particularly severe, and this is considered absolutely contraindicated as listed in the drug insert. In this case, one can continue cyclosporine (CsA) at a reduced dose, but it is recommended to stop sirolimus. A recent small retrospective study suggested that sirolimus and CsA can be given together if the CsA dose can be reduced to 10% of the original dose. This is preliminary data, and certainly 50% reduction is not adequate in this case.

References

Marty FM, et al. Voriconazole and sirolimus coadministration after allogeneic hematopoietic stem cell transplantation. Biol Blood Marrow Transplant. 2006;12:552–9.

Omero AJ. Effect of voriconazole on the pharmacokinetics of cyclosporine in renal transplant patients. Clin Pharmacol Ther. 2002;71:226–34.

Answer to question 9: C

Educational objective

To understand the etiologies of central nervous system (CNS) changes during stem cell transplantation, in particular the management of cyclosporine (CsA)/ tacrolimus toxicity

Critique

CNS toxicity is a recognized side effect for patients receiving the calcineurin inhibitors cyclosporine or tacrolimus, occurring in up to 5% of patients and highest in the first few months after transplant. The presenting features include headache, seizures, hypertension, confusion, or cortical blindness. Magnetic resonance imaging scans show changes suggestive of white matter diseases (T2 and fluid-attenuated inversion recovery sequence abnormalities with multifocal areas of signal hyperintensity). A computed tomographic scan can be normal. The only treatment available is to stop the medication. Phenytoin, as a P450 inducer, could decrease the serum level of CsA/tacrolimus and prevent further seizure. In this case, the tempo and clinical features are most consistent with CsA/tacrolimus CNS toxicity.

References

Bechstein WO. Neurotoxicity of calcineurin inhibitors: impact and clinical management [review]. Transpl Int. 2000;13:313–26.

Singh N. Immunosuppressive associated leukoencephalopathy in organ transplant recipients. Transplantation. 2000;69:467–72.

Answer to question 10: B

Educational objective

To understand the factors involved in the selection of donors in the transplant setting

Critique

HLA histocompatibility is the most important predictor for the transplant outcomes after a matched unrelated donor stem cell transplant. A younger donor age is associated with better outcome, and multiple pregnancies are associated with increased risk of chronic graft-versus-host disease. Cytomegalovirus (CMV) status does not affect the outcome in this setting. In this case, all the potential donors are matched in all alleles, so the donor should be chosen according to age of donor, parity, and CMV status, followed by blood group. Among the 4 donors, donor 2 is a male and the youngest and should be the preferred donor.

Reference

Kollman C, Howe CW. Donor characteristics as risk factors in recipients after transplantation of bone marrow from unrelated donors: the effect of donor age. Blood. 2001;98:2043–51.

Answer to question 11: D

Educational objective

To understand the potential etiology of pancytopenia as well as potential modifications in therapy

Critique

This young woman presents with clinical and laboratory findings consistent with bone marrow failure. If she is diagnosed with severe aplastic anemia, her best treatment option would be a matched related donor, and a syngeneic transplant would be ideal. The use of cyclophosphamide versus cyclosporine with antithymocyte globulin (CsA/ ATG) for individuals with severe aplastic anemia is currently under discussion. However, the individual in this question has a diagnosis of Fanconi anemia. Patients presenting with bone marrow failure should be evaluated for Fanconi anemia because there is a spectrum of morphologic presentations of the disorder even within a family. A diepoxybutane study can confirm the diagnosis in this patient. This patient does not have an autoimmune-based cause of her marrow failure, so immune modulation with cyclophosphamide or CsA/ATG will not improve her marrow status. The use of an ablative transplant would be too toxic for this patient. Modifications in both the dose of any alkylator therapy and radiation are required in this patient population.

References

Brodsky RA, Jones RJ. Aplastic anaemia. Lancet. 2005;365:1647–56.

Kook H. Fanconi anemia: current management. Hematology. 2005;10(suppl 1):108–10.

Tan PL, Wagner JE, Auerbach AD, et al. Successful engraftment without radiation after fludarabine-based regimen in Fanconi anemia patients undergoing genotypically identical donor hematopoietic cell transplantation. Pediatr Blood Cancer. 2006;46:630–6.

Answer to question 12: C

Educational objective

To understand the type of transplant for children with Hodgkin disease (HD)

Critique

The child has relapsed following standard therapy for HD. Although HD has been shown to be responsive to a graft-versus-leukemia/lymphoma effect, the benefit is outweighed by the risks of acute and chronic graft-versus-host disease. An autologous transplant provides this child with the best chance of long-term survival. If the patient has bone marrow involvement, he would be considered for an allogeneic transplant if he has a suitable donor.

References

Lieskovsky YE, Donaldson SS, Torres MA, et al. High-dose therapy and autologous hematopoietic stem-cell transplantation for recurrent or refractory pediatric Hodgkin's disease: results and prognostic indices. J Clin Oncol. 2004;22:4532–40.

Moskowitz CH, Kewalramani T, Nimer SD, et al. Effectiveness of high dose chemoradiotherapy and autologous stem cell transplantation for patients with biopsy-proven primary refractory Hodgkin's disease. Br J Haematol. 2004;124:645–52.

Answer to question 13: C

Educational objective

To understand the role of transplantation in children with acute myeloid leukemia (AML)

Critique

Children diagnosed with AML are treated with chemotherapy while HLA typing of family members is initiated. The presenting age and white blood cell count (WBC) does not alter the therapeutic options if no signs of leukostasis are seen. There are ongoing evaluations to determine if presenting WBC is a prognostic sign; however, there is no consensus at this time. Recently, the Children's Oncology Group has modified the current recommendation for transplantation in first complete remission (CR1) for patients with favorable cytogenetics including Inv(16) and t(8;21). For children without the designated favorable cytogenetics, transplantation with a matched related donor in CR1 is recommended; if there is not a related donor, they should proceed with chemotherapy. If the child relapses, then transplantation with an alternative donor is recommended.

Reference

Woods WG, Neudorf S, Gold S, et al. A comparison of allogeneic bone marrow transplantation, autologous bone marrow transplantation, and aggressive chemotherapy in children with acute myeloid leukemia in remission. Blood. 2001;97:56–62.

Answer to question 14: B

Educational objective

To understand the role of stem cell transplantation (SCT) in children with acute lymphoblastic leukemia (ALL)

Critique

A pediatric patient with ALL who relapses <18 months after attaining a remission should be offered SCT. Autologous transplant has not been shown to be effective in this situation. The duration of second complete remission (CR2) is likely to be shorter than CR1; however, the patient should be in a morphologic remission at the time of transplant. Therefore, she should be reinduced and not moved to transplant until remission is obtained. Although studies have demonstrated a role of graft versus leukemia, the benefit in ALL is limited.

References

Barrett AJ, Horowitz MM, Pollock BH, et al. Bone marrow transplants from HLA-identical siblings as compared with chemotherapy for children with acute lymphoblastic leukemia in a second remission. N Engl J Med. 1994;331:1253–8.

Eapen M, Raetz E, Zhang MJ, et al. Outcomes after HLA-matched sibling transplantation or chemotherapy in children with B-precursor acute lymphoblastic leukemia in a second remission: a collaborative study of the Children's Oncology Group and the Center for International Blood and Marrow Transplant Research. Blood. 2006;107:4961–7.

Gaynon PS, Harris RE, Altman AJ, et al. Bone marrow transplantation versus prolonged intensive chemotherapy for children with acute lymphoblastic leukemia and an initial bone marrow relapse within 12 months of the completion of primary therapy: Children's Oncology Group Study CCG-1941. J Clin Oncol. 2006;24:3150–6.

Answer to question 15: D

Educational objective

To understand long-term complications of stem cell transplantation (SCT)

Critique

Many long-term effects of SCT will be similar in adults and children. However, because children are still developing, the effects may be more marked or more obvious. Although children may be slightly smaller than what one would anticipate from their family members, there is not marked loss of height potential unless they develop growth failure secondary from the loss of growth hormone. All children who have received chemotherapy should be followed for long-term effects of their therapy. Children and adolescents who have received high-dose chemotherapy or total body irradiation (TBI) are at risk for additional problems and should be followed at least annually. The IQ of patients who have had an SCT does not fall; however, patients may need evaluation for potential learning problems. The exception to this is the concern regarding TBI in the very young child, resulting in many physicians using alternative preparative regimens.

This patient's new stem cells have not been exposed to etoposide or alkylators; therefore, she has a decreased risk for myelodysplastic syndrome or acute myeloid leukemia but an increased risk of solid tumors and skin cancers. Most young women develop ovarian dysfunction and require hormonal supplementation. Young adolescents who have not gone through puberty may require supplementation in order to develop secondary sexual characteristics. Young males generally are able to produce testosterone but are sterile. These individuals should be monitored closely and supplementation started because they are at a tenuous time in their psychosocial development.

Reference

Schmitz N, Eapen M, Horowitz MM, et al. Long-term outcome of patients transplanted with mobilized blood or bone marrow: a report from the International Bone Marrow Transplant Registry and the European Group for Blood and Marrow Transplantation. Blood. In press.

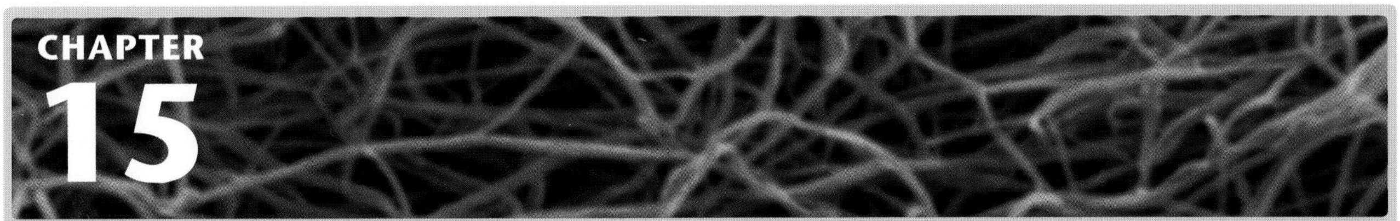

CHAPTER

15

Hemostasis and thrombosis

Answer to question 1: D

Educational objective

To understand the current recommendations for duration of anticoagulation after deep venous thrombosis (DVT)

Critique

This DVT occurs in the setting of a strong, transient risk factor (immobilization and surgery). In the absence of a family history of DVT, 3 months of anticoagulants would be sufficient. Her family history is, however, concerning and suggests a hypercoagulable state. The most likely hereditary thrombophilic state is factor V Leiden; this abnormality is known to predispose to DVT in the setting of orthopedic surgery. Although detection of factor V Leiden should not influence the optimal duration of therapy, its detection would inform the patient and her family about the cause of their thrombi. More important, detection of protein C, protein S, or antithrombin deficiency should probably prompt extended-duration anticoagulation because these abnormalities are likely associated with an increased risk of recurrent thrombosis after discontinuation of blood thinners (although this recommendation is not supported by good-quality prospectively acquired data). Furthermore, identification of these deficiencies would provide useful information to other family members who might be placed in situations (such as hip or knee replacement) known to predispose to DVT and who might benefit from intensified anticoagulant therapy.

Irrespective of the duration of her anticoagulant therapy, the patient should receive aggressive thromboprophylaxis when she is placed in situations of risk, and she should likely avoid all forms of hormonal therapy if she is not therapeutically anticoagulated.

References

Buller HR, Agnelli G, Hull RD, et al. Antithrombotic therapy for venous thromboembolic disease: the Seventh ACCP Conference on Antithrombotic and Thrombolytic Therapy. Chest. 2004;126(suppl 3):S401–28.

Ho WK, Hankey GJ, Quinlan DJ, et al. Risk of recurrent venous thromboembolism in patients with common thrombophilia: a systematic review. Arch Intern Med. 2006;166:729–36.

Answer to question 2: D

Educational objective

To understand the relationship between cancer-associated coagulopathy and thrombosis (venous or arterial)

Critique

Heparin administration could cause prolongation of both the international normalized ratio (INR) and activated partial thromboplastin time (APTT); however, the degree of prolongation of the APTT would be far in excess of that seen in this case if the INR is prolonged to 5.6. Gram-negative septicemia can certainly cause disseminated intravascular coagulation (DIC); however, the patient is too well. Surreptitious ingestion of warfarin should cause more marked prolongation of the INR if taken in quantities that would prolong the APTT to 84 seconds, and warfarin administration does not explain the thrombocytopenia. An acquired factor VIII inhibitor should not prolong the INR nor be associated with thrombocytopenia, and its usual presentation is with hemorrhage, not thrombosis. Transfusional coagulopathy requires massive blood replacement and does not cause arterial thromboembolism. The single unifying diagnosis in this case is chronic DIC associated with adenocarcinoma, in this case of the prostate. Classically, these patients can present with arterial thromboembolism in the setting of a marked coagulopathy. Investigation for malignancy is warranted, and low-dose intravenous heparin should be considered.

Reference

de la Fouchardiere C, Flechon A, Droz JP. Coagulopathy in prostate cancer. Neth J Med. 2003;61:347–54.

Answer to question 3: C

Educational objective

To understand the current role of computed tomographic (CT) pulmonary angiogram in the evaluation of patients with suspected pulmonary embolism

Critique

CT pulmonary angiogram has emerged as a valuable test in the assessment of patients with suspected pulmonary embolism over the last 5 years. In this case, a D-dimer assay is irrelevant to the evaluation of the patient because imaging of the lungs will be required to rule out the possibility of metastatic disease and because the negative predictive value of D-dimer for the evaluation of venous thromboembolism appears unacceptably low in patients with cancer. Traditional (direct) pulmonary angiography has been largely abandoned as a result of the availability of CT pulmonary angiogram. Additionally, it will not image the lung parenchyma with sufficient resolution to rule out the possibility of metastatic disease. Although bilateral leg compression ultrasounds may ultimately be required to evaluate this patient's symptomatology, at present they are unneeded because the initial evaluation can be limited to CT pulmonary angiogram. The most likely cause of this patient's presentation is metastatic disease; CT pulmonary angiography will both rule out acute pulmonary embolism (assuming it is performed in a facility with a validated algorithm CT pulmonary angiography) and will allow visualization of the lung parenchyma that, in this case, reveals evidence of metastatic disease. Although it is possible this patient suffered coincident pulmonary embolism as a result of the thrombophilic state associated with cancer, in this particular case the negative CT angiogram rules out acute pulmonary embolism with a negative predictive value in excess of 99%.

Reference

Roy PM, Colombet I, Durieux P, et al. Systematic review and meta-analysis of strategies for the diagnosis of suspected pulmonary embolism. BMJ. 2005;331:259.

Answer to question 4: D

Educational objective

To review the diagnosis of thrombotic thrombocytopenic purpura (TTP)

Critique

This patient's presentation is consistent with acute TTP. In many cases, this disorder is due to an autoantibody directed against ADAMTS13, a metalloproteinase involved in the normal processing of von Willebrand factor. In patients with autoantibody-mediated TTP, platelet activation leads to microvascular fibrin deposition and thrombocytopenia associated with hemolysis. Neurologic dysfunction, renal insufficiency, and fever are typical of this disorder. Treatment with plasmapheresis is curative in many cases and, in the absence of treatment, the disorder pursues a fulminant course often resulting in death.

Reference

Schech SD, Brinker A, Shatin D, et al. New-onset and idiopathic thrombotic thrombocytopenic purpura: incidence, diagnostic validity, and potential risk factors. Am J Hematol. 2006; 81:657–63.

Answer to question 5: A

Educational objective

To recognize those conditions that can cause bleeding despite normal screening laboratory

Critique

This child has demonstrated a positive bleeding history by manifesting bleeding from the heelstick blood sample and prolonged oozing from the umbilical cord. The fact that the family history is negative does not rule out a bleeding disorder, particularly in those who are autosomal recessive. Further specific testing as noted in the question will be helpful in determining a diagnosis. The screening test for factor XIII deficiency suggests this clot-stabilizing factor is present because there is no lysis of the clot in 5 M urea. Severe hemophilia, either A or B, is ruled out by a normal activated partial thromboplastin time. von Willebrand disease is a possibility but, as a platelet-vessel type of bleeding disorder, usually does not present with delayed bleeding such as seen with the prolonged oozing from the umbilical cord. The best answer is antiplasmin deficiency, which presents like hemophilia, has a normal screening laboratory, and has a short euglobulin lysis time due to unchecked plasmin degradation of the fibrin clot.

References

Griffin GC, Mammen EF, Sokol RJ, et al. Alpha 2-antiplasmin deficiency. An overlooked cause of hemorrhage. Am J Pediatr Hematol Oncol. 1993;15:328–30.

Miles LA, Plow EF, Donnelly KJ, et al. A bleeding disorder due to deficiency of alpha 2-antiplasmin. Blood. 1982;59:1246–51.

Answer to question 6: C

Educational objective

To understand the benign nature of postinfectious lupus anticoagulant (LA) in children

Critique

This case is a classic example of the LA in children and its benign nature. Postinfectious LA is usually directed against anionic phospholipids, but the pathogenic LA often requires a protein cofactor such as β_2-glycoprotein I. The family and personal bleeding history are clearly normal, ruling against an inherited bleeding disorder in this patient. Further, more detailed family history of bleeding might be helpful if it was not obtained at the outset, but it will not help to establish a diagnosis. The LA in children is usually defined by recent history of infection (usually viral) or administration of antibiotics. This is often seen in children who present to the ear, nose, and throat surgeon for possible tonsillectomy due to enlarged tonsils or repeated strep, sinus, ear, or other upper respiratory infections. The surgeon will usually perform an activated partial thromboplastin time (APTT), and its prolongation will prompt further evaluation from the hematologist. In this case, lack of correction of the APTT immediately and at 1 hour strongly suggests an inhibitor. A specific factor inhibitor is suggested by partial but not complete correction of the APTT immediately upon incubation and then prolongation to a greater degree at 1 hour. The best confirmatory test of an LA would be to demonstrate the phospholipid nature of the LA by performing a phospholipid neutralization of the APTT. If this test is positive, you have established the diagnosis of an LA. Repeating the APTT to rule against a laboratory error might be helpful but, if prolonged, will not shed further light on the diagnosis. Factor assays are helpful in determining a specific factor inhibitor or as an adjunct in the evaluation of an inhibitor that is difficult to discern (the so-called nonspecific or multiple-factor inhibitor).

Reference

Male C, Lechner K, Eichinger S, et al. Clinical significance of lupus anticoagulants in children. J Pediatr. 1999;134:199–205.

Answer to question 7: D

Educational objective

To recognize the factors underlying vitamin K deficiency in children

Critique

This child has late-onset hemorrhagic disease of the newborn (HDN). If the mother were on an anticonvulsant such as Dilantin, then possibly this medication could have contributed to early HDN but would be an unlikely culprit at 2 months of age. Undiagnosed cystic fibrosis could certainly contribute to malabsorption and resultant loss of fat soluble vitamins including vitamin K but would be low on the differential in this patient given she is thriving at 2 months. Breast-feeding can contribute to vitamin K deficiency but is extremely rare as a sole cause, without other contributing factors. The mother being a vegetarian would contribute to the possibility of vitamin B_{12} deficiency in the infant, not vitamin K deficiency where the vitamin is readily available in green leafy vegetables. The correct answer to this question is D, a combination of missing the vitamin K shot at birth, breast-feeding, and recent diarrhea decreasing vitamin K absorption in the diet.

Reference

Sutor AH, von Kries R, Cornelissen EA, et al. Vitamin K deficiency bleeding (VKDB) in infancy. ISTH Pediatric/Perinatal Subcommittee. International Society on Thrombosis and Haemostasis. Thromb Haemost. 1999;81:456–61.

Answer to question 8: D

Educational objective

To understand the diagnosis and management of acute immune thrombocytopenia purpura (ITP) in children

Critique

This case illustrates the common presentation of ITP in children and who should be treated. This child displays no mucosal bleeding symptoms, and his bleeding manifestations are purely cutaneous. Additionally, his bleeding is mild in presentation (a few scattered, small bruises and petechiae) and certainly not life threatening. From a laboratory perspective, his platelet count is >10,000/μL, the level that most pediatric hematologists now use as a treatment threshold (assuming no mucus membrane bleeding). Therefore, the most appropriate answer is to reassure the family about bleeding risk and then follow the patient closely, helping the family not to be unnecessarily focused on the platelet number. There should be no reason to perform a bone marrow aspiration to rule out leukemia because the child has no signs or symptoms of leukemia and his complete blood cell count (CBC) is completely normal other than the low platelet count and larger platelet size (suggesting increased destruction of platelets). Either of the treatment options in answers C and D would be appropriate if treatment is needed. Some would argue, however, that corticosteroids should not be utilized unless a bone marrow is performed first. But this concern appears appropriate only if there are findings from the history, physical examination, or CBC/peripheral blood smear that are concerning for other causes of thrombocytopenia.

Reference

Buchanan GR. Thrombocytopenia during childhood: what the pediatrician needs to know. Pediatr Rev. 2005;11:401–9.

Answer to question 9: A

Educational objective

To understand how to recognize and manage disseminated intravascular coagulation (DIC) in children

Critique

The main causes of DIC in children are infections (eg, meningococcemia), malignancy (eg, M3 acute myelogenous leukemia), massive tissue damage (eg, shock, burns), vascular disorders (eg, hemangioma), and immunologic issues (eg, transfusion reaction). Treatment should be focused on eliminating the inciting cause and providing supportive care and blood product support (if the laboratory or clinical findings warrant such support). Accordingly, the correct answer to this case is A. All of the other treatment options surround some element of controversy. Antithrombin III (AT-III) concentrates are certainly an adjunct to supportive care, but until clinical trials better define the role of AT-III in DIC, this treatment modality should be reserved for conditions where the AT-III level is documented to be low. Antifibrinolytic therapy such as aminocaproic acid can be very helpful in those cases of DIC where there is excessive fibrinolysis (such as certain snake bites and some cases of leukemia) but should not be used routinely due to risk of thrombosis. Finally, certain infections and malignancy are associated with excessive thrombin generation that leads to laboratory and clinical findings of thrombosis. In this setting, low-dose heparin has been utilized to interrupt excessive thrombin formation but should not be considered standard of care in most cases of DIC.

References

Levi M, ten Cate H. Disseminated intravascular coagulation. N Engl J Med. 1999;341:586–92.

Muller-Berghaus G, ten Cate H, Levi M. Disseminated intravascular coagulation: clinical spectrum and established as well as new diagnostic approaches. Thromb Haemost. 1999;82:706–12.

Answer to question 10: A

Educational objective

To interpret the laboratory features of Glanzmann thrombasthenia

Critique

Because flow cytometry can be used to make the diagnosis of GPIIa/IIIb deficiency, the focus of this question is meant to help the reader differentiate the types of platelet aggregation patterns seen in the various platelet-vessel bleeding disorders. Answer B is best seen in the Bernard–Soulier platelet function defect. This condition will also have mild thrombocytopenia, and the platelets will be larger than normal. Answer C is a normal aggregation tracing, and answer D is best seen in a failure-to-release (aspirin-like) platelet function defect. It is essential to rule out medication as a cause for this platelet function defect because over-the-counter medication use is a more likely culprit with this type of aggregation tracing. The correct answer is A because the platelet-to-platelet interaction is abnormal (via GP IIb/IIIa and fibrinogen) as measured by adenosine diphosphate or collagen, and the platelet-to-von Willebrand factor adhesion is normal (via GPIb) as characterized by normal aggregation to ristocetin.

References

Nurden AT. Qualitative disorders of platelets and megakaryocytes. J Thromb Haemost. 2005;3:1773–82.

White GC II. Congenital and acquired platelet disorders: current dilemmas and treatment strategies. Semin Hematol. 2006;43(suppl 1):S37–41.

Answer to question 11: D

Educational objective

To relate the proper first-line treatment of an acute bleed in a hemophiliac (factor VIII deficiency) with a high titer inhibitor

Critique

This patient presents in typical fashion for a new-onset high-titer inhibitor with a median FVIII exposure days (ED) = 10–12 ED. The bleed should be treated with recombinant FVIIa (rFVIIa) as described here. The long-term options for this patient are to utilize immune tolerance therapy (ITT) once the inhibitor titer drops below 10 BU. Answers A and B are the treatment options for the current international ITT trial, which randomizes between high-dose (200 IU/kg daily) and low-dose (50 IU/kg 3 times weekly) therapy. Although both dosing schedules are appropriate in the context of this randomized trial, it is best not to offer ITT until the BU drops below 10. If acute bleeds occur while waiting for the BU to drop to a lower level or while the patient is on ITT, the most appropriate treatment is to administer rFVIIa at a dose and interval as outlined in answer D. Although activated prothrombin complex concentrate is another treatment option for inhibitor patients, the interval suggested in answer C is not optimal unless there is close laboratory monitoring for possible disseminated intravascular coagulation. Additionally, this child has never been exposed to plasma-derived FVIII, and it would be best to utilize a bypassing agent, which is rFVIIa. It would not be appropriate to avoid treating the bleed, as suggested in answer E.

References

Abshire T, Kenet G. Recombinant factor VIIa: review of efficacy, dosing regimens and safety in patients with congenital and acquired factor VIII or IX inhibitors. J Thromb Haemost. 2004;2:899–909.

Key NS. Inhibitors in congenital coagulation disorders. Br J Haematol. 2004;127:379–91.

CHAPTER 16

Transfusion medicine

Answer to question 1: B

Educational objective

To diagnose an acute hemolytic transfusion reaction resulting from mislabeling of the type-and-crossmatch specimen

Critique

An acute hemolytic transfusion reaction is the most likely cause of the patient's decompensation for several reasons. First, febrile reactions, allergic transfusion reactions, and, especially, volume overload would not be expected to cause hypotension. Second, volume overload *per se* rarely causes fever, although all 4 of the other diagnostic possibilities can cause fever. A transfusion-induced acute lung injury reaction would not be expected to start so quickly but otherwise could closely resemble the case in question. The most common cause of acute hemolytic reactions is mislabeling of the specimens sent to the transfusion medicine service for type and crossmatch, most commonly due to labeling the tubes away from the bedside.

Another important consideration in managing this case is the possibility that at least one other patient on the same ward may be about to receive incorrectly identified blood as part of the same mislabeling error that resulted in the first reaction. Thus, the medical staff should obtain repeat bedside-labeled type-and-crossmatch specimens for each patient scheduled to receive transfusions and should not transfuse any additional blood until all patients have been definitively identified.

References

Goldfinger D. Acute hemolytic transfusion reactions: a fresh look at pathogenesis and considerations regarding therapy. Transfusion. 1977;17:85–98.

Sloop GD, Friedberg RC. Complications of blood transfusion. How to recognize and respond to noninfectious reactions. Postgrad Med. 1995;98:159–62.

Answer to question 2: D

Educational objective

To assess the relative importance of competing risk factors when selecting platelet products

Critique

With respect to both red blood cell (RBC) and platelet transfusions, major mismatches refer to situations in which the recipient is potentially capable of generating antibodies directed against the cellular component of the transfusion, whereas minor mismatches refer to situations in which the plasma component of the transfused product may contain antibodies directed against preexisting recipient-derived cells. Therefore, because platelet units contain significant amounts of plasma (more so than packed RBCs), most clinicians would prefer to administer ABO-*identical* (as opposed to ABO-matched or ABO-compatible) platelet products whenever possible. Such a strategy would (i) minimize the risk of donor-versus-recipient hemolytic reactions due to the isohemagglutinins that may be introduced by the plasma fraction of the platelet product and (ii) minimize the risk of recipient-versus-donor reactions manifested by reductions in platelet transfusion increments due to the fact that platelets express ABO antigens and may interact with host-derived isohemagglutinins. Furthermore, utilizing platelet products from donors who are Rh(D) identical would prevent Rh(D)-negative recipients from sensitization to Rh(D). Though platelets do not express Rh antigens, platelet units can contain milliliter amounts of contaminating donor RBCs that can immunize recipients to Rh(D).

However, in emergency situations such as this scenario, the first priority is to control the intracranial bleeding as rapidly as possible, and this priority must take precedence over the immunohematologic compatibility issues and clinical relevance of Rh(D) sensitization in a presumably postmenopausal female. Nevertheless, it is important for the clinician to be aware that analyses of large series of platelet transfusions have indicated that the mean platelet count increments following major ABO mismatches may be reduced by 50% or more in comparison with the increment that is achieved following ABO-identical transfusions, thus increasing the amount of time and number of platelet transfusions that may be required to obtain the desired peripheral blood platelet count increment. In the case of unavoidable transfusion of platelets derived from an Rh(D)-positive donor into an Rh-negative female of child-bearing age (for whom the risk of future hemolytic disease of the newborn is of concern), Rh(D)-immune globulin can be used to prevent sensitization from the red cells introduced by the platelet product.

In this scenario, every effort should be made to obtain a peripheral blood platelet count of 100,000/μL or more as quickly as possible and to maintain the platelet count in this range for 7–10 days following the neurosurgical procedure that is likely to be required in this patient. Achieving this goal is likely to require multiple infusions of platelets, each of which should be followed by a postinfusion platelet count to assess the response. Also, the scenario illustrates the fact that the incidence of spontaneous intracranial bleeding is particularly increased in patients with platelet counts <5,000/μL.

References

Bishop JF, McGrath K, Wolf MM, et al. Clinical factors influencing the efficacy of pooled platelet transfusions. Blood. 1988;71:383–7.

Klumpp TR, Herman JH, Innis S, et al. Factors associated with response to platelet transfusion following hematopoietic stem cell transplantation. Bone Marrow Transplant. 1996;17:1035–41.

Mair B, Benson K. Evaluation of changes in hemoglobin levels associated with ABO-incompatible plasma in apheresis products. Transfusion. 1998;38:51–5.

Answer to question 3: D

Educational objective

To diagnose the cause of failed erythroid recovery following allogeneic bone marrow transplantation

Critique

Unlike solid organ transplantation, in which donor–recipient ABO matching is of paramount importance, donor–recipient ABO mismatching is not considered to be a major contraindication in patients undergoing bone marrow or hematopoietic stem cell transplantation. However, a number of complications can occur following major or minor ABO-mismatched allogeneic hematopoietic stem transplantation, including immediate or delayed antibody-mediated alloimmune hemolytic anemia, delayed red cell engraftment, and pure red cell aplasia. There are numerous reports of posttransplant pure red cell aplasia developing after major, but not minor, ABO-mismatched transplants, and the pathophysiology is thought to involve the reaction of residual recipient-derived isohemagglutinins (anti-A or anti-B antibodies) against donor-derived erythroid progenitors such as **erythrocyte colony-forming units**, which are known to express the corresponding donor-derived ABO antigens. There are also occasional case reports of posttransplant pure red cell aplasia, apparently mediated by non-ABO, non-Rh antigen systems.

Donor–recipient gender mismatches, particularly the female-into-male mismatch depicted here, are associated with a notable increase in the risk of clinically significant graft-versus-host disease but are not generally thought to be associated with delayed red cell engraftment.

There have been a small number of reports of hemolytic anemia associated with Rh-mismatched allogeneic transplants. However, unlike the infusion of Rh-positive blood into Rh-negative immunocompetent individuals, most Rh-negative individuals who receive Rh-positive bone marrow do not acquire anti-Rh antibodies or experience any other negative sequela, apparently due to the profound immunodeficiency that characterizes the peritransplant period.

Both immediate and delayed alloimmune hemolytic anemia, sometimes severe enough to induce renal failure, have been occasionally reported following both major and minor ABO-mismatched allogeneic bone marrow transplantation. However, the normal lactate dehydrogenase and low reticulocyte count in this patient render this possibility much less likely.

Incompatibilities involving so-called non-HLA or minor histocompatibility loci are thought to account for the substantial incidence of graft-versus-host disease and the occasional occurrence of graft rejection among recipients of HLA-identical sibling bone marrow transplants, but these do not appear to play a major role in the development of posttransplant hemolysis or erythroid recovery.

Although not listed in this question, an additional recognized cause of inadequate red cell recovery following bone marrow transplantation is infection of the bone marrow erythroid progenitors with parvovirus B19.

There are conflicting data in the literature regarding the possible effect of donor–recipient ABO mismatches on overall survival following allogeneic transplant, but most of the larger studies have not demonstrated such a correlation.

References

Gandini G, Franchini M, Vassanelli A, et al. Immunohematological aspects of bone marrow transplantation. Hematology. 2002;7:89–93.

Klumpp TR. Immunohematologic complications of bone marrow transplantation. Bone Marrow Transplant. 1991;8:159–70.

Seebach JD, Stussi G, Passweg JR, et al. ABO blood group barrier in allogeneic bone marrow transplantation revisited. Biol Blood Marrow Transplant. 2005;11:1006–13.

Answer to question 4: C

Educational objective

To provide appropriate transfusion and anticoagulation support for a patient who suffers a major thrombotic event while severely thrombocytopenic

Critique

Acute venous thromboses, including thromboses of the lower extremities, upper extremities, superior vena cava, and other sites, are surprisingly common in patients with severe thrombocytopenia following high-dose myeloablative therapy and hematopoietic stem cell transplantation. It has been hypothesized that endothelial cell activation by high-dose chemotherapy may lead to an intrinsic prothrombotic state that—in combination with the apparent relative predominance of platelets in arterial, as opposed to venous, thrombosis and the fact that such patients often spend prolonged amounts of time relatively immobile in bed—allows such thromboses to develop. Although no randomized trials have been published regarding the optimal management of patients in this situation, most bone marrow transplant teams do not allow patients to remain severely thrombocytopenic in this situation due to the markedly increased risk of intracranial hemorrhage or other severe internal hemorrhage. Furthermore, as noted, thrombocytopenia does not appear to be particularly prophylactic against venous thrombosis in bone marrow transplant patients and would thus not be expected to be particularly therapeutic either. Administering full-dose heparin or streptokinase in the absence of platelets might maximize the rate of regression of the clot but would likely increase the risk of severe internal hemorrhage even further. Low-molecular-weight heparin (LMWH) simultaneously with so-called platelet hypertransfusion, ie, frequent transfusion of platelets to keep the trough peripheral blood platelet count about 50,000 or so, has been used in this setting, but in some patients it has been associated with severe hemorrhage due to the inability to rapidly reverse LMWH if bleeding does develop. Thus, the combination of unfractionated heparin and hypertransfusion of platelets appears to offer the best overall balance between protection against further thrombosis and protection against bleeding.

References

Gupta V, Keller A, Halliday W, et al. Cavernous sinus thrombosis presenting with diplopia in an allogeneic bone marrow transplant recipient. Am J Hematol. 2004;77:77–81.

Haire WD, Lieberman RP, Edney J, et al. Hickman catheter-induced thoracic vein thrombosis. Frequency and long-term sequelae in patients receiving high-dose chemotherapy and marrow transplantation. Cancer. 1990;66:900–8.

Answer to question 5: A

Educational objective

To diagnose the cause of acquired platelet transfusion refractoriness in a multiply transfused patient

Critique

Antibodies to HLA antigens have been found to be the most common cause of platelet transfusion refractoriness in both the transplant and the nontransplant setting. To rule out consumptive causes such as bleeding and D-dimers, it is often helpful to order 15–60 minute postinfusion platelet counts because broadly specific anti-HLA antibodies will typically result in an inadequate "immediate" increment as measured 15–60 minutes following the infusion, whereas consumptive causes more often leave the immediate increment at least somewhat intact despite the fact that the 24-hour increment is often markedly reduced. Lymphocytotoxic antibody screens incubate patient plasma with a panel of lymphocytes selected to represent many of the most common HLA antigens. These assays can yield not only an estimate of the percentage of common HLA antigens with which the patient's serum reacts, but also an estimate of the specificity of the antibodies, which can aid in the subsequent selection of HLA-matched donors in the refractory patient. Multiparous females, such as the patient depicted in this scenario, are at increased risk for platelet transfusion refractoriness, apparently as a result of sensitization to nonself paternally derived HLA antigens during pregnancy.

In contrast to HLA antigens, which are expressed on nearly every tissue in the body, platelet-specific antigens such as HPA-1 (formerly Pl^{A1}) are expressed only on platelets. Antibodies directed against platelet-specific antigens can also result in refractoriness to transfusion but are less commonly detected than antibodies directed against HLA antigens.

Splenomegaly is also an important cause of platelet transfusion refractoriness, but marked splenomegaly is significantly less common in patients with acute myelogenous leukemia, compared with patients with other types of leukemia such as chronic myelogenous leukemia or chronic lymphocytic leukemia, and is thus less likely to be present in this patient.

Disseminated intravascular coagulation (DIC) can also contribute to platelet transfusion refractoriness, but DIC more frequently occurs during the first few days of acute leukemia induction during the "tumor lysis" phase and would thus be expected to appear early in the induction course. In contrast, this patient responded well initially and only later developed refractoriness.

The absence of high-molecular-weight von Willebrand factor multimers would suggest the possibility of thrombotic thrombocytopenic purpura (TTP). However, TTP is less commonly diagnosed in patients who are already very sick and more commonly occurs as a *de novo* phenomenon in previously healthy patients.

References

Klumpp TR, Herman JH, Innis S, et al. Factors associated with response to platelet transfusion following hematopoietic stem cell transplantation. Bone Marrow Transplant. 1996;17: 1035–41.

Murphy S, Varma M. Selecting platelets for transfusion of the alloimmunized patient. Immunohematology. 1998;14:117–23.

Answer to question 6: C

Educational objective

To evaluate prospective blood donors in bone marrow transplant recipients

Critique

The first and most important point illustrated by this case is that the clinician should always request γ-irradiated, leukoreduced red cells when providing transfusion support to a patient who is about to undergo, or who has recently undergone, hematopoietic stem cell transplantation. γ-Irradiation is required because the markedly impaired recipient immune system is sometimes unable to reject the small but clinically significant number of so-called passenger leukocytes that are present in essentially all red cell and platelet products, which can result in fatal transfusion-induced graft-versus-host disease in susceptible recipients but can be almost completely prevented by γ-irradiation of blood products. Leukoreduction is required to reduce the incidence of recipient sensitization to HLA antigens and to reduce the incidence of transfusion-transmitted cytomegalovirus (CMV) infection, which can lead to life-threatening refractoriness to platelet transfusions or life-threatening pulmonary or gastrointestinal infections, respectively.

A second important point in this setting is to avoid pretransplant exposure to blood products obtained from family members due to the risk of inducing recipient-derived T-cell responses against major or minor histocompatibility antigens, which increases the risk of subsequent graft rejection.

Although there is obviously no risk of hemolytic disease of the newborn occurring during pregnancy in a male recipient, the development of anti-Rh antibodies as a result of exposure to Rh-positive red cells could complicate subsequent compatible blood product acquisition, especially in an emergency setting, and is thus best avoided.

Reactivation of latent CMV infection is a major cause of morbidity and mortality following allogeneic bone marrow transplant, and thus the selection of CMV-negative blood donors, if available, is theoretically desirable. However, many authorities believe that the leukopoor blood products provide adequate protection against CMV transmission in bone marrow transplant recipients as long as proper quality management controls are in place to ensure that the leukocyte content of such products meets Food and Drug Administration standards.

References

Bowden RA, Slichter SJ, Sayers M, et al. A comparison of filtered leukocyte-reduced and cytomegalovirus (CMV) seronegative blood products for the prevention of transfusion-associated CMV infection after marrow transplant. Blood. 1995;86: 3598–603.

Klumpp TR. Immunohematologic complications of bone marrow transplantation. Bone Marrow Transplant. 1991;8:159–70.

Nichols W, Garrett W, Price TH, et al. Transfusion-transmitted cytomegalovirus infection after receipt of leukoreduced blood products. Blood. 2003;101:4195–200.

Trial to Reduce Alloimmunization to Platelets Study Group. Leukocyte reduction and ultraviolet B irradiation of platelets to prevent alloimmunization and refractoriness to platelet transfusions. N Engl J Med. 1997;337:1861–9.

Answer to question 7: B

Educational objective

To diagnose and treat disseminated intravascular coagulation (DIC) characterized by simultaneous bleeding and thrombosis

Critique

Although the simultaneous onset of mental status changes, fever, schistocytosis, thrombocytopenia, and thrombosis should raise the possibility of thrombotic thrombocytopenic purpura (TTP), there are a number of clues that the correct diagnosis is DIC rather than TTP. First, the patient clearly has acute bacterial sepsis, which is one of the most common antecedents of DIC but is rarely seen as a lead-up to TTP because the latter more commonly occurs in previously well patients. Second, the markedly abnormal coagulation parameters are typical of DIC and almost never seen in isolated TTP. Third, multicentric bleeding in combination with thrombosis is common in severe DIC but rarely seen in TTP. Fourth, most patients with full-blown TTP have striking schistocytosis, whereas this patient is described as having only mild to moderate schistocytosis.

The cornerstone of the management of DIC is to identify and treat the precipitating cause. However, as this case illustrates, the latter is often not sufficient to avert life-threatening DIC, so blood product support often becomes necessary. A common problem in DIC is to avoid further fluid overload and potential noncardiogenic pulmonary edema in patients who are often already suffering from systemic capillary leak. As a result, cryoprecipitate, which is a concentrated solution containing primarily prothrombotic elements such as fibrinogen, von Willebrand factor, and factor XIII, is commonly administered to patients with severe hemorrhagic DIC. However, it is important to recall that patients with DIC, and particularly those who are already manifesting active thrombosis, are typically suffering from substantial depletions of both naturally circulating procoagulants and anticoagulants. Thus, repleting only the procoagulants, ie, by administering cryoprecipitate alone, has the potential to induce or exacerbate thrombosis. Therefore, most authorities recommend including at least some fresh frozen plasma (FFP) in the initial therapeutic cocktail for patients with severe DIC, even in patients who are not yet manifesting overt thrombosis. In severely thrombotic patients, heparin may be indicated, and there is evidence that infusion of activated protein C reduces mortality in patients with sepsis-associated DIC.

Steroids and plasma exchange would be appropriate for TTP but are not indicated in patients with DIC, whereas choices C and D omit the important components of FFP and cryoprecipitate, respectively.

References

Levi M, Ten Cate H. Disseminated intravascular coagulation. N Engl J Med. 1999;341:1937–8.

Toh CH, Dennis M. Disseminated intravascular coagulation: old disease, new hope. BMJ. 2003;327:974–7.

Answer to question 8: D

Educational objective

To understand the proper use and indications for Rh(D)-immune globulin in the obstetrical patient

Critique

Rh(D) immune globulin (RhIg) is indicated for immune prophylaxis, ie, for the prevention of sensitization to the Rh(D) antigen. Once an individual has mounted an immune response to Rh(D), the administration of RhIg will not shut off anti-Rh(D) production. For Rh(D)-negative individuals who do not show evidence of sensitization to Rh(D), the standard of care is to administer 1 vial of RhIg at 28 weeks of pregnancy and another at delivery. If, after birth, it is found that the newborn is Rh(D)-negative, then the postdelivery dose is not necessary. RhIg should also be given to unsensitized Rh(D)-negative women following a spontaneous or therapeutic abortion, or following any kind of trauma during a pregnancy in which a fetal–maternal bleed may have occurred. Though platelets do not express the Rh(D) antigen, doses of pooled whole blood-derived platelets as well as apheresis platelets collected from Rh(D)-positive donors can contain quantities (a few milliliters) of Rh(D)-bearing red blood cells (RBCs) sufficient to induce sensitization to Rh(D). For this reason, the administration of 1 vial of RhIg, which is sufficient to cover ~15 mL of RBCs, is recommended for Rh(D)-negative patients who may have received platelet products from Rh(D)-positive donors.

It would appear that this patient has been exposed to Rh(D) at some point in her past, either from an inadvertent transfusion of Rh(D)-positive RBCs or through a previous pregnancy with an Rh(D)-positive fetus (carried to term or not) for which she did not properly receive RhIg prophylaxis. Had the patient not been so sure that she had never received RhIg, it is possible that the anti-Rh(D) detected in her serum was actually passively acquired from a dose of RhIg given within the past 3 months, following, eg, a miscarriage, though a titer of 1:16 is quite high for passively acquired anti-Rh(D).

Dosing of RhIg to unsensitized Rh(D)-negative individuals is based on an estimate of the degree of fetal Rh(D)-positive cells in the maternal circulation, and a 300-μg vial is administered for every 15 mL of fetal RBCs. To assess the degree of fetal–maternal hemorrhage, most blood banks initially employ an agglutination-based assay known as the "rosette test," which, if positive, indicates that there is more of a bleed than can be covered by 1 vial of RhIg. To quantify the bleed and determine how many vials to administer, assays are used that rely on distinguishing

RBCs by their content of fetal versus adult hemoglobin. Classically, fetal–maternal hemorrhage was quantified using the Kleihauer–Betke test, which relied on the precipitation of fetal hemoglobin under acid conditions on a blood smear of maternal blood. Due to inherent inaccuracies in this approach, the use of antifetal hemoglobin antibodies and flow cytometry have replaced the Kleihauer–Betke test in many laboratories.

References

American College of Obstetricians and Gynecologists. Prevention of Rh D Alloimmunization. Washington, DC: ACOG; May 1999. ACOG Practice Bulletin No. 4.

Chen JC, Davis BH, Wood B, et al. Multicenter experience with flow cytometric method for fetomaternal hemorrhage detection. Cytometry. 2002;50:285–90.

Answer to question 9: D

Educational objective

To understand proper transfusion practice with respect to the ABO blood group system and to recognize and appreciate the possible etiologies for forward and reverse typing discrepancies

Critique

The forward and reverse typing reactions for patients 1, 2, and 4 represent straightforward results for patients with ABO blood group types O, A, and AB, respectively. Patient 3 has a forward/reverse typing discrepancy in which the forward reaction would indicate blood group B but the reverse reaction is what one would expect to find in a blood group O individual.

Though one refers to blood group O red blood cells (RBCs) as "universal donor" red cells because they lack A and B antigens and blood group AB patients as "universal recipients" of RBCs because they lack anti-A and anti-B isohemagglutinins, just the opposite can be said with respect to the transfusion of plasma. Blood group O individuals are universal recipients of plasma because their cells lack both A and B antigens, and blood group AB plasma is the universal donor plasma because it lacks both isohemagglutinins. For this reason, though all patients can be transfused with AB plasma, blood group AB patients such as patient 4 can be safely transfused with plasma donated only by a blood group AB donor.

The serologic results found for patient 3 are most consistent with those of a blood group B individual whose serum contains cold-reactive antibodies that can agglutinate both the A and B reagent RBCs used for the reverse typing reactions. The fact that the blood bank had to wash the patient's cells with warm saline before testing of the cells could proceed suggests that the patient's cells had "autoagglutinated" due to some endogenous antibody that apparently loses its ability to bind to RBCs at warmer temperatures. This effect of temperature combined with the ability of these agglutinins to directly agglutinate RBCs and deposit complement on their surfaces (the direct antiglobulin test results) suggests that these agglutinins are of the immunoglobulin M (IgM) isotype (choice A). Given that the patient reports never having been transfused with RBCs, it is unlikely that he would have had a reason to develop RBC alloantibodies, much less those to a commonly expressed alloantigen, and, in any case, alloantibodies by definition would not agglutinate the patient's own cells (choice B). Though it is possible that the patient received blood group O platelets and passively acquired anti-A and anti-B isohemagglutinins (choice C), it is extremely unlikely that they would be present in sufficient titer to cause autoagglutination and a clinically significant hemolytic anemia. Paroxysmal cold hemoglobinuria is a type of autoimmune hemolytic anemia caused by cold-reactive, complement-fixing autoantibodies, but the hallmark of this disease is that the autoantibodies are IgG, not IgM, and such IgG antibodies would not be expected to directly agglutinate the patient's own cells and the reagent cells. Given the association of cold agglutinin disease with B-cell lymphoma, the clinical, laboratory, and serologic findings are most consistent with a diagnosis of IgM-mediated cold autoimmune hemolytic anemia.

Reference

American Association of Blood Banks. Technical Manual. 15th ed. Bethesda, MD: AABB Press; 2005.

Answer to question 10: A

Educational objective

To understand proper transfusion practice with respect to the ABO blood group system and to recognize and appreciate the possible etiologies for forward and reverse typing discrepancies

Critique

The forward and reverse typing reactions for patients 1, 2, and 4 represent straightforward results for patients with ABO blood group types O, A, and AB, respectively. Patient 3 has a forward/reverse typing discrepancy in which the forward reaction would indicate blood group B but the reverse reaction is what one would expect to find in a blood group O individual.

Though one refers to blood group O red blood cells (RBCs) as "universal donor" red cells because they lack A and B antigens and blood group AB patients as "universal recipients" of RBCs because they lack anti-A and anti-B isohemagglutinins, just the opposite can be said with respect to the transfusion of plasma. Blood group O individuals are universal recipients of plasma because their cells lack both A and B antigens, and blood group AB plasma is the universal donor plasma because it lacks both isohemagglutinins. For this reason, though all patients can be transfused with AB plasma, blood group AB patients such as patient 4 can be safely transfused with plasma donated only by a blood group AB donor.

The serologic results found for patient 3 are most consistent with those of a blood group B individual whose serum contains cold-reactive antibodies that can agglutinate both the A and B reagent RBCs used for the reverse typing reactions. The fact that the blood bank had to wash the patient's cells with warm saline before testing of the cells could proceed suggests that the patient's cells had "autoagglutinated" due to some endogenous antibody that apparently loses its ability to bind to RBCs at warmer temperatures. This effect of temperature combined with the ability of these agglutinins to directly agglutinate RBCs and deposit complement on their surfaces (the direct antiglobulin test results) suggests that these agglutinins are of the immunoglobulin M (IgM) isotype (choice A). Given that the patient reports never having been transfused with RBCs, it is unlikely that he would have had a reason to develop RBC alloantibodies, much less those to a commonly expressed alloantigen, and, in any case, alloantibodies by definition would not agglutinate the patient's own cells (choice B). Though it is possible that the patient received blood group O platelets and passively acquired anti-A and anti-B isohemagglutinins (choice C), it is extremely unlikely that they would be present in sufficient titer to cause autoagglutination and a clinically significant hemolytic anemia. Paroxysmal cold hemoglobinuria is a type of autoimmune hemolytic anemia caused by cold-reactive, complement-fixing autoantibodies, but the hallmark of this disease is that the autoantibodies are IgG, not IgM, and such IgG antibodies would not be expected to directly agglutinate the patient's own cells and the reagent cells. Given the association of cold agglutinin disease with B-cell lymphoma, the clinical, laboratory, and serologic findings are most consistent with a diagnosis of IgM-mediated cold autoimmune hemolytic anemia.

Reference

American Association of Blood Banks. Technical Manual. 15th ed. Bethesda, MD: AABB Press; 2005.

Answer to question 11: C

Educational objective

To recognize the signs and symptoms of a delayed hemolytic transfusion reaction and to understand appropriate blood bank workup and interpretation of results

Critique

This clinical scenario is typical of what one would see in a patient undergoing a delayed hemolytic transfusion reaction (DHTR). In such a reaction, a patient has become sensitized to a foreign red blood cell (RBC) alloantigen in the past, but the titer of that antibody then drops below the limit of detection using standard serologic techniques. Consequently, it is not known that blood for transfusion needs to be screened for the absence of the corresponding alloantigen. If, by chance (and the chance will depend on the prevalence of that particular alloantigen in the donor population), the transfused RBC unit carries that alloantigen, the patient can experience an anamnestic immune response in which the somewhat dormant alloantibody-producing B-cell clones undergo a resurgence of production of that particular alloantibody. This process takes a few days to occur, after which the transfused cells bearing the alloantigen can be gradually destroyed. Because this is a secondary immune response, ie, one in which immunoglobulin G (IgG), not IgM, antibodies would be the major isotype, destruction of the transfused cells can go somewhat unnoticed, rarely leading to severe complications like acute renal failure or disseminated intravascular coagulation. One notable exception is DHTRs involving alloantibodies to the Kidd blood group antigens. Besides being notorious for dwindling in titer over time and becoming undetectable prior to subsequent transfusions, anti-Kidd antibodies, though IgG, are capable of fixing complement and can cause an intravascular hemolysis that may become significantly problematic.

With respect to the serologic workup of this patient, the blood bank would perform a series of tests to rule out the possibility that a mistake was made the week before, eg, (i) repeating the patient's pretransfusion type and screen to make sure that no additional alloantibodies were missed besides the 4 that had been identified, (ii) retyping the transfused units to make sure that they indeed lacked those 4 alloantigens (choice A), and (iii) repeating the crossmatches of those units with the patient's pretransfusion specimen to make sure they were indeed compatible (choice B). Retyping the patient's RBCs in the pretransfusion sample for the absence of the 4 alloantigens (choice D) would probably not be repeated—it would have been performed at the time of the first workup as a check to see that the patient's phenotype was consistent with an individual whose immune system could make alloantibodies to those 4 alloantigens.

Although the preceding tests rule out the possibility that a laboratory error had occurred during the first blood bank workup, another set of serologic tests would focus on the analysis of the patient's current blood sample. The most informative tests in the workup of a DHTR would be the antibody screen/panel (choice C) and direct antiglobulin test (DAT, "direct Coombs test"). In this hypothetical case, now approximately 7 days out from the transfusion, the patient's serum not only shows the presence of alloantibodies to K1, E, Fy^a, and S, but also demonstrates an anti-Jk^a alloantibody (Jk^a being a member of the Kidd blood group system). In addition, the patient's DAT is positive for both IgG and C3 (a DAT is then performed on the pretransfusion RBCs and is found to be negative). An eluate is then performed in which the IgG responsible for the positive DAT is stripped from the cells by any one of a number of methods (eg, low pH), and then the eluted IgG is run against a panel of reagent RBCs to identify its specificity. In this case, the eluate contains anti-Jk^a IgG. To close the loop in this post-DHTR workup, retained aliquots of cells from the transfused units are typed for Jk^a. One of them is found to be Jk^a-positive, explaining why the drop in the patient's hemoglobin is consistent with the loss of nearly all of 1 U of cells. If crossmatches are repeated with aliquots from the transfused units and the patient's current serum, one of the units would now appear crossmatch incompatible.

Reference

American Association of Blood Banks. Technical Manual. 15th ed. Bethesda, MD: AABB Press; 2005.

Answer to question 12: D

Educational objective

To understand the serologic workup for a recently transfused patient with pan-reactive autoantibodies

Critique

The physician is correct in that units of blood that will be eventually issued by the blood bank for this patient will be crossmatch incompatible. This is because the autoantibodies in autoimmune hemolytic anemia (AIHA) are nearly always specific for "public" antigens, ie, antigens present not only on the patient's own cells, but also on all donor cells. The issue here is that, before releasing units to this patient whom one knows *a priori* will be incompatible because of the autoantibodies, it is necessary to first determine whether the patient's serum also contains any underlying alloantibodies. If the patient's serum does contain alloantibodies, then blood that lacks those particular alloantigens should be provided so as not to compound the immunologic incompatibility. Because the serum of patients with AIHA contain autoantibodies that agglutinate all panel cells, the ability to identify the specificity of underlying alloantibodies by differential reactivity against panel cells is obscured. To get around this, autoabsorptions can be performed in which patient cells are used to absorb out the autoantibody component but leave behind any alloantibodies (choice B). Autoabsorbed serum is then run against a set of panel cells to determine if there are any alloantibodies present.

However, in a patient such as this one who has recently been transfused and has allogeneic cells circulating with her own cells, absorbing with cells drawn from the patient could remove not only the autoreactivity, but the alloreactivity as well. In this case, a more complex series of differential absorptions are required using a carefully selected set of reagent red blood cells (RBCs) of varying phenotype (choice D). Each reagent cell is designed to remove the autoantibodies but will differ in what alloantibodies it can leave behind. For optimal management of this patient, it would ideally be desirable to know the patient's extended phenotype (choice C) so units that most closely match the patient's phenotype (and thereby incapable of inducing further alloantibody formation) could be issued to this patient. However, given that the patient was recently transfused, a pure preparation of just her cells is unavailable at this time. Extended phenotyping of patients with AIHA is best performed when the patient first presents and has not yet been transfused. Choice A, the result of which would be of academic interest, would, at best, indicate that perhaps there is an extremely rare type of RBC that lacks the "public" antigen to which this patient's autoantibodies are directed, yet finding multiple units of this blood sufficient for supporting the transfusion needs of this patient in real time would be totally impractical.

References

American Association of Blood Banks. Technical Manual. 15th ed. Bethesda, MD: AABB Press; 2005.

Petz LD. A physician's guide to transfusion in autoimmune hemolytic anemia. Br J Haematol. 2004;124:712–6.

Answer to question 13: B

Educational objective

To provide appropriate blood product support in immunoglobulin A (IgA)-deficient individuals

Critique

Although the absence of plasma IgA occurs in approximately 1 in 700 individuals in the general population, anaphylactoid reactions to IgA are much less common, occurring in approximately 1 in 30,000 transfusions. Nevertheless, it is important for the hematologist to be aware of this complication. The reaction itself is usually due to the development of IgG antibody directed against IgA that is normally present in the plasma in the supernatant of transfused red cells or platelets and thus is usually characterized as anaphylactoid rather than truly anaphylactic. Because the reaction is to a plasma component, the administration of irradiated or leukofiltered blood products will not prevent the reaction. In theory, other IgA-deficient individuals could be used as donors, but in most situations this is not practical due to the relative scarcity of IgA-deficient individuals in the population. The latter would be a particular issue in a patient undergoing acute leukemia induction, in which it is likely that many units of blood products will be required during the course of his induction, consolidation, and maintenance therapy. Even if an IgA-deficient family member were available, the use of his or her blood products would be relatively contraindicated because the transfusion of blood from family members may increase the risk of subsequent graft rejection if an allogeneic bone marrow transplant from a matched family member becomes necessary.

Prevention of transfusion-transmitted cytomegalovirus (CMV) infection is a very important issue in patients with hematologic malignancies, a high percentage of whom will go on to require bone marrow transplantation, but it is very unlikely that CMV transmission could account for the acute reaction depicted here. In contrast, a recurrence of such reactions can usually be prevented by the use of washed red cells, ie, red cells that have been resuspended in saline rather than plasma. In IgA-deficient individuals who have had true anaphylactic reactions to prior blood product transfusion and urgently require *plasma* products, judicious administration of plasma products obtained from IgA-deficient individuals may be the only solution. Though platelets can be washed free of plasma proteins like red blood cells, platelet quantity and quality are more adversely affected by the washing process. Consequently, platelet products derived from IgA-deficient individuals, if available within a reasonable time frame, would be the platelet product of choice for the IgA-deficient patient.

References

Lilic D, Sewell WAC. IgA deficiency: what we should – or should not – be doing. J Clin Path. 2001;54:337–8.

Sandler SG. How I manage patients suspected of having had an IgA anaphylactic transfusion reaction. Transfusion. 2006; 46:10–3.

Sandler SG, Eckrich R, Malamut D, et al. Hemagglutination assays for the diagnosis and prevention of IgA anaphylactic transfusion reactions. Blood. 1994;84:2031–5.

Answer to question 14: D

Educational objective

To diagnose transfusion-induced graft-versus-host-disease in an immunosuppressed patient who receives non-γ-irradiated blood products

Critique

Transfusion-induced graft-versus-host-disease is a usually lethal complication of the administration non-γ-irradiated blood products to markedly immunosuppressed individuals. The risk appears to be the highest in recent allogeneic bone marrow transplant recipients and patients with T-cell immunodeficiency syndromes, but other risk factors include patients with hematologic malignancies in general and the administration of transfusions from close family members. The classic triad of *transplant*-induced graft-versus-host disease is skin itching, diarrhea, and abnormal liver function tests, but patients with *transfusion*-induced graft-versus-host disease typically develop severe pancytopenia in addition to the classic triad just listed. The severe pancytopenia is probably due to the fact that the hematopoietic stem cells are recipient derived rather than donor derived. Unfortunately, the case-fatality rate for transfusion-induced graft-versus-host disease is very high, due primarily to the severe refractory pancytopenia.

The development of viral hepatitis or cytomegalovirus disease only 14 days after transfusion would be unusual and would not readily explain all of the extrahepatic manifestations.

The timing of the anemia would be about right with regard to a delayed hemolytic transfusion reaction or marrow suppression by antibiotics, but again these diagnoses would not explain all of the other features of the child's illness.

References

Anderson K. Broadening the spectrum of patient groups at risk for transfusion-associated GVHD: implications for universal irradiation of cellular blood components. Transfusion. 2003;43:1652–4.

Orlin JB, Ellis MH. Transfusion-induced graft-versus-host disease. Curr Opin Hematol. 1997;4:442–8.

Answer to question 15: D

Educational objective

To understand the serologic workup of a case of suspected hemolytic disease of the newborn (HDN)

Critique

This is a case of ABO-mediated HDN. Fetal–maternal ABO incompatibility is usually not high on the differential as a cause of HDN because anti-A and anti-B isohemagglutinins are classically thought of as IgM antibodies, which cannot cross the placenta. However, blood group O individuals make an IgG form of isohemagglutinin typically referred to as anti-A,B because it cross-reacts with both A and B blood group antigens. In blood group O mothers, such IgG can cross the placenta; bind to fetal red blood cells (RBCs) that are blood group A, B, or AB; and induce hemolysis. Usually, the hemolysis, if any, is mild, though severe cases of ABO HDN are well documented and are best treated with exchange transfusion with blood group O RBCs. One of the main reasons why ABO HDN is usually not clinically significant is because, unlike Rh(D), ABO blood group antigens are expressed on nearly all tissues of the body so that much of the maternal antibody can be absorbed by fetal cells other than RBCs. Also, ABO blood group antigens can be present in a soluble form in plasma and can compete with RBCs for binding. In cases of active HDN, bilirubinemia can actually increase following birth (as in this case) because the mother's liver is no longer able to help the infant's rather immature liver conjugate all of the bilirubin that results from the ongoing destruction of the antibody-coated cells postdelivery.

A key to understanding the serologic workup in this case is the recognition that, by convention, all screening cells and panel cells used for alloantibody specificity determination are intentionally selected to be blood group O so that a patient's isohemagglutinins will not confound the interpretation of results. That is why the baby's anti-A,B-containing eluate was nonreactive unless incubated with blood group A and B cells (choice D). Performing the tests in choices A and C would not reveal anything new because at birth essentially all serum antibody in the newborn is derived from the maternal circulation. Therefore, the baby's serum would be nonreactive with maternal RBCs (choice C) and would either be negative on an antibody screen (choice A) or positive for passively transferred anti-D from the mother. If it were to turn out that the eluate was negative for anti-A,B, then the possibility would exist that the baby has sensitized the mother to a low-frequency (ie, rare) antigen that she inherited from her father. All screening tests are negative in this case because standard sets of reagent RBCs do not generally express low-frequency antigens. To address this, many blood bank laboratories have frozen stocks of RBCs with rare phenotypes that can be used for determining the specificity of antibodies to low-frequency antigens (choice B). However, such an extensive workup may be more for academic interest because knowledge of the offending antibody would not be needed to find compatible blood for the baby as nearly every donor unit, by definition, would lack the corresponding low-frequency antigen.

Reference

Judd WJ. Practice guidelines for prenatal and perinatal immunohematology, revisited. Transfusion. 2001;41:1445–52.

CHAPTER 17

Laboratory hematology

Answer to question 1: D

Educational objective

To recognize cold agglutinin through effect on complete blood cell count

Critique

At first glance, this appears to be a macrocytic anemia, but there is a discrepancy in the hemoglobin and hematocrit values, and the mean corpuscular hemoglobin concentration (MCHC) is markedly elevated. This is the artifactual pattern typically caused by the presence of cold agglutinins, which are often seen in lymphoplasmacytic lymphoma (Waldenstrom macroglobulinemia). The 3 direct measurements performed by automated counters are number of cells, size of cell, and hemoglobin content of the sample. All other values are calculated. Cell counters are actually particle counters, so the presence of agglutination or rouleaux formation may cause clumps of cells to be counted and sized as if they are one cell. Hereditary spherocytosis causes elevated MCHC, but the hemoglobin and mean corpuscular volume (MCV) values should be low. Pernicious anemia causes macrocytic anemia with elevated MCV, but again there is no anemia present, and the other cell lines are normal. Myelodysplasia may cause elevated MCV and a refractory anemia, but the hemoglobin is too high and the MCHC would not be elevated. The anemia of renal failure is normocytic and not macrocytic.

Reference

Stone MJ, Merlini G, Pascual V. Autoantibody activity in Waldenstrom's macroglobulinemia. Clin Lymphoma. 2005;5:225–9.

Answer to question 2: E

Educational objective

To interpret impairment of platelet aggregation testing

Critique

There is normal platelet aggregation induced by all agonists except ristocetin. This is present in most types of von Willebrand disorder (vWD), although type IIB and platelet-type vWD may have hyperresponsiveness to ristocetin. Reduced ristocetin-induced aggregation is also the classic finding in Bernard–Soulier syndrome (BSS), due to the absence of membrane glycoprotein Ib, which participates in ristocetin-mediated von Willebrand factor (vWF) binding. Replacing the plasma used in the aggregation assay with plasma that has normal vWF and ristocetin cofactor will correct the defect in vWD but not in BSS. In addition, BSS platelets are usually thrombocytopenic, both because of a lower than normal number as well as a much higher mean platelet volume that interferes with accurate counting. Glanzmann thrombasthenia is caused by absence of the membrane glycoprotein IIb/IIIa complex, and causes diminished responses to most agonists with the exception of ristocetin. Aspirin effect and storage pool defects usually have normal ristocetin-induced aggregation, although a variety of abnormal responses to the other agonists can be present.

Reference

Zhou L, Schmaier AH. Platelet aggregation testing in platelet-rich plasma: description of procedures with the aim to develop standards in the field. Am J Clin Path. 2005;23:172–83.

Answer to question 3: B

Educational objective

To interpret significance of rouleaux on blood smear

Critique

This is rouleaux formation, with the typical linear "stack of coins" alignment that distinguishes it from agglutination. It is seen when increased levels of asymmetrically charged serum proteins, chiefly γ globulins or fibrinogen, alter the electrostatic charge of the red cell. Although the increased amount of monoclonal γ globulin in myeloma (and some lymphoma) can lead to rouleaux, autoimmune and inflammatory diseases also cause this. Protein electrophoresis would be the best way to determine the presence of a paraprotein, polyclonal gammopathy, or elevated inflammatory globulins. Rouleaux is not mediated through red cell-specific antibodies, as detected by the direct antiglobulin test. Fibrinogen levels may be elevated in inflammation, but rouleaux is not limited to elevations of this acute phase reactant. Skeletal surveys are helpful in making the diagnosis of myeloma but would be premature in the workup at this point, as would a computed tomographic scan.

Reference

Anderson KC. Multiple myeloma: how far have we come? Mayo Clin Proc. 2003;78:15–7.

Answer to question 4: C

Educational objective

To characterize pseudothrombocytopenia

Critique

This is pseudothrombocytopenia caused by platelet clumping, and it shows the clustering effect around neutrophils known as platelet satellitism. This is from EDTA-dependent antibodies that cause platelet aglutination as an artifact in the collection tube, but not true thrombocytopenia in the patient. There is no mention of signs or symptoms of sepsis, and this patient probably has an unchanged platelet count *in vivo*. The time course is not consistent with the usual presentation of heparin-induced thrombocytopenia (HIT), and although HIT antibodies cause primary platelet activation, this leads to platelet destruction and true thrombocytopenia, not *in vitro* platelet clumping. In similar fashion, clopidogrel has been reported to cause thrombotic thrombocytopenic purpura, which is also a condition with primary platelet activation, but there is no evidence of microangiopathy on smear. In some series, one third or more of patients with antiphospholipid antibody have autoimmune thrombocytopenia, but these antibodies do not cause clumping. The finding in this patient underscores the importance of examining the smear in any case of suspected thrombocytopenia.

Reference

Gschwandtner ME, Siostrzonek P, Bodinger C, et al. Documented sudden onset of pseudothrombocytopenia. Ann Hematol. 1997;74:283–5.

Answer to question 5: B

Educational objective

To distinguish lupus anticoagulant from acquired factor inhibitor

Critique

This patient has an acquired bleeding problem associated with a prolonged partial thromboplastin time (PTT) that does not correct with mixing, and the picture is most consistent with an acquired factor deficiency. The most common are inhibitors to factor VIII, and many cases are seen in elderly patients with occult malignancy, often colon cancer. Her gastrointestinal (GI) symptoms may be indicative of this. Lupus anticoagulant (antiphospholipid antibodies) is also an acquired condition that causes a prolonged PTT that does not correct with mixing, but it is associated with hypercoagulability rather than bleeding. Factor XI deficiency is an autosomal defect associated with variable rates of bleeding and can affect women, and it does cause a prolonged PTT. However, it would correct to normal during a mixing study and is unusual in ethnic populations other than Ashkenazi Jews. Warfarin ingestion would affect the prothrombin time (PT) more than the PTT and unless quite severe would correct with mixing. The history of GI disease may indicate acquired vitamin K deficiency, but again the PT rather than the PTT would be the most affected test, and the deficiency would correct with mixing.

References

Baudo F, de Cataldo F, Gaidano G. Treatment of acquired factor VIII inhibitor with recombinant activated factor VIIa: data from the Italian registry of acquired hemophilia. Haematologica. 2004;89:759–61.

Sallah S, Aledort L. Treatment of patients with acquired inhibitors. J Thromb Haemostasis. 2005;3:595–7.

Answer to question 6: B

Educational objective

To distinguish α thalassemia trait effect on hemoglobin electrophoresis

Critique

The predominant hemoglobin (Hb) present is Hb A, with a smaller amount of Hb S. This defines sickle cell trait, rather than a sickle cell hemoglobinopathy syndrome. Although transfusion may obscure the percentages in sickle cell disease patients, there is neither transfusion history nor any history consistent with a sickle cell syndrome. The diagnostic feature of this patient's laboratory findings is a reduction in the amount of Hb S compared with the expected 40–45% in most sickle cell trait individuals. This is the typical effect of α thalassemia, which limits the number of α chains available for heterodimerization with non-α gene products. As the number of functional α chains decreases from the typical number of 4, lower percentages of non-A Hb are observed because of preferential binding to Hb A chains during hemoglobinization of red cell precursors. This "skewing" effect has been known since the 1970s, and α thalassemia genes (both the single- as well as double-deletion type) are present in approximately equal numbers to the Hb S gene in African American populations. If a β thalassemia gene were present, there should be elevated levels of Hb A_2. The presence of 2 functioning non-α hemoglobin genes is clearly demonstrated by the presence of both Hb A and Hb S. β^+ mutations of the Hb A gene would allow both non-α genes to be expressed, but the level of Hb A would be well below the Hb S level. β^0 mutations would allow only Hb S to be expressed. This patient has a mild anemia with marked hypochromia and microcytosis, but with a higher number of red cells than normal. This is most consistent with the effect of a thalassemia gene rather than iron deficiency or other less common causes of microcytic, hypochromic anemia. Besides, the patient has been on oral iron for some time, without improvement. The patient could have an undiagnosed underlying inflammatory condition (perhaps her irritable bowel syndrome is really inflammatory disease?) and so could have anemia of chronic disease, which can sometimes give a microcytic appearance to red cells. However, anemia of chronic disease would not elevate the red cell count nor skew the percentages of Hb A and Hb S.

References

Steinberg MH. Predicting clinical severity in sickle cell anaemia. Br J Haematol. 2005;129:465–81.

Wambua S, Mwacharo J, Uyoga S, et al. Co-inheritance of alpha+-thalassaemia and sickle trait results in specific effects on haematological parameters. Br J Haematol. 2006;133:206–9.

Answer to question 7: A

Educational objective

To distinguish heparin effect from dysfibrinogenemia

Critique

Prolongation of the thrombin time with a normal reptilase time indicates the effect of heparin, heparinoids, or similar thrombin inhibitor. Presumably, there was a cumulative heparin effect from this patient's chronic dialysis. The thrombin time is performed by adding thrombin to the sample and measuring clot formation. The venom of the snake used in the reptilase time directly cleaves fibrinogen at sites other than thrombin cleavage sites but also measures fibrin formation. Both tests are relatively insensitive to other factor deficiencies, even prothrombin deficiency. Vitamin K deficiency may give abnormal prothrombin time and partial thromboplastin time results, but fibrinogen levels are not vitamin K dependent. Disturbances in either the amount or function of fibrinogen will prolong both the thrombin time and the reptilase time. Increased fibrin degradation products will prolong both tests, as will fibrinogen levels much below 100 mg/dL, as in the case of hypofibrinogenemia or afibrinogenemia. This patient's fibrinogen level is well above 100. Dysfibrinogenemia from impaired hepatic synthesis due to liver disease will also cause both tests to become prolonged, even at levels that approach normal values. Dysfibrinogenemia may give markedly discrepant results between functional fibrinogen assays and immunoassays. Paraproteins and amyloidosis may prolong both tests as well through interference with fibrin formation but will not give a prolonged thrombin time and a normal reptilase time.

References

Cunningham MT, Brandt JT, Laposata M, et al. Laboratory diagnosis of dysfibrinogenemia. Arch Pathol Lab Med. 2002;126:499–505.

Van Cott EM, Smith EY, Galanakis DK. Elevated fibrinogen in an acute phase reaction prolongs the reptilase time but typically not the thrombin time. Am J Clin Pathol. 2002; 118:263–8.

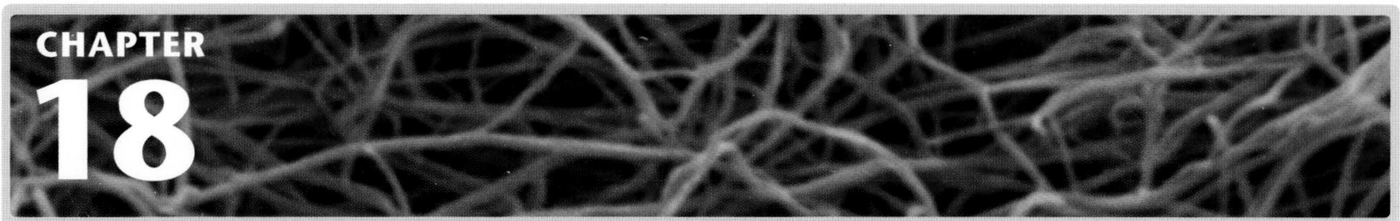

CHAPTER 18

Consultative hematology

Answer to question 1: D

Educational objective

To recognize and initiate appropriate treatment for delayed-onset heparin-induced thrombocytopenia (HIT)

Critique

This patient presented with symptomatic coronary artery disease and underwent cardiac catheterization, at which time she was exposed to heparin. Seven days later, she was reexposed to heparin during cardiac bypass surgery and developed moderate thrombocytopenia immediately afterward. However, her platelet count was increasing at the time of her discharge. Three weeks later, she returned with a pulmonary embolism and thrombocytopenia. A diagnosis that ties the thrombocytopenia together with a new thromboembolic event is delayed-onset HIT. This disorder may develop weeks after heparin exposure, and its development in the postbypass setting is well described. A further fall in the platelet count and worsening of symptoms upon reinstitution of heparin therapy is consistent with this diagnosis. Thus, the appropriate treatment of this patient is to discontinue heparin and initiate therapy for the pulmonary embolism with a direct thrombin inhibitor (D). Discontinuation of the heparin without replacement by an alternative anticoagulant (C) would not be an acceptable approach, given the pulmonary embolism, nor would replacement of heparin with low-molecular-weight heparin (B), because more than 80% of unfractionated heparin-platelet factor 4 antibodies cross-react with low-molecular-weight heparin-platelet factor 4 complexes. Corticosteroid therapy (E) would be appropriate therapy for a primary immune thrombocytopenia such as idiopathic thrombocytopenic purpura, but the presentation is not consistent with this diagnosis. Finally, increasing the heparin dosage, despite worsening symptoms, would not be appropriate in a patient with HIT (A).

References

Warkentin TE, Greinacher A. Heparin-induced thrombocytopenia and cardiac surgery. Ann Thorac Surg. 2003;76:638–48.

Warkentin TE, Kelton JG. Delayed-onset heparin-induced thrombocytopenia and thrombosis. Ann Int Med. 2001;135: 502–6.

Warkentin TE, Kelton JG. Temporal aspects of heparin-induced thrombocytopenia. N Engl J Med. 2001;344:1286–92.

Answer to question 2: E

Educational objective

To diagnose and initiate appropriate treatment for thrombotic thrombocytopenic purpura (TTP) in a pregnant patient

Critique

This patient presents in the third trimester of pregnancy with malaise, fever, and thrombocytopenia. The peripheral blood film reveals a striking microangiopathic hemolytic anemia. There is neither hypertension nor significant proteinuria, allowing the exclusion of preeclampsia. Likewise, the alanine aminotransferase and aspartate aminotransferase are normal, allowing the exclusion of the HELLP (hemolysis, elevated liver enzymes, low-platelet count) syndrome. Hence, it appears that this patient has microangiopathic hemolytic anemia, thrombocytopenia, and fever, with her inability to concentrate perhaps representing a neurologic symptom as well. This constellation of symptoms is consistent with TTP/hemolytic uremic syndrome (TTP/HUS). In any case, the optimal therapy for this patient would be daily plasma exchange (E), which induces remission of TTP in more than 80% of cases. Expeditious delivery would not change the course of TTP/HUS; thus, answer (A) is not correct. Pulse dexamethasone (B) or rituximab (C) are useful therapies for idiopathic thrombocytopenic purpura (ITP), but ITP is not the correct diagnosis in this patient because thrombocytopenia in ITP is not accompanied by microangiopathic hemolytic anemia. Rituximab is an emerging therapy for TTP/HUS but at this point cannot be considered first line; moreover, its safety in pregnancy has not been established. Finally, obtaining the fetal platelet count (D) would not be optimal because it is associated with a complication rate of approximately 1%, even in patients without an acute, life-threatening illness, and would not affect therapy delivered to the mother.

References

George JN. How I treat patients with thrombotic thrombocytopenic purpura-hemolytic uremic syndrome. Blood. 2000;96:1223–9.

Karim R, Sacher RA. Thrombocytopenia in pregnancy. Curr Hematol Rep. 2004;3:128–33.

McCrae KR. Thrombocytopenia in pregnancy: differential diagnosis, pathogenesis and management. Blood Rev. 2003; 17:7–14.

Answer to question 3: A

Educational objective

To understand the appropriate anticoagulant management in a patient contemplating pregnancy with a history of a prior venous thromboembolic event associated with an identifiable cause

Critique

This patient has a history of a prior thrombotic event at a young age. However, this event was associated with an easily identifiable risk factor, ie, a fractured ankle that required immobilization in a cast. Moreover, subsequent screening for an underlying thrombophilic state revealed no abnormalities. Current guidelines of the American College of Chest Physicians recommend that a patient such as this be followed with close clinical surveillance during pregnancy and receive anticoagulation during the postpartum period (A). Coumadin is also safe in nursing mothers. There is no need to repeat genetic testing for thrombophilia (B) or testing for antiphospholipid antibodies (C), particularly because the patient's thrombotic event was several years earlier and she has experienced no recurrences. Likewise, antepartum therapy with either low-molecular-weight heparin (D) or coumadin (E) is not indicated, as noted previously. Coumadin is associated with an embryopathy, particularly during weeks 6–12 of pregnancy, though it may probably be used safely during the first few weeks of pregnancy.

References

Bates SM, Greer IA, Hirsh J, et al. Use of antithrombotic agents during pregnancy. The seventh ACCP conference on antithrombotic and thrombolytic therapy. Chest. 2004;126: S627–44.

Brill-Edwards P, Ginsberg JS, Gent M, et al. Safety of withholding heparin in pregnant women with a history of venous thromboembolism. Recurrence of clot in this Pregnancy Study Group. N Engl J Med. 2000;343:1439–44.

James AH, Abel DE, Brancazio LR. Anticoagulants in pregnancy. Obstet Gynecol Surv. 2005;61:59–69.

Answer to question 4: B

Educational objective

To recognize and provide proper management for the HELLP (hemolysis, elevated liver enzymes, low-platelet count) syndrome

Critique

This patient is in the latter half of the third trimester of pregnancy and presents with thrombocytopenia, microangiopathic hemolytic anemia (see peripheral blood film), hypertension, and 3+ proteinuria accompanied by increased transaminases. Although she would meet criteria for a diagnosis of preeclampsia, the increased transaminases values and right upper quadrant pain are characteristic of the HELLP syndrome. Subcapsular hematomas may also occur in approximately 5% of patients with HELLP. This overlap in criteria between the 2 disorders is not uncommon. The most appropriate management of this patient is to stabilize her medically (ie, ensure normal fluid and electrolyte status, control hypertension) and after fetal lung maturity is confirmed initiate expeditious delivery (B). Daily plasma exchange would be considered for thrombotic thrombocytopenic purpura/hemolytic uremic syndrome, and although the patient clearly has a microangiopathic hemolytic anemia, her other symptoms should lead to a diagnosis of HELLP. Because plasma exchange is not the standard therapy for HELLP, answer (A) is not correct. Rituximab has not been shown to be of any benefit in HELLP or preeclampsia, and its safety in pregnancy has not been established. Though the elevated level of D-dimers suggests some degree of activation of the coagulation system, the prothrombin time and activated partial thromboplastin time are normal, and there is no indication for the use of fresh frozen plasma in this patient (D). Although right upper quadrant pain may also occur in acute cholecystitis, the constellation of symptoms here are consistent with HELLP rather than a primary gastrointestinal illness; thus, there is no indication for cholecystectomy (E).

References

George JN. How I treat patients with thrombotic thrombocytopenic purpura-hemolytic uremic syndrome. Blood. 2000;96:1223–9.

Karim R, Sacher RA. Thrombocytopenia in pregnancy. Curr Hematol Rep. 2004;3:128–33.

McCrae KR. Thrombocytopenia in pregnancy: differential diagnosis, pathogenesis and management. Blood Rev. 2003;17: 7–14.

Answer to question 5: E

Educational objective

To diagnose a congenital thrombocytopenia in a pregnant patient with isolated thrombocytopenia

Critique

This patient presents with isolated thrombocytopenia of unknown duration. When seen previously by another hematologist, she was presumed to have idiopathic thrombocytopenic purpura (ITP) and was treated with corticosteroids, but she did not respond. She believes she has a sister with ITP, though there are no confirmatory records available. The patient's thrombocytopenia is isolated, with normal red and white counts, and there is no history of significant bleeding, although it does not appear that she has faced significant hemostatic challenges.

Review of the patient's peripheral blood smear reveals large platelets as well as Döhle bodies in the leukocytes. This appearance would be very atypical for ITP. Likewise, ITP is not an inherited disorder and, given its low incidence, its occurrence in other first-degree relatives would be atypical. Finally, the majority of cases of ITP respond, at least initially, to corticosteroids, unlike this patient. The mild increase in platelets after intravenous immunoglobulin is probably nonsignificant and representative of normal variability in the platelet count.

The most likely diagnosis in this patient is a congenital thrombocytopenic disorder, specifically the May–Hegglin anomaly, which is characterized by mild to moderate thrombocytopenia, large platelets, and Döhle bodies in leukocytes. This disorder belongs to the *MYH9* gene-related congenital macrothrombocytopenias, which display autosomal dominant inheritance. Other members of this family include the Fechtner and Sebastian syndromes. This individual has had a relatively benign course and is not bleeding, and no specific intervention is indicated at the present time other than close observation. Comparison of the blood films of other family members is the most efficient and cost-effective means to confirm her diagnosis (E).

Bone marrow examination in this disorder is not diagnostic and therefore would not be helpful (A). She has already failed one course of corticosteroids, and additional treatment with corticosteroids would not raise the platelet count and would also increase the risk of pregnancy-related complications (B). Rituximab would not be of benefit in this nonimmune-mediated thrombocytopenia, and its safety in pregnancy has not been clearly established (C). Because the *MYH9*-related disorders represent primarily problems in platelet production, splenectomy is not a recognized treatment of these disorders (D).

References

Balduini CL, Iolascon A, Savoia A. Inherited thrombocytopenias. Haematologica. 2002;87:860–80.

Drachman JG. Inherited thrombocytopenia: when a low platelet count does not mean ITP. Blood. 2004;103:390–8.

Answer to question 6: C

Educational objective

To evaluate a preoperative patient with a prolonged activated partial thromboplastin time (APTT)

Critique

The preoperative hemostatic assessment of a patient without medical comorbidities or suspicious bleeding history who is undergoing a moderate- or high-risk surgical procedure should be limited to the prothrombin time (PT), APTT, and platelet count. Patients with normal screening tests and negative history, and even patients with a negative history and mildly abnormal screening tests, do not have increased perioperative bleeding or greater need for postoperative transfusions. Abnormal preoperative hemostatic tests that correlate with postprocedure bleeding are most commonly found in patients with a history of abnormal bleeding from any source (skin, mucous membranes, gastrointestinal tract, menses, and childbirth); family history of bleeding disorders; current use of antiplatelet, anticoagulant, or other medications that can affect hemostasis (eg, chronic antibiotics); prior bleeding associated with hemostatic challenges (surgery, trauma, and dental procedures); and/or known medical comorbidities associated with bleeding diathesis (eg, renal failure, hepatic failure, moderate to severe thrombocytopenia). More extensive evaluation of these patients is required to characterize the defect and to plan for perioperative hemostatic support. This patient's negative history of bleeding or oozing strongly suggests that the moderately prolonged APTT is due to a lupus anticoagulant. A lupus anticoagulant would not impart a risk of bleeding but could possibly predispose to postoperative thromboembolism. A moderately prolonged APTT due to any of the other disorders would reflect a significant defect in secondary hemostasis and likely would correspond to a history or signs of spontaneous or trauma-induced bleeding. A repeat APTT with a 1:1 mixing study would further characterize the abnormality. If the 1:1 mix fully corrects, it would suggest a factor deficiency, such as von Willebrand disease or inherited factor XI deficiency. A 1:1 mixing study that does not correct after 1–2 hours incubation would suggest a lupus anticoagulant or acquired inhibitor to factor VIII. Given the greater likelihood of a lupus anticoagulant, the next step should be a specific assay to determine whether the prolonged clotting time is corrected by provision of excess phospholipid (eg, dilute Russell viper venom time with phospholipid titration). If that is negative, a factor VIII activity level would then be appropriate.

Reference

Smetana GW, Macpherson DS. The case against routine preoperative laboratory testing. Med Clin N Am. 2003;87:7–40.

Answer to question 7: A

Educational objective

To manage postoperative hemorrhage after orthotopic liver transplantation

Critique

Liver transplantation is associated with bleeding risks due to temporary cessation of coagulation factor synthesis and enhanced fibrinolysis. Similar to other surgeries, postoperative hemorrhage can result from coagulopathy of hypertransfusion to treat massive hemorrhage, dilutional thrombocytopenia, disseminated intravascular coagulopathy (DIC), and underlying hemostatic defects. Surgical bleeding due to a vascular or tissue defect can often be differentiated from a hemostatic defect in that the former is typically associated with localized and brisk bleeding within the surgical bed whereas the latter often manifests as slow oozing from multiple sites. The initial evaluation requires an assessment of the laboratory coagulation profile to identify defects that will guide the replacement of factors and/or platelets to hemostatic levels. Severe acidosis and hypothermia should also be ruled out as a cause of bleeding.

In this case, the severely low fibrinogen and high D-dimer levels reflect a combination of fibrinolysis, deficient liver fibrinogen production, and inadequate fibrinogen replacement during transfusion support. Perioperatively, the thromboelastogram can be another useful assay to differentiate fibrinolysis from the other hemostatic derangements. The prolonged prothrombin time (PT) and activated partial thromboplastin time (APTT) in this patient may be due to the low fibrinogen level rather than a reflection of multiple factor deficiencies. Cryoprecipitate should be given to achieve a fibrinogen level of at least 1 g/L. After fibrinogen is repleted, a follow-up coagulation profile should be assessed to determine whether fresh frozen plasma might be required to achieve a PT/international normalized ratio (INR) of $\leq$1.5 and an APTT of $\leq$1.5 times control. If the patient has not received antiplatelet agents and is not uremic, a platelet count of $\geq$50,000/μL should be adequate for primary hemostasis and would not indicate a need for platelet transfusion.

Although recombinant factor VIIa (rFVIIa) showed promise as an effective prophylactic agent in early nonrandomized trials of liver transplantation, 2 recent randomized, double-blind, placebo-controlled trials observed no decreases in the number of perioperative red blood cell units transfused to patients who had received either a single preoperative dose of rFVIIa or multiple perioperative doses. Although rFVIIa may be beneficial for selected bleeding patients with severe liver failure and coagulopathy, this off-label usage carries the potential risk of inducing thrombosis. Antifibrinolytic agents, such as aprotinin or lysine anologues (ie, aminocaproic acid and tranexamic acid), are commonly used for bleeding prophylaxis in liver transplantation. In this postoperative patient with very low fibrinogen, aminocaproic acid would likely not offer additional benefit beyond that provided by correcting the coagulopathy with cryoprecipitate. However, like rFVIIa, aminocaproic acid could be considered for highly selected patients with persistent or uncontrolled bleeding after factor replacement.

References

Dagi TF. The management of postoperative bleeding. Surg Clin N Am. 2005;85:1191–213.

Lodge JP, Jonas S, Jones RM, et al. Efficacy and safety of repeated perioperative doses of recombinant factor VIIa in liver transplantation. Liver Transpl. 2005;11:973.

MacLaren R, Weber LA, Brake H, et al. A multicenter assessment of recombinant factor VIIa off-label usage: clinical experiences and associated outcomes. Transfusion 2005;45:1434–42.

Planinsic RM, van der Meer J, Testa G, et al. Safety and efficacy of a single bolus administration of recombinant factor VIIa in liver transplantation due to chronic liver disease. Liver Transpl. 2005;11:973–9.

Answer to question 8: D

Educational objective

To diagnose posttransplant lymphoproliferative disorder (PTLD)

Critique

The most important features in this case are the abnormal lymph node in the supraclavicular region, a possible new mass or lymphadenopathy in the left hilum of the transplanted lung, and recent fever with weight loss. Together, these are highly suggestive of a PTLD. Excisional biopsy of the pathologic node is the next step to assess for PTLD and alternative inflammatory, reactive, or infectious etiologies. If PTLD is found, immunohistochemistry, cytofluorometry, cytogenetics, and/or molecular studies will be important to classify the clonality status and histologic subtype of PTLD. Lung transplant patients have a roughly 60-fold relative risk of developing PTLD. Not uncommonly, the disease may present with masses or nodules in or near the transplanted organ. Most PTLD cases occur in the first year after a solid organ transplant, but the risk persists for many years. Most cases are associated with active Epstein–Barr virus (EBV) replication, which is thought to play an important role in disease pathogenesis. EBV seronegative recipients of organs from seropositive donors are, therefore, particularly susceptible to this complication. Although very high EBV DNA copy numbers are often found in the blood of patients with PTLD, this is not an adequate diagnostic test. Also, although extranodal disease is common with PTLD, the bone marrow is infrequently involved. A bronchoscopy would be a diagnostic option if an endobronchial mass was suspected and a pathologic peripheral lymph node was not available for biopsy. Bronchoalveolar lavage fluid has a low yield for PTLD diagnosis but might be helpful to rule out opportunistic infections. Anemia and thrombocytopenia in a posttransplant patient on a calcineurin inhibitor (ie, cyclosporine or tacrolimus) should raise the suspicion of drug-induced thrombotic microangiopathy (TMA)/ hemolytic uremic syndrome (HUS). However, in general, the ADAMTS13 protease activity is not causally associated with posttransplant TMA (the exception being patients with pretransplant thrombotic thrombocytopenic purpura [TTP]/HUS). Therefore, an assay for blood ADAMTS13 activity is not helpful. The anemia and thrombocytopenia in this patient are most likely due to azathioprine, which causes cytopenias in over 10% of posttransplant patients.

Reference

Taylor AL, Marcus R, Bradley JA. Post-transplant lymphoproliferative disorders (PTLD) after solid organ transplantation. Crit Rev Oncol Hematol. 2005;56:155–67.

Answer to question 9: D

Educational objective

To manage venous thromboembolism in a postoperative patient with cancer

Critique

When venous thromboembolism occurs in the immediate postoperative period, the bleeding risks associated with therapeutic anticoagulation must be quickly assessed. Absolute and relatively strong contraindications to anticoagulation include active bleeding, recent major hemorrhage (eg, gastrointestinal bleeding), recent hemorrhagic stroke, uncontrolled hypertension, underlying coagulopathy, thrombocytopenia (ie, $<50{,}000/\mu L$) or platelet dysfunction, ophthalmologic surgery, invasive procedures in the spinal canal or central nervous system, and indwelling or recent spinal catheters. The surgeon must estimate the risk for recurrent bleeding in the surgical bed based on the nature of the procedure and the integrity of the residual tissues and repair. For most low-risk procedures, full anticoagulation can be safely initiated within 12–24 hours after surgery. By the third postoperative day after uncomplicated surgery, the risks of anticoagulation are comparable to those in a nonsurgical patient. In this case, with stable hemodynamic parameters and stable hematocrit at 48 hours after surgery, therapeutic anticoagulation would be considered relatively safe. However, because of lingering concerns about bleeding in this setting, continuous-infusion unfractionated heparin (UFH) would be preferable to low-molecular-weight heparin (LMWH) because of the short half-life and ability to rapidly and fully reverse the drug with protamine.

If an absolute contraindication to anticoagulation existed, or if bleeding developed on heparin, an inferior vena cava filter would be indicated. Thrombolytic therapy with tissue plasminogen activator (tPA) is contraindicated in this patient because of major surgery 2 days previously and risk of bleeding. Independent of recent surgery, tPA would also not be a strong consideration in this case because of the limited extent of thrombosis and the recommendation that thrombolysis be reserved for more extensive and/or limb-threatening deep venous thrombosis (DVT). The choice of agent for long-term anticoagulation is between warfarin and LMWH. A recent large randomized controlled trial of cancer-associated venous thromboembolism (DVT and/or pulmonary embolism) revealed that 6-month therapy with the LMWH dalteparin was associated with a 2-fold lower rate of recurrent thromboembolism compared with secondary prophylaxis with warfarin. No difference was seen in bleeding risk between the 2 groups. A follow-up study subsequently revealed an improvement in survival among patients without metastatic disease who received dalteparin compared with those who received warfarin. Thus, the American College of Chest Physician's evidence-based guidelines recommend the use of LMWH for long-term treatment (ie, at least 3 to 6 months or as long as the cancer is active) for patients with cancer-associated venous thromboembolism. Given the high cost of LMWH agents compared with warfarin and the limitations of insurance coverage, this option may not be available for all patients.

References

Buller HR, Agnelli G, Hull RD, et al. Antithrombotic therapy for venous thromboembolic disease: the Seventh ACCP Conference on Antithrombotic and Thrombolytic Therapy. Chest. 2004;126(suppl):S401–28.

Lee AY, Levine MN, Baker RI, et al. Low-molecular-weight heparin versus a coumarin for the prevention of recurrent venous thromboembolism in patients with cancer. N Engl J Med. 2003;349:146–53.

Lee AY, Rickles FR, Julian JA, et al. Randomized comparison of low molecular weight heparin and coumarin derivatives on the survival of patients with cancer and venous thromboembolism. J Clin Oncol. 2005;23:2123–9.

Answer to question 10: B

Educational objective

To manage pregnancy-associated Hodgkin disease

Critique

Hodgkin disease (HD) is the most common hematologic malignancy diagnosed during pregnancy, affecting 0.1% to 0.06% of women who carry to term. Roughly 70% of cases are diagnosed with stage I or II disease. HD does not appear to adversely affect pregnancy outcomes, and pregnancy does not compromise the response rates of HD to treatment or overall long-term survival. When possible, chemotherapy should be delayed until at least the second trimester or until after delivery in a woman with stable, low-stage disease. Symptomatic or aggressive supradiaphragmatic disease can be treated with tumoricidal doses of radiation, with abdominal shielding, without undue risk to the fetus. One recent study suggests, however, that breast cancer risk is higher among women who received radiotherapy for HD around the time of pregnancy, compared with nonpregnant women who received similar radiotherapy. Women with aggressive disease should receive multiagent chemotherapy with curative intent. Strong consideration should be given to elective termination of the pregnancy if treatment is required in the first trimester because of the high risk of spontaneous abortion, fetal death, and major malformations. Antimetabolites (especially methotrexate and cytarabine) are highly teratogenic; however, the agents in standard HD therapy regimens, including mechlorethamine, vincristine, prednisone and procarbazine or doxorubicin, bleomycin, vinblastine, and dacarbazine, have been administered with acceptable risk. Chemotherapy should not be administered shortly before delivery because fetal elimination of the drugs depends heavily on the placenta. Retrospective and long-term follow-up studies of children exposed to chemotherapy in utero have shown relatively few congenital malformations and very few late occurrences of hematologic malignancies and cardiac dysfunction (among those exposed to anthracyclines). In this case, the low-stage and nonthreatening disease burden provide the option of delaying therapy without compromising the safety of the patient or limiting her chances for an excellent overall outcome with curative therapy. Because rare cases of HD have been reported to metastasize to the placenta, it should be closely inspected at delivery. No cases of transmission of maternal HD to a neonate have been reported.

References

Cardonick E, Iacobucci A. Use of chemotherapy during human pregnancy. Lancet Oncol. 2004;5:283–91.

Chen J, Lee RJ, Tsodikov A, et al. Does radiotherapy around the time of pregnancy for Hodgkin's disease modify the risk of breast cancer? Int J Radiat Oncol Biol Phys. 2004;58:1474–9.

Hurley TJ, McKinnell JV, Irani MS. Hematologic malignancies in pregnancy. Obstet Gynecol Clin N Am. 2005;32:595–614.

Answer to question 11: D

Educational objective

To recognize that certain coagulation factor levels are normally significantly lower in newborns than in older children and adults

Critique

Although circumcision is occasionally associated with significant complications such as infection or bleeding, most of newborns undergoing circumcision do so uneventfully. With modern techniques, even children with unrecognized severe hemophilia may not bleed, whereas for others, bleeding with circumcision leads to the diagnosis. Nevertheless, for such an elective procedure, the onus is on the physician to do it as safely as possible, and obtaining a family history for potential inheritable bleeding disorders is important. This infant's prothrombin time (PT) and partial thromboplastin time (PTT) are prolonged compared with adult norms but are within normal limits for term newborns. In particular, the vitamin K-dependent factors are physiologically low in normal neonates, despite the administration of vitamin K. In contrast, factor VIII levels are indistinguishable from adult levels at birth. In the absence of a family history or clinical bleeding, the PT and PTT values in this infant would not warrant further workup. However, given the positive family history, because mild hemophilia might result in a factor level low enough to cause a bleeding risk but not necessarily low enough to prolong the PTT (especially for factor IX), it is reasonable to perform factor levels (although factor VII would generally not be ordered in this situation, especially given its autosomal recessive inheritance). In this infant, the 19% factor IX level is within the newborn normal range of 15–50% and does not suggest hemophilia B. Similarly, the factor VII level, as a vitamin K-dependent factor, is normal for a newborn (28–78%). Thus, the factor levels in this infant are within normal limits and do not suggest a hemostatic abnormality nor a missed vitamin K dose, so circumcision could proceed as planned.

References

Andrew M, Paes B, Milner R, et al. Development of the coagulation system in the full-term neonate. Blood. 1987;70: 165–72.

Reverdiau-Moalic P, Delahousse B, Body G, et al. Evaluation of blood coagulation activators and inhibitors in the healthy human fetus. Blood. 1996:88;900–6.

Answer to question 12: A

Educational objective

To understand that lupus anticoagulants are usually not associated with an increased risk of thrombosis or bleeding in children

Critique

The fact that this patient's partial thromboplastin time (PTT) does not correct with a 1:1 mix with normal plasma rules out hemophilia A, B, or other factor deficiency; thus, factor VIII and IX levels are not indicated. Lupus anticoagulants (LAs) can be identified in children in 3 clinical situations. In the first, during evaluation for a thrombotic event, the finding of an LA or other antiphospholipid antibody has the same implications as in adult patients and is generally presumed to have contributed to clot formation. In the second, an LA is identified during the workup for symptomatic bleeding that is usually of recent onset. In that group of patients, not only do the bleeding complaints themselves suggest a functionally significant impairment of hemostasis, but also the prothrombin time (PT) is usually prolonged in addition to the PTT, reflecting the fact that prothrombin levels are often markedly depressed. In such cases, even the administration of fresh frozen plasma is unlikely to improve hemostasis enough to proceed safely to tonsillectomy. For such patients with dangerous levels of bleeding, immunosuppression with prednisone may hasten the resolution of the acquired inhibitor. However, this case presents a classic scenario for an acquired lupus-like inhibitor that does not pose a risk of bleeding and requires no special intervention. The key is that this lupus anticoagulant has been identified in an asymptomatic child, who has had neither bleeding nor thrombosis, a PTT that is only mildly prolonged, and a normal PT. In a study of 95 children found to have LA during evaluation in a hemostasis clinic, 84% were free of symptoms and the LA was found incidentally, usually during preoperative screening (54 patients prior to adenotonsillectomy). None of these went on to develop subsequent problems with bleeding, thrombosis, or autoimmune disease. All available data suggests that surgery can be performed without special intervention, without excess risk of bleeding. Given the lack of associated morbidity with these incidental LAs, immunosuppression is not warranted in asymptomatic patients.

References

Briones M, Abshire T. Lupus anticoagulants in children. Curr Opin Hematol. 2003;10:375–9.

Male C, Lechner K, Eichinger S, et al. Clinical significance of lupus anticoagulants in children. J Pediatr. 1999;134:199–205.

Mizumoto H, Maihara T, Hiejima E, et al. Transient antiphospholipid antibodies associated with acute infections in children: a report of three cases and a review of the literature. Eur J Pediatr. 2006;165:484–8.

Answer to question 13: E

Educational objective

To understand the presentation and management of neonatal alloimmune thrombocytopenia

Critique

To make the best treatment decision for this infant, it is important to understand the most likely diagnosis. In thrombocytopenic infants, the critical initial distinction is whether the infant is "well" or "ill." In this otherwise well infant whose physical examination abnormalities reflect only his thrombocytopenia, the most likely etiology for his thrombocytopenia is antibody-mediated destruction. With normal to large platelets, and no obvious congenital abnormalities such as absent radii or thumb defects, a production defect such as thrombocytopenia with absent radii or Fanconi anemia is unlikely, and congenital amegakaryocytic thrombocytopenia is extremely uncommon. Newborns make little antibody themselves, so antiplatelet antibody would be transmitted transplacentally from mother. If the mother's platelet count was low, maternal idiopathic thrombocytopenic purpura (ITP) would be most likely. However, with a normal maternal platelet count, the most likely diagnosis is neonatal alloimmune thrombocytopenia (NAITP), which results from the production of maternal antibody directed against a paternally derived antigen expressed by the infant's platelets. NAITP can occur in first pregnancies because the small size of the platelet allows access to the maternal circulation during gestation. NAITP can and should be confirmed by parental studies of platelet antigen expression/discrepancy and maternal antibody; in 80% of affected infants, mother's platelets will express HPA-1B, whereas father's and infant's express HPA-1A.

However, management should *not* await results of these studies, which often require sendout to a specialized laboratory. Although platelet transfusions are rarely given to older children with antibody-mediated destruction (ie, ITP), neonates who have recently undergone the physical stresses of delivery are at significant risk of intracranial hemorrhage and thus warrant emergent platelet transfusion. Without platelet antigen study results, the only way to be certain that transfused platelets will not express the paternal, "incompatible" antigen is to use maternal platelets, which can be collected if mother is readily available and physically able to donate. It is critical that the platelets be washed of excess maternal plasma to avoid infusion of additional antiplatelet antibody. If mother is not able to donate, random-donor platelets have been shown to result in at least a temporary platelet increment even if they are antigen incompatible, and their life span after transfusion may be increased by the infusion of intravenous immunoglobulin. Prednisone will be of limited utility given that the antibody has been passively transmitted. In situations where the specific antigen incompatibility is known, many blood banks have an identified group of antigen-specific platelet donors (eg, donors known to be HPA-1B positive) who can be called in for longer term platelet support, especially when mother's ability to donate is limited. This can be particularly helpful for second pregnancies. It should be noted that confirmation of the diagnosis is important not only for management of the affected infant, but also for subsequent pregnancies, where infants can develop severe thrombocytopenia and even intracranial hemorrhage as early as the second trimester.

References

Kaplan RN, Bussel JB. Differential diagnosis and management of thrombocytopenia in childhood. Pediatr Clin N Am. 2004;51:1109–40.

Roberts I, Murray NA. Neonatal thrombocytopenia: causes and management. Arch Dis Child Fetal Neonatal Ed. 2003;88: F359–64.